Recent Advances in
ORTHOPAEDICS

B. McKIBBIN MD MSc(Surg) FRCS
Professor of Traumatic and Orthopaedic Surgery,
The Welsh National School of Medicine, Cardiff

Recent Advances in
ORTHOPAEDICS

EDITED BY
B. McKIBBIN

NUMBER FOUR

CHURCHILL LIVINGSTONE
EDINBURGH LONDON MELBOURNE AND NEW YORK 1983

CHURCHILL LIVINGSTONE
Medical Division of Longman Group Limited

Distributed in the United States of America by
Churchill Livingstone Inc., 1560 Broadway, New York,
N.Y. 10036, and by associated companies, branches
and representatives throughout the world.

© Longman Group Limited 1983

All rights reserved. No part of this publication
may be reproduced, stored in a retrieval system,
or transmitted in any form or by any means,
electronic, mechanical, photocopying, recording
or otherwise, without the prior permission of the
publishers (Churchill Livingstone, Robert Stevenson
House, 1–3 Baxter's Place, Leith Walk,
Edinburgh EH1 3AF).

First published 1983

ISBN 0 443 02627 0
ISSN 0308-4914

Library of Congress Cataloging Card Number: 79-40019

Printed in Great Britain at The Pitman Press, Bath

Preface

In previous volumes in this series the Preface has largely been given over to the semantic problem of reconciling the title with the contents and that need is no less in this present volume.

Both the terms 'Recent' and 'Advance' are relative and their assignment therefore depends on individual judgement. However, editorial policy has been based on the perception that by any reasonable definition there are in fact very few subjects which qualify under both headings and therefore one has been deemed sufficient provided that the topic is one of current interest to orthopaedic surgeons.

The topic of knee replacement can scarcely be regarded as 'recent' in terms of the speed of present developments in the speciality, but an appraisal of the extent to which it represents an 'advance' was thought timely and these considerations apply to several other topics. Conversely the various uses of carbon fibre are undoubtedly recent and hopefully therefore of interest, but an estimate of their ultimate usefulness, if any, lies many years ahead. Other articles lie in a somewhat intermediary position and the reader may decide for himself under which heading they best qualify, although in some instances the individual authors have given their own opinions.

As before, an attempt has been made to cover as wide a variety of topics as possible and to make the contributions as worldwide as could be. Although the balance, this time, has come out weighted more heavily in favour of Europe and North America than in previous editions this is quite fortuitous.

Once more the Editor would like to thank all the contributors for their patience and forbearance. All are busy men and their success in meeting the various deadlines varied. It is unfortunate that the punctual are punished by the delays of the more dilatory in that their contributions are not so recent as they otherwise might have been, but such problems are unfortunately inseparable from a venture such as this.

Cardiff, 1983   B. McK.

Contributors

HARLAN C. AMSTUTZ MD
Professor and Chief, Division of Orthopaedic Surgery, UCLA School of Medicine, Center for the Health Sciences, Los Angeles, California, USA

SHERMAN S. COLEMAN MD BS MS
Professor of Orthopaedic Surgery, University of Utah, Salt Lake City. Chief of Staff, Shriners Hospital for Crippled Children, Salt Lake City, Utah, USA

DAVID J. DANDY MA MB BChir FRCS
Consultant Orthopaedic Surgeon, Newmarket General Hospital and Addenbrooke's Hospital, Cambridge. Associate Lecturer, Faculty of Clinical Medicine, University of Cambridge, UK

PATRICK J. KELLY MD
Consultant in Orthopaedics, Mayo Clinic/Foundation. Professor of Orthopaedic Surgery, Mayo Medical School, Rochester, Minnesota, USA

B. McKIBBIN MD MSc(Surg) FRCS
Professor of Traumatic and Orthopaedic Surgery, The Welsh National School of Medicine, Cardiff, UK

PAUL G. J. MAQUET MD
Orthopaedic Surgeon, Clinique Ste Elisabeth, Liège, Belgium

H. MILLESI MD
Head of the Department of Plastic and Reconstructive Surgery, University of Vienna Medical School. Director of the Ludwig-Boltzmann-Institute for Experimental Plastic Surgery, Vienna, Austria

JOSEPH WATSON BSc SM PhD CEng FIEE
Reader in Electrical and Electronic Engineering, University of Wales, Swansea, UK

WILLIAM WAUGH MA MChir FRCS
Professor of Orthopaedic and Accident Surgery, University of Nottingham, UK

LEON L. WILTSE MD
Clinical Professor of Orthopaedic Surgery, University of California, Irvine, California, USA

Contents

1. Microsurgery of peripheral nerves *H. Millesi* — 1

2. Reconstructive procedures in congenital dislocation of the hip *S. S. Coleman* — 23

3. Knee replacements *W. Waugh* — 45

4. The surgical treatment of osteoarthritis of the hip by reduction of articular pressure *P. Maquet* — 65

5. Arthroscopy and arthroscopic surgery of the knee *D. J. Dandy* — 87

6. Chemonucleolysis in the treatment of lumbar disc disease *L. L. Wiltse* — 103

7. Chronic osteomyelitis in adults *P. J. Kelly* — 119

8. The electrical stimulation of bone healing in cases of nonunion and delayed union *J. Watson* — 131

9. Recent advances in total hip resurfacing *H. C. Amstutz* — 155

10. New materials in orthopaedics: carbon fibre *B. McKibbin* — 179

Index — 205

1. Microsurgery of peripheral nerves

H. Millesi

INTRODUCTION

The experiments of Cruikshank (1795) demonstrated that regeneration was possible after transection of a peripheral nerve by the sprouting of nerve fibres from the proximal to the distal stump. In spite of this observation, surgeons did not dare to suture transected nerves, being afraid of 'convulsions' and sought to achieve copatation indirectly by apposition of the soft tissues ('cum carne'). In 1871 Hueter suggested the restoration of the continuity of a resected nerve by epineural stitches. Thus surgeons utilised their anatomical knowledge by employing the external (epifascicular) layers for anchoring their stitches without touching the nerve tissue itself.

The technique of epineural nerve repair proved to be very successful. It was the technique of choice for nearly one hundred years and it still meets the requirements in many cases. The technique was steadily improved by the introduction of less reactive and atraumatic suture material and it was performed by many surgeons under optical magnification using a loup. The peak of development of this technique was reached in the years after World War II, and although many other distinguished surgeons were involved this development is inextricably linked with the outstanding personality of Sir Herbert Seddon.

There would be no need for further development if all nerve lesions were clean transections, and if all nerves consisted of only one fibre type — sensory or motor — and if motor, of only one basic function. Unfortunately, even in the hands of extremely experienced surgeons, the percentage of moderate or poor results from this technique is high. Björkesten (1947) achieved a fair or better result in 50 of 77 cases with ulnar lesions (65%) but in only six of them (7.8%) did interosseus function return (Table 1.1). Nicholson & Seddon (1957) using Highets scheme for evaluation

Table 1.1 Björkesten 1947 — Ulnar nerve N = 77

Interosseous function	6 (7.8%)	50 (65%)
Medium and good	44 (57.2%)	
Poor and bad	27 (35.0%)	

reported results of M 3 or better in 147 of 255 peripheral ulnar lesions (57.6%) with 108 patients (42.4%) remaining below this level. In proximal lesions of the ulnar nerve on the other hand 35 of 55 cases (67.3%) remained below M 3 (Tables 1.2, 1.3).

In cases where there was actual loss of nerve tissue the results worsened significantly if the defect was between 2.5 and 5 cm (Nicholson & Seddon, 1957) and defects of more than 5 cm were regarded as incompatible with a useful recovery (Peripheral nerve injury report, 1954).

Table 1.2 Nicholson & Seddon, 1957 — Ulnar nerve — Nerve sutures

	Distal lesions N = 255	
M 4 or better	64 (25.1%)	
M 3	83 (32.5%)	147 (57.6%)
Less than M 3	108 (42.4%)	

Table 1.3 Nicholson & Seddon, 1957 — Ulnar nerve — Nerve sutures

	Proximal lesions N = 52	
M 4 or better	3 (5.8%)	
M 3	14 (26.9%)	17 (32.7%)
Less than M 3	35 (67.3%)	

In the early sixties many surgeons felt that something had to be done to improve the results of nerve repair and, in fact, during this period of time many new approaches were suggested but some of these were merely revivals of old ideas using new materials, such as wrapping the suture site with millipore (Campbell et al, 1961; Böhler, 1962), with collagen membranes (Braun, 1964; Kline & Hayes, 1964), and silastic membranes (Ducker & Hayes, 1968; Midgley & Woodhouse, 1968).

Based on experimental observations of the fibre distribution in the peripheral portions of nerves, Langley and Hashimoto had suggested, as early as 1917 the suture of separate nerve bundles in a nerve trunk. Sir Sydney Sunderland studied the intraneural topography (Sunderland, 1945; Sunderland & Ray, 1948; Sunderland et al, 1959) and discussed the possibility of fascicular repair (Sunderland, 1952, 1953). He thought, however, that this approach would only have a limited application (Sunderland, 1978). A heated discussion about the relative merits of epineural or fascicular (perineural) nerve repair was thus initiated.

Another new development was the application of optical magnification by the use of the operating microscope (Smith, 1964; Kurze, 1964; Michon & Masse, 1964). This technique was met with scepticism at first and many surgeons could not understand, that surgery performed under the microscope, should yield better results than without it. They could see no difference between utilising the microscope or a loup and indeed many still cannot do so. In fact, Braun (1967) and Ellis (1966) were unable to show any differences in comparative studies. However, if the whole approach to peripheral nerve surgery is modified in such a way as to make maximal use of the optical magnification, a significant difference can be seen both experimentally as well as clinically (Millesi, Ganglberger & Berger, 1967). The microsurgery of peripheral nerves does not mean the performing under optical magnification of what was formerly done without it. Rather it represents a shift from a mechanistic to a more biological approach. Tissue layers have become accessible to surgery which were indistinguishable before. The tissue reaction is taken into account more than formerly and as a result all manipulations have become more delicate and less traumatic.

SOME REMARKS ON HEALING AND REGENERATION AFTER PERIPHERAL NERVE LESIONS

The first axon sprouts can be seen proximal to the gap between the two stumps as early as 24 hours after injury (Hudson et al, 1970). It would be ideal if all axons in the proximal stump produced one or two axon sprouts, and all of them safely reached the distal stump approximately at a corresponding site. It is evident that they can do so only if they originate very close to the end of the proximal stump. The axon sprout will be delayed if it has to work its way across fibrous tissue within the proximal stump. This means that an adequate resection of the two stumps to reach normal nerve tissue is of extreme importance and Mackenzie & Woods (1961) went so far as to suggest that the surgeon should convince himself by frozen section that he had performed an adequate resection. During the first day epineural fibroblasts proliferate and advance into the gap between the two stumps. Schwann cells, perineurial and endoneurial fibroblasts follow en suite during the next few days (Jurecka, Ammerer & Lassmann, 1975). The proliferation of Schwann cells is extremely important because the axon sprouts cross the gap in contact with them.

Too many fibroblasts impede the outgrowth of Schwann cells and the progress of the axon sprouts, especially if they have started to produce collagen. Ramón y Cajal stated in 1928 that the axon sprouts may cross the suture line and reach the distal stump under favourable conditions on the third day, but if this is not achieved may be delayed up to 40 or 50 days due to the slow advancement across the scar tissue. Huber (1895) regarded nerve regeneration across a gap as a struggle between proliferating connective tissue and advancing axon sprouts. In fact, all authors describe the gap between the two stumps as a zone of disorganised tissue. The axon sprouts struggle across this zone, divide into many branches to bypass obstacles and deviate into the tissues outside the nerve, or return forming Perroncito's spirals (Seddon, 1972). This junctional scar is not only an obstacle to proceeding axon sprouts, but it may damage axons which have already reached the distal stump if the scar becomes distracted or hypertrophic (Millesi, Berger & Meissl, 1970; Millesi, Berger & Meissl, 1972; Millesi, 1977). It is interesting to note that the formation of the junctional scar was accepted as inevitable as in the past was callus formation in fracture healing although attempts were made to reduce the amount of fibroblastic proliferation and its consequences. Unfortunately, although the wrapping of the suture site with any material tends to minimise the ingrowth of fibroblasts from the surrounding tissues, since the main source of such fibroblasts is the epineural tissue which remains *inside* the tube, no significant effect can be expected. Hastings & Peacock (1973) tried to improve the results of experimental nerve repair by interference with collagen synthesis by introducing vitamin C avitmaninosis. Pleasure et al (1974) reduced collagen production by the application of D-penicillamine but Bucko et al (1981) were unable to see any effect of this treatment on nerve regeneration. Tissue culture studies provided the explanation (Bunge & Bunge, 1978; Bunge, 1980, 1981) by revealing that the presence of a few fibroblasts was essential for the production of a fascicle-like structure.

It has been demonstrated by comparative studies (Millesi et al, 1970; Millesi et al, 1972; Millesi, 1977) that beyond a certain limit the zone of junctional scar tissue increases with the amount of tension at the suture site. If tension is completely avoided, only minimal scar tissue is formed. Tension at the suture site, if it passes a critical value, which may differ between individuals and species, increases fibroblast proliferation and scar tissue formation and the junctional zone between the two stumps becomes expanded.

The amount of fibroblastic proliferation at the suture site can be reduced and retarded by local resection of the epineurial tissue (Millesi, 1968). By this procedure the risk of coapting fascicles with non-fascicular tissue from the opposing stump is reduced. It is evident that this applies only to nerve segments which consist of many fascicles containing a high percentage of non-fascicular tissue. Connective tissue proliferation can also be reduced by minimising surgical trauma and by the burying of foreign material (sutures, etc.).

In summary

Attempts to influence nerve regeneration on a biochemical level have so far failed. Nerve healing with minimal tissue reaction can be achieved by proper resection, exact fascicular coaptation, with minimal surgical trauma and without tension. Of course, in cases of extended trauma to the nerve, these conditions cannot be achieved by end to end neurorrhaphy. Sufficient resection of the stumps means a longer defect and more tension and the utilisation of a graft is the answer to this problem if a critical value is exceeded.

LESION IN CONTINUITY AND NEUROLYSIS

Sir Herbert Seddon differentiated nerve lesions into three types:
 Neuropraxia
 Axonotmesis
 Neurotmesis

Sir Sydney Sunderland (1951) distinguished five degrees:

1st degree. The trauma caused an interruption of conduction. The axon might be thinner than normal, but its continuity is preserved. Eventually there is segmental demyelination (i.e. neurapraxia).
2nd degree. The trauma caused disintegration of the axon with Wallerian degeneration distal to the site of the lesion (i.e. axonotmesis).
3rd degree. The trauma caused a disorganisation of the internal structure of the fascicle by haemorrhage, vascular stasis or ischaemia. Fibrosis may develop within the fascicle, which can form a serious obstacle to regeneration.
4th degree. The trauma caused a disorganisation of the bundles. They are no longer sharply demarcated from the epineurium and the trunk is ultimately converted into a strand of connective tissue.
5th degree. Loss of continuity (i.e. neurotmesis).

This scheme fits very well with the immediate consequences of a traction lesion but it recognises the reaction of the epineurium only partially. By definition in a 1st, 2nd and 3rd degree lesion the epineurium should be intact. However, epineurium is a very reactive tissue, it responds to trauma and chronic irritation with fibrosis of different degrees leading to shrinkage and constriction and it may react in a different way in different locations. In some cases limited fibrosis of the superficial (epifascicular) epineurium can be observed and as a result of shrinkage it becomes too tight and compresses the fascicles like an overtight stocking. In other cases the fibrosis extends between the fascicle groups, including also the interfascicular epineurium. These two types of epineurial fibrosis occur in 1st-, 2nd- and 3rd-degree lesions and make spontaneous recovery, which would otherwise be expected, impossible. In all cases of 3rd-degree lesions some degree of fibrosis of the endoneural tissue occurs. Severe endoneural fibrosis transforms the fascicle into a hard inelastic strand, a situation in which recovery is not likely to occur.

In a 3rd-degree lesion with severe endoneural fibrosis or in a 4th-degree lesion internal neurolysis will not solve the problem. However, in a 3rd-degree lesion without such fibrosis and in a 1st- and 2nd-degree lesion decompression by internal neurolysis may assist in accelerating spontaneous regeneration.

The following procedures can be distinguished:

External neurolysis. The nerve is liberated from adhesions to the surrounding tissue which compress the nerve or restrict its mobility so that it is unable to adjust itself to joint motion.

Internal neurolysis: is performed if epineural fibrosis compresses the fascicles and impedes movement of the fascicles against one another.

In *epifascicular epineurotomy*: the epifascicular epineurium is split longitudinally along the site of the lesion from sound tissue to sound tissue.

In *epifascicular epineurectomy*: the epifascicular or superficial circumferential epineurium is excised if epineurotomy alone does not provide sufficient decompression.

Interfascicular epineurectomy (partial): is performed if massive fibrosis extends between the fascicles and epifascicular epineurectomy alone did not provide sufficient decompression. Interfascicular epineurectomy is performed only partially, because it is not necessary to excise all the fibrous tissue between the fascicles, it being sufficient to remove only enough to achieve decompression. If fascicles have suffered a 3rd-degree lesion with severe endoneurial fibrosis or if fascicle groups or nerve segments have suffered 4th-degree damage these will form obstacles to regeneration even after neurolysis. In such conditions these fascicles or nerve portions should be completely excised and continuity restored by nerve grafts. This may be necessary for the whole nerve segment but should be confined to individual fascicles or fascicle groups if the remaining part of the nerve is not damaged to the same degree.

Thus, internal neurolysis is a stepwise procedure. Its extension is dictated by the amount of damage the nerve has suffered and where that damage is extreme it progresses to resection with restoration of continuity.

Strong objections have been raised to internal neurolysis; it is argued that in performing this procedure, more scar tissue might be produced than before thus jeopardising any possible benefit, in addition many interfascicular connections might actually be divided. It has been further argued that interfascicular vessels may be damaged or excised thus impairing the nutrition of the fascicles.

These arguments might be valid if in all cases the internal neurolysis was carried to the extreme of isolating each individual fascicle. However, in clinical practice this is never actually done. The surgical procedure is complete as soon as the aim, namely decompression, has been achieved. Since the interfascicular epineurectomy is only partial the majority of interfascicular connections are preserved as well as interfascicular vessels, especially within fascicle groups. In any case where there has been extreme interfascicular fibrosis the interfascicular connections and the longitudinal vessels have already been damaged. Rydevik et al (1976) and Lundborg (1980, 1981) demonstrated that internal neurolysis was not harmful so long as the perineurium remained intact. In a recent paper Villes (1981) showed that the deprivation of extrafascicular vascularisation did not cause an endoneurial vascular deficit.

Internal neurolysis is indicated in selected cases of entrapment syndromes. Curtis &

Eversman (1973) were able to improve the results of simple decompression in carpal tunnel syndrome by this procedure. In all cases of this condition in which a constriction of the nerve does not expand after release of the tourniquet because of fibrosis step-wise internal neurolysis, starting with epifascicular epineurotomy is indicated. Thus optical magnification and microsurgical techniques not only allow the performing of internal neurolysis without significant risk of damaging fascicles but also allow the possibility, by careful dissection, layer by layer, of isolating the median nerve without destroying the parietal lining of the carpal tunnel above the nerve and without opening a communication to the part of the carpal tunnel which contains the flexor tendons and which is separated from the median nerve by a distinct layer.

NEURORRHAPHY

Timing

Ever since peripheral nerve repairs have been undertaken there has been an argument about the relative merits of primary or secondary repair and this controversy will probably continue indefinitely. A controlled study in human beings cannot be performed for obvious reasons and comparing different clinical series cannot solve the problem since the cases having had primary or secondary repair represent different statistical populations in relation to the severity of the damage and the other important factors concerned.

There is no question that a clean transection without severe lesions of other tissues should be treated by a primary repair. Since there is no scar tissue nor restriction by fibrosis the patient needs only one procedure and therefore primary repair offers an economic but not necessarily a biological advantage. From the latter point of view early secondary repair is preferable. By this time the nerve segment proximal and distal to the level of transection which has suffered severe damage during the accident has become fibrotic and the amount of necessary resection can be estimated much more accurately. In cases of doubt therefore our preference is for an early secondary repair.

In early secondary repair it is the loss of elasticity of the nerve stump which makes end-to-end approximation difficult if there is a defect and for many years it has been our practice to use nerve grafts in the majority of secondary repairs. Similar experience was published recently by Chanson et al (1979). The series of Geldmacher & Albers (1981) is difficult to assess. The cases selected for secondary repair by neurorrhaphy achieved much better results (83.4% good and very good) than cases selected for primary repair by neurorrhaphy (72.8%) so far as motor function was concerned. Cases selected for secondary repair and grafting also did better (75.8% good and very good) than the cases selected for primary repair, in spite of the fact that these cases apparently were the ones which were involved in the most severe trauma and the longest time intervals. On the other hand sensory function was best in primary neurorrhaphy (77.4% good and very good), followed by the series of secondary repair by grafts (58.1%) while secondary repair by neurorrhaphy was worse (52.1%), an outcome which was attributed to the existence of too much tension.

Selection of technique

As mentioned above, for various reasons, fascicular neurorrhaphy with perineural stitches was favoured by many surgeons (Bora et al, 1976; Goto, 1967; Ito, 1969; Grabb et al, 1970). Tupper went to the extreme of uniting each small fascicle independently, even in polyfascicular nerves and digital nerves. However, his results were not rewarding (Tupper, 1977). Wise et al (1969), Bora et al (1976), Cabaud et al (1976) published experimental data showing better results following epineural repair. However, these contradictory results are in part due to a failure to compare like with like.

The great advantage of fascicular repair, is that by reduction of the non-fascicular tissue fascicular coaptation is guaranteed and by partial resection of the epineurium the amount of fibroblastic proliferation reduced. It is evident that this applies only to nerve segments in which a high percentage of the cross-section consists of epineural tissue and the number of fascicles is neither too small nor too large. If the nerve segment consists of only a few fascicles, there is inevitably only a small amount of non-fascicular tissue present and fascicular coaptation can therefore be easily achieved by epineural stitches. In such instances the surgical trauma involved in isolating the fascicles and resection of the epineurium is not justified. On the other hand if there are six, eight or ten fascicles in the major nerve trunk, fascicular coaptation cannot always be achieved by epineural stitches because of the large amount of non-fascicular tissue between the bundles. In such instances isolation and resection of the epineurium and individual fascicular coaptation is the better solution.

At the other extreme, if the cross-section consists of many fascicles the surgical trauma in isolating these and resecting all the epineurium becomes counterproductive. In addition it is more difficult to identify the individual fascicles. Thus, epineural and fascicular (perineural) repairs are not to be seen as optional alternatives; each technique has its particular indications.

These modern developments cause problems in terminology. The terms epineural and perineural nerve repair do not really describe the procedure which was performed, rather they refer to the tissue layer where the stitches have been anchored (epineural or perineural) or to the type of coaptation (trunk-to-trunk or fascicle-to-fascicle) respectively. From the surgical point of view four basic fascicular patterns can be distinguished:

The *monofascicular pattern* Here the nerve trunk contains only one large fascicle.

In this instance trunk-to-trunk coaptation is automatically a fascicular coaptation and there is no interfascicular epineurium involved. The stump is prepared by transverse section.

The *oligofascicular pattern* Here the nerve trunk consists of a limited number of rather large fascicles.

If there are only a few fascicles present — 3 to 5, the amount of interfascicular tissue is still limited. The stump can therefore be prepared easily by resection, and coaptation of the fascicles can be controlled by epineural stitches opposing the cross section of the two trunks. If there are more fascicles than this — 7 to 10 — the increased amount of non-fascicular tissue dictates that isolation of the fascicles, dissection of the epineurium and fascicular coaptation is preferred.

The *polyfascicular pattern without group arrangement*
Here the cross section consists of many small fascicles in diffuse distribution with a

large amount of interfascicular epineurium. Although isolation of the fascicles and resection of the epineurium is desirable it is difficult to achieve and involves a lot of surgical trauma. In these circumstances trunk-to-trunk coaptation with interfascicular guide sutures is still justified as being the less traumatic method. In the case of nerve grafting, the grafts are coapted with corresponding sectors in the cross section.

The polyfascicular pattern with group arrangement
Again the cross section consists of many fascicles of different sizes, but these are arranged in groups. Again there is a great deal of non-fascicular epineural tissue between them and although resection of the whole epineurium and isolation of the fascicles would be desirable this would again mean too much surgical trauma. The optimal solution to this problem at present is resection of the epifascicular epineurium and the isolation of the individual fascicle groups by dissecting into the spaces between them. It cannot be too strongly emphasised that in this situation the fascicle groups are pre-formed and the isolation is carried out by following natural cleavage planes between them. The fascicles are not 'dissected free from epineurium and then formed into groups or arranged into groups' (Sunderland, 1978). The fascicle groups are not only present just before the branching of a nerve, but can be followed for quite a distance proximally (Williams 1979, Jabaley 1980).

Neurorrhaphy consists of four basic steps

Preparation of the stumps
This is performed by resection or by interfascicular dissection to isolate large fascicles or fascicle groups starting in normal tissue and proceeding towards the site of the lesion.

Approximation
This is permissible under slight tension and can be achieved by mobilisation and the flexion of adjacent joints. Alternatively, the joints may be maintained in neutral position with only minor mobilisation of the nerve but in this case a nerve graft will have to be used if the defect exceeds certain limits.

Coaptation
One can coapt the cross sections of nerve trunks, isolated fascicles or fascicle groups. Regardless of the type of coaptation every effort should be made to coapt the cross section of the fascicles as accurately as possible. If there was a clean transection, the two stumps will contain the same number of fascicles and under ideal circumstances a perfect fascicular coaptation might be possible. However, if there is even a small defect, the number of fascicles will not correspond in the two cross sections so that a perfect fascicular coaptation cannot be achieved. This applies also to the coaptation of fascicle groups where the changing size and number of fascicles within it prevents perfect coaptation. Fortunately the axon sprouts are able to find their way within certain limits as Lundborg (1979), Lundborg & Hansson (1980), demonstrated so well with their tissue chamber technique. Clinical experience has also shown that nature provides a certain amount of tolerance in this regard (Millesi, 1980).

It is, of course, extremely important to coapt corresponding fascicles. Retrograde tracing of the fascicles from the division of a nerve back to the cross section of the distal stump provides a good idea of the fascicular pattern of this stump. By comparing the cross section of the distal and proximal stump a guess can be made as to the orientation in the proximal stump. Hakstian (1968) used electrical stimulation to get an idea of the fascicular pattern while Freilinger et al (1975) applied the staining technique developed by Gruber & Zenker (1973), which allows differentiation between motor and sensory fibres based on the different content of acetylcholinesterase. Unfortunately this technique needs two days before one gets the result. Engel et al (1980), published a staining technique based on acetylcholinetransferase, which gives the result within 60 minutes but clinical experience with this technique has not yet been published.

Maintenance of the Coaptation. This can be done by sutures or by adhesives. Matras & Kuderna (1975) used a concentrated fibrinogen solution for the latter but the final results were not satisfactory (Kuderna, 1979). Sutures are anchored in the epifascicular (circumferential) epineurium in the case of trunk-to-trunk coaptation, or in the interfascicular epineurium in the case of group-to-group coaptation. The suture may be fixed in the perineurium or it can catch the epi- and perineurium at the same time (Michon & Masse, 1964). If there is tension, more sutures will have to be used, and if there is no tension at all very few are sufficient and we do not believe that the number of sutures is decisive in determining the result as suggested by Guegan (1979) and Foucher et al (1978). There is also good evidence to believe that the close apposition of the perineurium in fascicular coaptation is not important (Millesi, 1980).

How much tension can be accepted?
This question will be answered by different surgeons in different ways according to their background and experience. Nowadays all surgeons would consider nerve grafting if there is a defect of 5 cm or more. Conversely, all surgeons would consider a neurorrhaphy if the defect were less than 1.5 to 2.5 cm. Between these extremes the point of decision will vary but it should be recognised that these figures apply to nerve trunks in average patients and are in no way to be regarded as absolute values. To restore the continuity of the finger nerve the writer would use a nerve graft in a much shorter defect than that quoted. If one has to restore the continuity of the palmar branch of the median nerve because of a painful neuroma a defect of only a few millimetres may be enough to constitute an indication for grafting. However, whatever decision a surgeon makes in an individual case he must be aware of the fact that if he accepts a certain amount of tension he must employ a technique which is capable of resisting that tension and undoubtedly the strongest bond is provided by the conventional epineurial repair. More sophisticated techniques such as the coaptation of fascicle groups or individual fascicles can only be performed if there is virtually no tension.

NERVE GRAFTING

The effective distance between two nerve stumps is the sum of the following factors:

1. The real nerve defect (the amount of nerve tissue actually lost during the accident).

2. The resection necessarily performed at the time of repair to remove damaged and potentially fibrotic segments.
3. The retraction due to elasticity of the nerve which eventually becomes fixed due to slight fibrosis.
4. Differences due to alteration of joint position.

The actual loss of nerve tissue as a result of the accident and any subsequent resection obviously has to be accepted. Elastic retraction on the other hand may be overcome completely by traction during primary repair while fixed retraction can only be partially overcome at secondary repair. This traction represents the actual tension at the suture site and can obviously be minimised by extreme joint flexion and maximised by joint extension. Unfortunately, minimising the tension by joint flexion only postpones the problem because the site of coaptation will come under tension when mobilisation commences. Even if such mobilisation is performed very carefully and the axon sprouts have already crossed the line of coaptation there is still the possibility of axon damage due to traction on scar tissue and hypertrophy.

There are two basic approaches to nerve grafting
1. By attempting to minimise the distance to be bridged by mobilisation and traction.

This approach is based on the belief that the results would be better if the nerve graft was shorter. However, in reality this combines both the disadvantage of grafting — requiring the axon sprouts to cross two sites of coaptation together with the disadvantages of tension at the sites of coaptation.

2. To measure the defect with the joints in neutral position without traction on the stumps and adding 10%. In this way the nerve graft will be fully relaxed. It is true that one has to utilise a longer graft but the two sites of coaptation are ideal, and do not present obstacles to the advancing axon sprouts. The result in fact does not depend on the length of the graft but rather on the length of the defect produced by the trauma and subsequent resection. By increasing the length of the defect we have to deal with a different fascicular pattern and the definition of corresponding fascicle groups becomes more difficult. Undoubtedly a graft of 20 cm will yield an inferior result to a graft of 2 cm, but within certain limits whether it be 6, 8 or 10 centimeters long does not matter provided that the nerve defect is the same.

NERVE GRAFT VERSUS NEURORRHAPHY

Theoretically, nerve grafting might be expected to be inferior to neurorrhaphy because of its two suture sites and this opinion was generally accepted in spite of remarkably good results published by Foerster (1916), Seddon (1947, 1963, and 1972), and Brooks (1955). Certainly it is true if nerve grafting and neurorrhaphy are performed under identical conditions. However, based on the principle of avoiding tension as outlined above, and utilising the interfascicular grafting technique, useful results have been obtained in cases whose defects were inimical to recovery and better results have been obtained using nerve grafts compared with direct suture under tension (Millesi, Ganglberger & Berger, 1967; Millesi, 1968; Millesi, Berger & Meissl,

1972; Millesi, Meissl & Berger, 1972; Millesi, Meissl & Berger, 1976). Our results have been supported by experimental studies by Samii & Wallenborn (1972), Terzis et al (1975), Bratton et al (1979). McCarroll et al (1977 and 1980) also performed experimental studies in which neurorrhaphy was compared with nerve grafts under slight to moderate tension. They found that recovery across the grafts was slower than with neurorrhaphy but ultimately reached similar levels. The authors therefore concluded that grafts are no better than neurorrhaphies but at the same time did not demonstrate that they were any worse. With increasing tension the advantages of the graft would have become more and more significant.

Allografts and xenografts do not offer an alternative to autografts at present. Only time will tell whether the combination of an allograft framework plus cultivated Schwann cells from the host as proposed by Aguayo (1980 and 1981) will become a clinically applicable method.

With any nerve graft there is always the possibility of a block occurring at the distal suture site due to scar tissue formation preventing further advancement of the axons, although with modern techniques this happens infrequently. It may be detected clinically by the failure of the Tinnel Hoffmann sign to advance beyond the distal end of the graft. In these circumstances the distal site of coaptation should be resected at a second operation and a new suture carried out. The planning of a grafting procedure as a two-stage operation from the beginning leaving the distal end of the graft open and performing this distal coaptation at a subsequent stage has recently been suggested again by Bosse (1979, 1980, and 1981), but has not been found to be justified in our own clinical experience.

Technique of free cutaneous nerve grafting (Fig. 1.1)

The exposure is performed using generous incisions; these are planned in such a way as to avoid crossing the graft by scar lines. The exposure and preparation of the stumps is done under tourniquet but the grafting itself is performed without a bloodless field.

The two stumps are prepared by interfascicular dissection, isolating large fascicles or fascicle groups in oligofascicular or polyfascicular nerves respectively.

The local epineurium is resected. Grafts are provided by excision of the sural nerve through several transverse incisions. Surgeons who are not familiar with atraumatic techniques for this procedure may alternatively use a longitudinal incision exposing the whole nerve. In its proximal portion, the sural nerve is a mono- or oligofascicular nerve while towards the periphery the pattern becomes more and more polyfascicular. The nerve defect is measured with the joint held in neutral position and without mobilisation of the stumps. Ten per cent of the length is then added. Appropriate segments of the sural nerves are then selected which fit best between the individual fascicle groups of the two stumps. The fascicular pattern of the distal stump is clarified by retrograde tracing from the next division of the nerve. Sketches are made of the two cross-sections although the identification of the corresponding fascicles of the proximal stumps has to be arrived at by guesswork. The selected segments of the sural nerves are approximated to the fascicle or fascicle group by a single stitch. Since there is no tension usually one suture, if placed correctly, is sufficient to achieve adequate contact between the cross sections. Otherwise a second, or even a third suture might have to be used, but the aim is to keep the number of sutures to a

12   RECENT ADVANCES IN ORTHOPAEDICS

Fig. 1.1 This series of photographs of a median nerve lesion at the wrist demonstrates the technique of exploration, preparation of stumps and nerve grafting using a microsurgical approach.

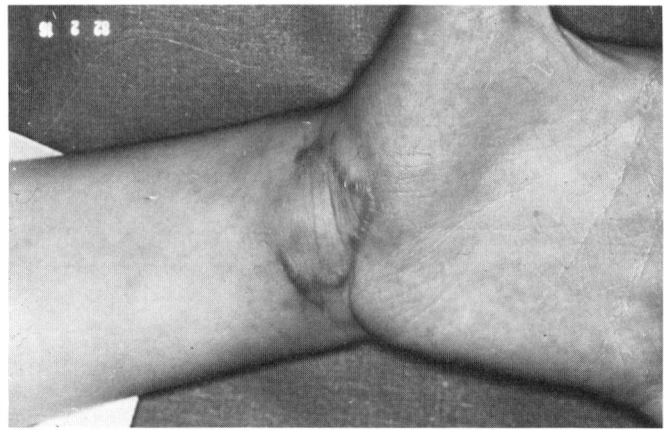

(A)

A: A seven-year-old patient suffered an injury from glass splinters at the left wrist two months previously.

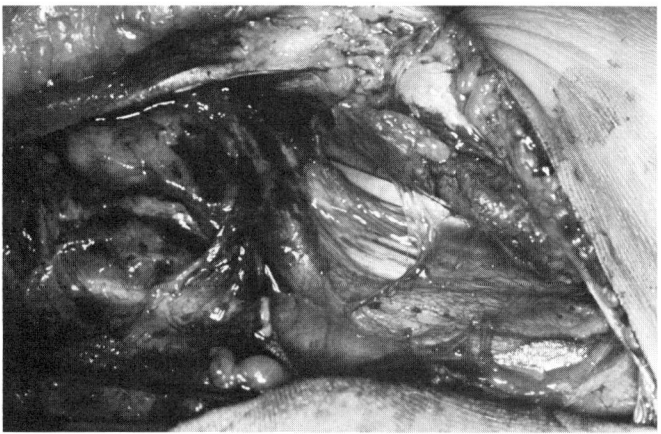

(B)

B: The site of the lesion just proximal to the carpal tunnel is exposed. The flexor retinaculum has been divided and a parietal layer of loose connective tissue covering the nerve can be clearly recognised.

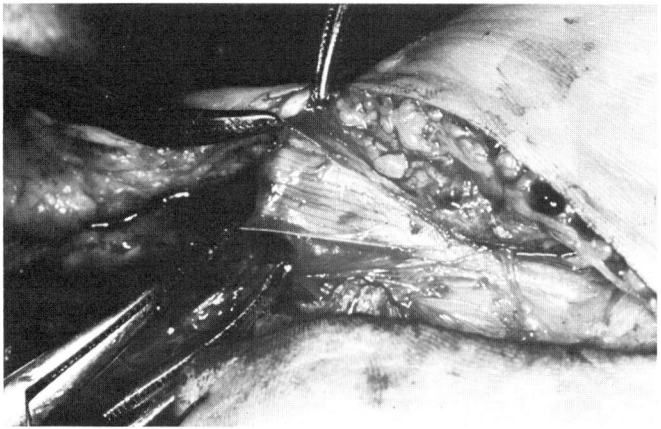

(C)

C: Even after division of this layer the nerve is still enveloped in a special sheath external to the epineurium.

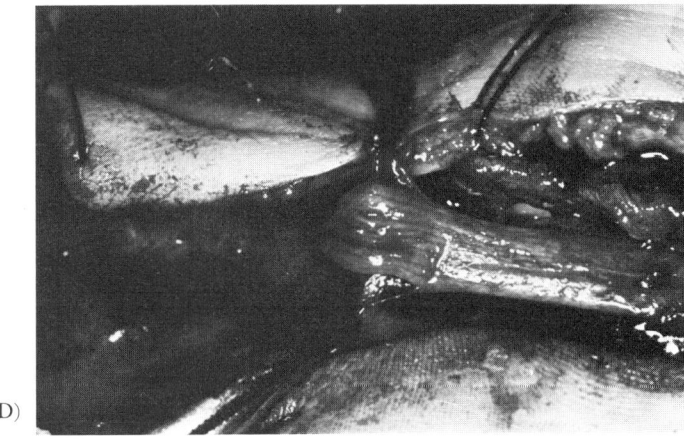

(D)

D: The distal stump after complete isolation. The external layer of epifascicular epineurium has been partially divided but the fascicles are still covered by a second layer of epifascicular epineurium. Individual fascicles can be recognised, some closer to each other forming groups.

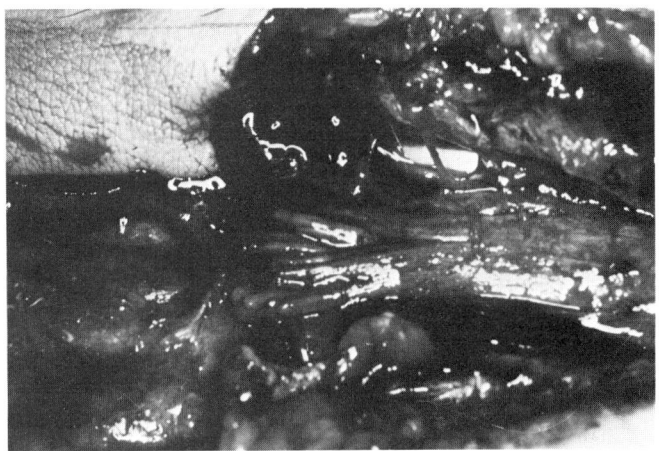

(E)

E: After resection of the epifascicular epineurium five fascicle groups can be distinguished.

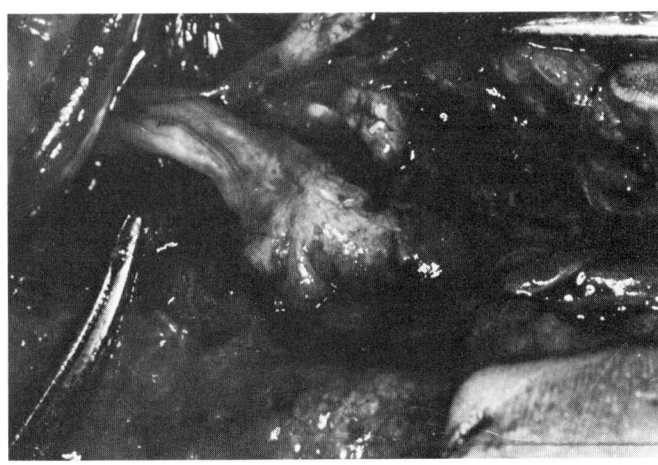

(F)

F: Illustrates the appearance of the proximal stump.

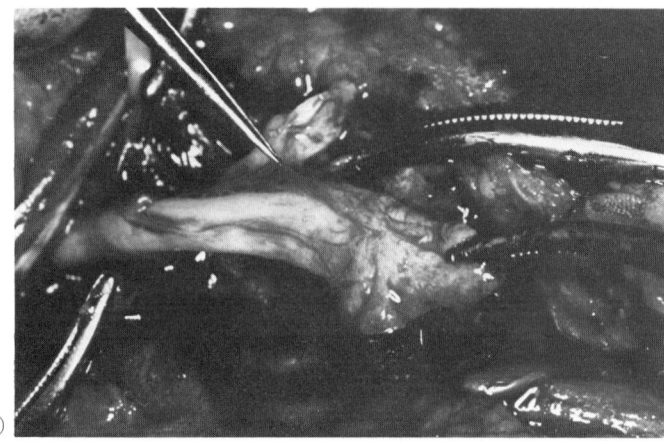

(G)

G: The group arrangement of fascicles in the proximal stump is revealed after removal of the epifascicular epineurium.

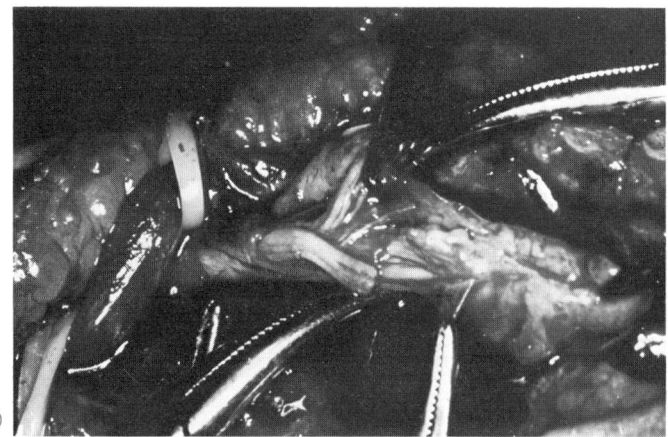

(H)

H: Isolation of the groups.

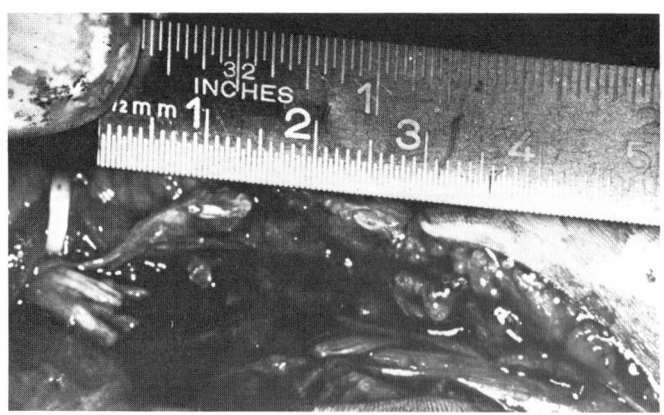

(I)

I: The two stumps after preparation. The defect is between 2 and 2.5 cm

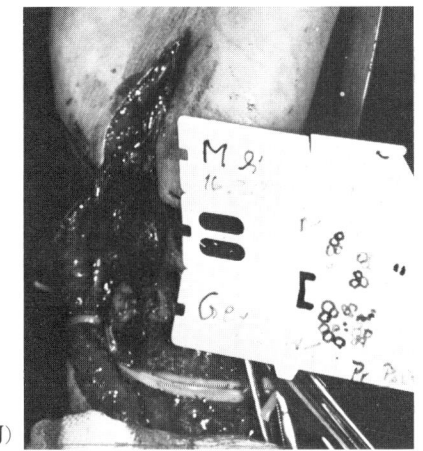 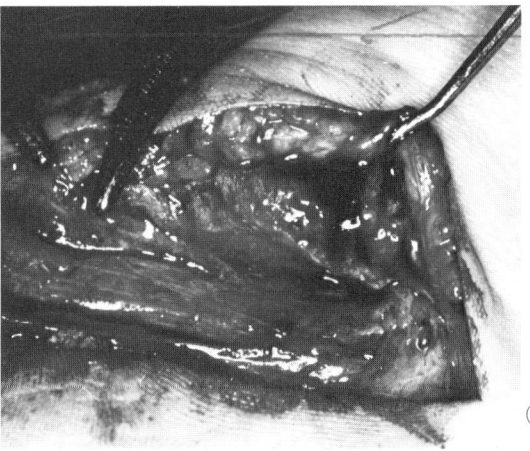

J: Sketches are made of the fascicular structure of the two stumps. The fascicular group containing the motor fibres is defined by retrograde tracing and marked 'M' in the distal sketch. A guess is made as to which is the corresponding fascicle group in the proximal stump and is marked 'W' in the mirror-like reverse sketch of the proximal stump.

K: Here is illustrated how the motor thenar branch ascends around the distal end of the flexor retinaculum.

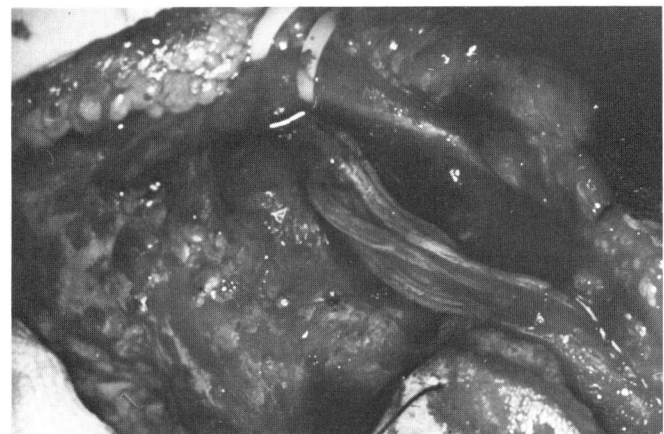

L: Five strands of one sural nerve are used to restore continuity between individual fascicle groups.

minimum. The transection of the fascicles or fascicle groups will have been performed at different levels. This leads to an interdigitation between the fascicles or fascicle groups increasing the stability of the junction. During wound closure extreme care is necessary to avoid shearing forces with separation of the grafts. The limb is then immobilised exactly in the same position as it was held during the operation for a period of 10 days. In addition to the sural nerves the medial cutaneous nerve of forearm and the lateral cutaneous nerve of thigh can also be used as donors.

In the case of a monofascicular stump, several grafts are united with the one large fascicle (fascicular grafting 1:2, 1:3, etc.). If there is a polyfasicular pattern without group arrangement interfascicular dissection is not possible and the grafts are applied to corresponding sectors of the cross section. No attempt should be made to combine several cutaneous nerve segments to achieve something like a cable graft, because survival of the grafts might be impaired by the decreased contact with the recipient side. Trunk grafts are not suitable for free grafting, they are too thick and they will suffer ischaemic damage leading to fibrosis before circulation is re-established. If a trunk graft is to be utilised as a free graft, as for example the ulnar nerve in brachial plexus lesions, the epifascicular epineurium is resected and the graft split into minor units.

If the location of the proximal or the distal stump is known from a previous operation, minimal exposure by transverse incisions may suffice. A tunnel is created across which the grafts are introduced and the coaptations performed within this limited exposure.

Vascularised nerve grafts
Taylor & Ham (1976), developed a technique of grafting nerve trunks by establishing neurovascular anastomosis to provide an immediate blood supply. Different nerve trunks have been used successfully. For obvious reasons these can only be obtained from limbs amputated at the same operation and this is one of the main limitations of this technique. A second problem is the fact that a vascularised trunk graft is associated with all the disadvantages of trunk-to-trunk coaptation. Due to the change in fascicular pattern along the graft one is not able to predict which fascicle group of the proximal end will correspond with a given fascicle group at the distal end. An alternative application for this technique is a brachial plexus lesion in which the ulnar nerve can be used as a graft. However, before excising the ulnar nerve, avulsion of the eighth cervical and first thoracic roots must be demonstrated surgically.

The superficial branch of the radial nerve has also been used as a vascularised nerve graft. Because of its small diameter it was combined with free nerve grafts (Biemer, 1978) and recent techniques have been developed to utilise the sural nerve as a vascularised graft (Fachinelli et al, 1981; Townsend, 1981).

Results
Comparing results is always difficult. An objective study would require the comparison of a prospective series with cases assigned to a particular technique at random and for obvious reasons this is not possible in clinical practice. Tables 1.4 and 1.5 present

Table 1.4 Ulnar nerve

Nerve grafts	
Proximal lesions N = 21	
M 4 or better	9 (42.9%)
M 3	3 (14.2%) — 12 (57.1%)
(×) Less than M 3	9 (42.9%)
(×) Length of defect: (cm) 6, 6, 6, 10, 13, 15, 16, 19, 20	

Table 1.5 Ulnar nerve — Nerve grafts

Distal lesions N = 21	
M 4 or better	12 (57.1%)
M 3	8 (38.1%) — 20 (95.2%)
Less than M 3	1 (4.8%)

MICROSURGERY OF PERIPHERAL NERVES 17

our own results obtained by free cutaneous nerve grafts utilising the interfascicular grafting technique performed between 1964 and 1976. The evaluations were performed according to Highet's scheme as used by Nicholson & Seddon (1957). A good example is shown in Figure 1.2.

The results obtained in cases where a favourable result might well have been anticipated, as for example in children, do not differ very much from the results of cases operated on in the conventional way. However, in more unfavourable cases we

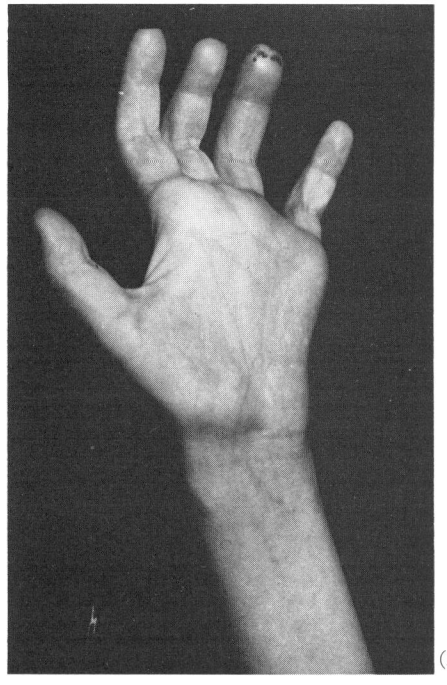

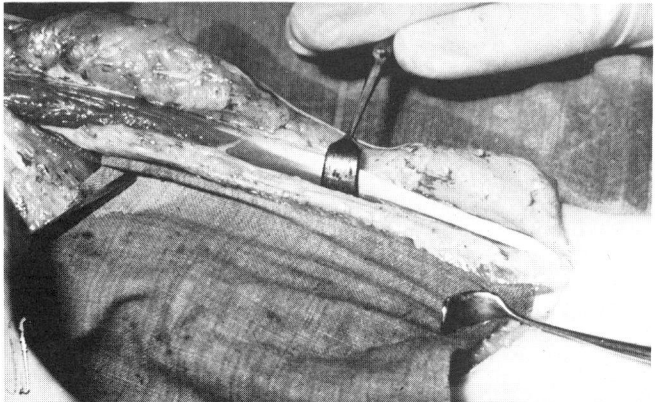

Fig. 1.2 Median and ulnar nerve lesions in a ten-year-old boy. A defect of 12 cm in the median nerve and 6 cm in the ulnar nerve was bridged by a sural nerve graft in 1966.

A: Pre-operative appearance.
B: Seven months later an opportunity was taken during an operation for other reasons, to inspect the nerves grafts bridging the median nerve defect.
C: see over.

18   RECENT ADVANCES IN ORTHOPAEDICS

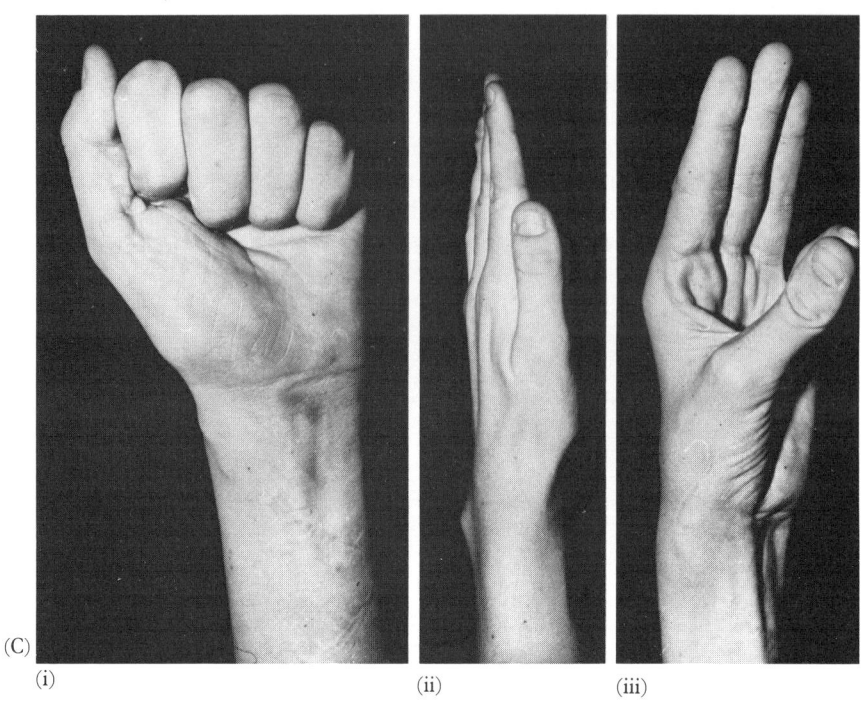

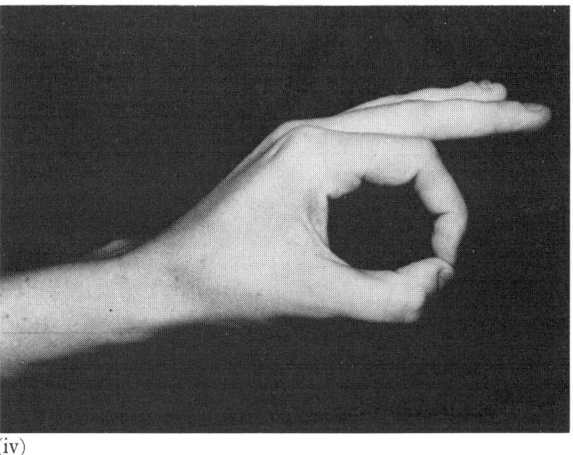

C: (i), (ii), (iii) and (iv) demonstrating the excellent function after 10 years.

think that there is considerable improvement. This applies particularly to patients with large defects which are quite impossible to bridge by neurorrhaphy, proximal lesions, nerve lesions in older patients and ones in which there has been a long time interval before reconstruction.

The surgical management of brachial plexus injuries has been improved considerably by the development of microsurgery. Intraneural neurolysis performed under the microscope permits an attack on lesions in continuity without too great a risk of damaging fascicles with spontaneous recovery potential. Divided roots or trunks may be treated by nerve grafting to restore continuity since neurorrhaphy is not usually possible because of the length of the defect. In cases where there has been avulsion of several roots, repairs have been achieved by nerve transfers using intercostal nerves as donors or motor parts of the cervical plexus or parts of the accessory nerve. Again, nerve grafts provide the link between the proximal and the distal stump.

Summary

The development of microsurgical techniques has initiated a significant change in the philosophy of nerve repair — a process which started years ago and is still continuing. Surgery has become more and more delicate and the possibility has been acquired of dealing with layers of nerve tissue which were inaccessible before. The results have been improved considerably, especially in those cases previously associated with poor prospects of recovery.

REFERENCES

Aguayo A J 1980 Myelinated and Unmyelinated Nerve Fibres, International Symposium on Post-Traumatic Nerve Regeneration, Padua 1980. In: Gorio A, Millesi H, Mingrino S (eds) Posttraumatic Peripheral Nerve Regeneration (Experimental Basis and Clinical Implications) 1981, Raven Press, New York p 165

Biemer E, Freie E 1978 Rippentransplantation mit mikrovaskulärem Gefässanschluss. Paper: 1st Ann. Meeting of the Deutschsprachige Arbeitsgemeinschaft für Mikrochirurgie der peripheren Nerven und Gefässe, Vienna, Dec. 7–9, 1978

Björkesten G 1947 Suture of war injuries to peripheral nerves: Clinical studies of results. Acta chirurgia scandinavica 95: 119, I

Böhler J 1962 Nervennaht und homoioplastische Nerventransplantation mit Milliporeumscheidung. Langenbeck's Archiv für Chirurgie 301: 900

Bora F W, Pleasure D E, Didzian N A 1976 A study of nerve regeneration and neuroma formation after nerve suture by various techniques. The Journal of Hand Surgery 1,2: 138

Bosse J P 1976 Personal Communication at the 5th International Symposium on Microsurgery in Guaruja, May 15–18, 1979

Bosse J P 1980 Discussion remark at the International Symposium on Post-Traumatic Peripheral Nerve Regeneration, Padua 1980. In: Gorio A, Millesi H, Mingrino S (eds) Posttraumatic Peripheral Nerve Regeneration (Experimental Basis and Clinical Implications) 1981, Raven Press, New York p 347

Bratton B R, Kline D G, Coleman W, Hudson A R 1979 Experimental interfascicular nerve grafting. Journal of Neurosurgery 51/3: 323

Braun R M 1964 Experimental peripheral nerve repair. Surgical Forum 15: 452

Braun R M 1966 Comparative studies of neurorrhaphy and sutureless peripheral nerve repair. Surgery, Gynecology and Obstetrics 122: 15

Brooks D 1955 The place of nerve grafting in orthopaedic surgery. Journal of Bone and Joint Surgery 37-A: 299

Bucko C D, Yoynt R L, Grabb W C 1981 Peripheral Nerve Regeneration in Primates During D-Penicillamine-Induced Lathyrism. Plastic and Reconstructive Surgery 67: 23

Bunge R, Bunge M 1978 Evidence that contact with connective tissue is required for normal interaction between Schwann cells and nerve fibres. Journal of Cell Biology 78: 943

Bunge R 1980 Contributions of tissue culture studies to our understanding of basic processes in peripheral nerve regeneration. Int. symposium on post-traumatic nerve regeneration, Padua, 1980. In: Gorio A, Millesi H, Mingrino S (eds) Posttraumatic Peripheral Nerve Regeneration (Experimental Basis and Clinical Implications) 1981, Raven Press, New York p 105

Cabaud H E, Rodkey W G, McCarroll Jr. H R, Mutz St. B, Niebauer J J 1976 Epineural and perineural fascicular nerve repair: A critical comparison. The Journal of Hand Surgery 1,2: 110

Campbell J B, Andrew C J, Husby J, Thulin C, Feringa E 1961 Microfilter sheathing in peripheral nerve surgery. Journal of Trauma 1: 139

Chanson L, Michon J, Merle M 1979 Etude des résultats de la réparation de 85 nerfs dont 49 gros troncs. In: Michon J, Moberg E (eds) Monographies du G.E.M.: Les lésions traumatiques des nerfs périphériques, 2nd edn. Expansion Scientifique Française, Paris p 139

Cruikshank W 1795 Experiments on the nerves, particularly on their reproduction and on the spinal marrow of living animals. Phylos. Trans 85: 1777

Curtis R M, Eversmann W W 1973 Internal neurolysis as an adjunct to the treatment of the carpal-tunnel syndrome. Journal of Bone and Joint Surgery 55A: 733
Ducker T B, Hayes G 1968 Experimental Improvement in the Use of Silastic Cuff of Peripheral Nerve Repair. Journal of Neurosurgery 28,6: 582
Ellis J S 1967 Technical aspects of peripheral nerve surgery. The British Club for Surgery of the Hand. The London Hospital Medical College Nov 17, 1967, 11
Engel J, Ganel A, Melamed R, Russon S, Farnie I 1980 Choline Acetyl Transferase for Differentiation between Human Motor and Sensory Nerve Fibres. Ann of Plastic Surgery 41: 376
Fachinelli A, Masquelet A, Restrepo J, Gilbert A 1981 The vascularized sural nerve. Anatomy and surgical approach. International Journal of Microsurgery 3,1: 57
Foerster O 1916 Paper read at the Außerordentliche Tagung der Deutschen Orthopädischen Gesellschaft Berlin, Februar 2–6, 1916 Münchener medizinische Wochenschrift 63: 283
Freilinger G, Gruber H, Holle J, Mandl H 1975 Zur Methodik der 'sensomotorisch' differenzierten Faszikelnaht peripherer Nerven. Handchirurgie 7: 133
Geldmacher J, Albers W 1981. The microsurgical restoration of peripheral nerves. Technique, results, problems in evaluation. Paper read at the 4th Congress of the European Section of the International Confederation for Plastic and Reconstructive Surgery, Athens, May 10–14, 1981
Goto Y 1967 Experimental study of nerve autografting by funicular suture. Arch. jap. chir. 36: 478
Grabb W C, Spencer L B, Koepke G H, Green R A 1970 Comparison of Methods of Peripheral Nerve Suturing in Monkeys. Plastic and Reconstructive Surgery 46: 31
Gruber H, Zenker W 1973 Acetylcholinesterase: Histochemical differentiation between motor and sensory nerve fibres. Brain Research 51: 207
Guegan Y 1979 Intérêt de points de suture dans la réalisation fasciculaires. Etude expérimentale. In: Michon J, Moberg E (eds) Les lésions traumatiques des nerfs périphériques. Monographies du G.E.M., Expansion Scientific Française Paris p 47
Hakstian R W 1968 Funicular orientation by direct stimulation, an aid to peripheral nerve repair. Journal of Bone and Joint Surgery 50A: 1178
Hastings J C, Peacock E E J 1973 Effect of injury, repair, and ascorbic acid deficiency on collagen accumulation in peripheral nerves. Surgical Forum 241: 516
Huber G C 1895 A study of the operative treatment for loss of nerve substance in peripheral nerves. Journal of Morphology 11: 629
Hudson A, Morris J, Weddel G 1970 An electron microscopic study of regeneration in sutured rat sciatic nerves. Surgical Forum 21: 451
Hueter K 1873 Die allgemeine Chirurgie. Vogel Verlag, Leipzig
Ito T 1969 The repair of severed peripheral nerves by funicular suture. Excerpta Medica Foundation, ICS 192 (60)
Jabaley M E, Wallace W H, Heckler F R 1980 Internal topography of major nerves of the forearm and hand: A current view. Journal of Hand Surgery 5: 1
Jurecka W, Ammerer H P, Lassmann H 1975 Regeneration of a transected peripheral nerve. An autoradiographical and electronmicroscopic study. Acta Neuropathologica (Berl.) 32: 299
Kline D G, Hayes G C 1964 The use of resorbable wrapper for peripheral nerve repair. Experimental studies in chimpanzees. Journal of Neurosurgery 21: 737
Kuderna H 1979 Ergebnisse und Erfahrungen in der klinischen Anwendung des Fibrin-Klebers bei der Wiederherstellung durchtrennter peripherer Nerven. Paper read at 17th Ann. Meeting of the Deutsche Gesellschaft für Plastische und Wiederherstellungschirurgie, Heidelberg, November 1–3, 1979
Kurze T 1964 Microtechnique in neural surgery. Chir. Nrosurg 11: 128
Langley J N, Hashimoto M 1917 On suture of separate nerve bundles in a nerve trunk and on internal nerve plexus. Journal of Physiology London 51: 318
Lundborg G, Hansson H H 1979 Regeneration of a peripheral nerve through a preformed tissue space. Brain Research 178: 573–576
Lundborg G, Hansson H H 1980 Nerve Lesions with Interruption of Continuity: Studies on the Growth Pattern of Regenerating Axons in the Gap Between the Proximal and Distal Nerve Ends. Int. Symp. on Post-Traumatic Nerve Regeneration, Padua 1980. In: Gorio A, Millesi H, Mingrono S (eds) Posttraumatic Peripheral Nerve Regeneration (Experimental Basis and Clinical Implications) 1981, Raven Press, New York p 229
Mackenzie I G, Woods C G 1961 Case of Failure after Repair of Median Nerve. Journal of Bone and Joint Surgery 43B: 465
Matras Helene, Kuderna H 1976 The principle of nervous anastomosis with clotting agents. In: Transactions of the 6th International Congress of Plastic and Reconstructive Surgery, Paris, August 24–29, 1975. Masson, Paris New York Barcelone Milan, p 143
McCarroll H R Jr, Rodkey W G, Cabaud D 1980 Results of suture of cat ulnar nerves: A comparison of surgical techniques. Symposium San Francisco 1977. In: Jewett D L, McCarroll Jr H R (eds) Nerve

Repair and Regeneration — Its clinical and experimental basis. The C V Mosby Company, Saint Louis, p 228

Michon J, Masse P 1964 Le moment optimum de la suture nerveuse dans les paies du membre supérieur. Revue Chirurgicale et Orthopédique 2, 205: 212

Midgley R, Woodhouse F 1968 Silicone rubber sheathing as an adjunct to neural anastomosing. Canadian Medical Journal 98: 550

Millesi H 1968 Zum Problem der Überbrückung von Defekten peripherer Nerven. Wiener medizinische Wochenschrift 118: 182

Millesi H 1977 Healing of Nerves. Clinics in Plastic Surgery 4 (3): 459

Millesi H 1980 Looking Back on Nerve Surgery. International Journal of Microsurgery 2 (3–4): 143

Millesi H 1980 How Exact Should Coaptation Be?. Int. Symposium on Post-Traumatic Nerve Regeneration, Padua 1980. In: Gorio A, Millesi H, Mingrino S (eds) Posttraumatic Peripheral Nerve Regeneration (Experimental Basis and Clinical Implications). Raven Press, New York, 1981, p 301

Millesi H, Ganglberger J, Berger A 1967 Erfahrungen mit der Mikrochirurgie der peripheren Nerven. Chirurgia plastica 3: 47

Millesi H 1970 Probleme der Wiederherstellung bei ausgedehnten Weichteildefekten an der oberen Extremität. Handchirurgie 2, 2: 80

Millesi H 1972 Die operative Wiederherstellung verletzter Nerven. Langenbecks Archiv für Chirurgie 332: 347

Millesi H, Berger A, Meissl G 1970 Razvoj Reparatorno Operativnih Postupaka Kod Ozijeda Periferinih Zivaca. Drugi Simpozij O Bolestima I Ozljedama Sake 161

Millesi H, Berger A, Meissl G 1972 Experimentelle Untersuchungen zur Heilung durchtrennter peripherer Nerven. Chirurgia plastica 1: 174

Millesi H, Meissl G, Berger A 1972 The interfascicular nerve-grafting of the median and ulnar nerves. Journal of Bone and Joint Surgery (Am) 54: 727

Millesi H, Meissl G, Berger A 1976 A further experience with interfascicular grafting of the median, ulnar and radial nerves. Journal of Bone and Joint Surgery (Am) 58: 209

Nicholson O R, Seddon H J 1957 Nerve repair in civil practice. Results of treatment of median and ulnar nerve lesions. British Medical Journal 2: 1065

Peripheral Nerve Injury Report 1953 In: Sir Zachary Cope (ed) History of the Second World War. United Kingdoms Medical Series Her Majesty's Stationery Office, London

Pleasure D, Bora F W, Lane J, Prockop D 1974 Regeneration after nerve transsection: Effect of inhibition of collagen synthesis. Experimental Neurology 45: 72

Ramón y Cajal S 1928 Degeneration and Regeneration of the Nervous System. Oxford University Press, London Vol. I

Rydevik B, Lundborg G, Nordborg C 1976 Intraneural Tissue Reactions Induced by Internal Neurolysis. Scandinavian Journal of Plastic and Reconstructive Surgery 10: 3

Samii M, Wallenborn R 1972 Tierexperimentelle Untersuchungen über den Einfluss der Spannung auf den Regenerationserfolg nach Nervennaht. Acta Neurochirurgia (Vienna) 27: 87

Seddon H J 1943 Three types of nerve injury. Brain 66: 237

Seddon H J 1963 Nerve grafting. Journal of Bone and Joint Surgery 45B: 447

Seddon H J 1972 Surgical disorders of the peripheral nerves 1st edn. and 1975 2nd edn. Churchill Livingstone, Edinburgh, London, New York, p 15

Smith J W 1964 Microsurgery of peripheral nerves. Plastic and Reconstructive Surgery 33: 317

Sunderland S 1945 The intraneural topography of the radial, median and ulnar nerves. Brain 68: 243

Sunderland S, Ray L N 1948 The intraneural topography of the sciatic nerve and its popliteal division in man. Brain 71: 242

Sunderland S 1952 Factors influencing the course of regeneration and quality of the recovery after nerve suture. Brain 75: 19

Sunderland S 1953 Funicular suture and funicular exclusion in the repair of severed nerves. British Journal of Surgery 40: 580

Sunderland S, Marshall R D, Swaney W E 1959 The intraneural topography of the circumflex musculocutaneous and obturator nerves. Brain 82: 116

Sunderland S 1978 Nerves and Nerve Injuries, 2nd edn. Churchill Livingstone, Edinburgh, London, New York. ch 14, p 212

Sunderland S 1978 Nerves and Nerve Injuries, 2nd edn. Churchill Livingstone, Edinburgh, London, New York. ch 49, p 593

Sunderland S 1951 A classification of peripheral nerve injuries producing loss of function. Brain 74: 491

Taylor G I, Ham F J 1976 The free vascularized nerve graft. Plastic and Reconstructive Surgery 57: 413

Terzis J F, Faibisoff R, Williams H B 1975 The nerve gap: Suture under tension versus graft. Plastic and Reconstructive Surgery 56: 166

Townsend P 1981 Microvascular nerve grafts. Personal communication at the 4th Congress of the European Section of the International Confederation for Plastic and Reconstructive Surgery, Athens, May 10–14, 1981
Tupper J W 1977 Fascicular nerve repair. Symposium at San Francisco, 1977. In: Jewett D L, McCarroll Jr H R (eds) Nerve Repair and Regeneration: Its clinical and experimental basis. The C. V. Mosby Company, Saint Louis, 1980 p 320
Wise A J, Topuzlu C, Davis P, Kaye I S 1969 A comparative analysis of macro- and microsurgical neurorrhaphy techniques. American Journal of Surgery 117: 566
Williams H B 1979 Intraneural topography. Personal communication at 5th International Symposium on Microsurgery, Guaruja, May 15–18, 1979

2. Reconstructive procedures in congenital dislocation of the hip

S. S. Coleman

INTRODUCTION

Successful treatment of congenital dislocation of the hip, even when the diagnosis is made in early infancy, occasionally requires a reconstructive procedure on either the acetabular or femoral side of the hip joint sometime during the child's growth. In some rare circumstances, both sides may need a corrective operation. It is the purpose of this section to discuss these procedures as they are currently being employed in the treatment of congenital dislocation of the hip and its sequelae.

It is essential that there is agreement upon what constitutes a *reconstructive* operation on the hip in a child or an adolescent. It is also necessary to separate them, conceptually at least, from those operations that have become established as 'salvage' operations. In order to do so, brief allusion to these latter operations is required, because there is a very basic difference between reconstructive and salvage procedures. In the former, the intent is to achieve an anatomical result that ultimately is, or very nearly approaches, normal; whereas, in the latter a temporary solution to a problem in congenital dislocation of the hip is all that can be expected to be achieved.

Reconstructive procedures on the acetabular side consist of the pericapsular iliac osteotomy (Pemberton, 1965), the innominate redirectional osteotomy (Salter, 1961), the double innominate osteotomy (Sutherland, 1977), the triple innominate osteotomy (Steel, 1973), and the spherical (Wagner, 1978) or 'dial' (Eppright, 1981) procedures that are more or less complete pericapsular acetabuloplasties. All have one thing in common, namely, that their ultimate goal is to place the bone of the acetabulum, with its hyaline articular cartilage, into a more anatomically normal position over the weight-bearing portion of the femoral head.

On the other hand, salvage procedures on the acetabular side consist of the Chiari osteotomy, the 'shelf' procedure, the Colonna capsular arthroplasty, the trochanteric arthroplasty; and, lastly, implant arthroplasty. This latter operation should never be done in a skeletally immature patient; and is only mentioned at this time for completeness. The former procedures, except for the trochanteric arthroplasty, an operation that is rarely indicated in congenital dislocation of the hip, have one major accomplishment in common; namely, that in different ways they utilize in varying degrees the joint capsule as the weight-bearing surfaces for the femoral head. This is an extremely important concept to grasp, because fibrocartilaginous metaplasia of the capsule is necessary in order for any of these salvage procedures to provide an acceptable result, and even then it must be considered a temporary 'compromise' solution.

The need for reconstructive procedures on the femoral side of the hip joint in congenital dislocation of the hip is much easier to establish than for reconstructive operations on the pelvic side. The reason for this is that the morphology of the femur, as compared to the acetabulum, is relatively easy to characterize; and any substantial abnormalities in rotation or angulation can be demonstrated rather accurately, if the three radiographic views discussed in the subsequent section are appropriately utilized. Thus, the need for either a rotational or an angulation osteotomy should be based upon a clearly defined radiographic abnormality in the configuration of the proximal femur. More specifically, a proximal femoral osteotomy that is accomplished in treatment of congenital dislocation of the hip, should be directed towards achieving *correction* of an abnormality in the femur rather than producing a *compensatory* skeletal abnormality (abnormal varus or rotation) that is indirectly designed to accomplish some improvement in the hip joint relationship and development of the acetabulum. The argument for this concept is based upon my observation that there is little scientific data to prove that a varus or a varus-rotational osteotomy of the proximal femur, accomplished in the femur of *normal* configuration, can effect any substantial change in the development of the acetabulum, wherein there is a stable, concentric hip reduction. This will be discussed in greater detail in a subsequent section.

As implied in the foregoing paragraph, reconstructive proximal femoral osteotomies consist of either angular (varus or valgus) or rotational (usually outward rotation of the distal fragment), or both. Each has the same indication; namely, the need for correction of a defined deformity, and each has its own prerequisites which, from a practical point of view, are identical to those established for pelvic osteotomy, a subject to be covered in depth in later sections.

One can summarize the foregoing discussion by concluding that reconstructive procedures about the hip joint in congenital dislocation of the hip should be directed towards correcting proven deformity and establishing normal acetabular-femoral anatomy as well as possible. To what extent this may require an operative procedure on the acetabulum, the proximal femur, or both will depend substantially upon the diagnostic skill and acumen of the surgeon. In addition, the effectiveness of the surgical treatment usually will be governed not only by the technical expertise with which the corrective operations are accomplished, but also by the age of the patient at the time of surgery as well as the ability of the hip joint to respond to the surgical procedures by means of growth and remodelling.

Pelvic reconstructive procedures

As noted above, the basic accomplishments these procedures have in common is rotation of the roof of the acetabulum in such a way so as to utilize the hyaline articular cartilage for weight bearing. All of them have (or should have) the same fundamental indications and prerequisites in order to achieve the most optimal results. On the other hand, there are substantial differences in the technique by which they are accomplished, as well as in their contraindications and complications. The prerequisites can be discussed as a general issue, but the specific indications, the techniques, the contraindications, and the potential hazards and complications will be discussed separately.

Prerequisites and indications for a reconstructive
PELVIC OSTEOTOMY

Prerequisites: There are at least *three* conditions (or prerequisites) that must be fulfilled before a reconstructive pelvic osteotomy can be effectively accomplished. These include (1) a normal or near-normal range of hip motion, (2) congruent relationships between the femoral head and acetabulum, with a concentrically reduced femoral head, and (3) a normal, or reasonably normal, cartilage or 'clear' space in the hip joint.

Because the prime purpose of these osteotomies is to rotate the cartilage covered roof of the acetabulum so as to provide a more normal and effective weight-bearing relationship to the femoral head, it is obvious that the femoral head must move freely in the acetabulum. Thus, normal or near-normal ranges of hip motion are an essential prerequisite. It is especially important that the motions of flexion, abduction and inward rotation be normal, because anterior and lateral deficiencies of the femoral head coverage are almost always the directions in which the acetabulum is rotated. Substantially restricted hip motion will not permit such rotation and, in fact, any effort to accomplish acetabular rotation may simply cause the femoral head to be pushed more laterally rather than become better covered.

The femoral head and acetabular joint surfaces *must* be *reasonably* congruent, and the femoral head *must* be concentrically situated within the acetabulum. These prerequisites are just as critical as the need for a normal range of motion of the hip. The same principles apply; namely, when there is a non-spherical femoral head-acetabular relationship, or where the hip joint is inadequately reduced, effective rotation of the acetabular roof over the femoral head cannot be satisfactorily achieved. Again, the effect of the acetabular rotation will simply be a more lateral, and perhaps downward, displacement of the femoral head, without really improving its weight-bearing coverage by the acetabulum.

It is preferable that the cartilage or 'clear' space of the hip joint be of reasonably normal thickness. This will almost always exist *if* the earlier prerequisites have been fulfilled. In other words, in the presence of a normal range of motion, a congruent femoral head-acetabular relationship, and a concentric reduction, there should be very little reduction in the thickness of the cartilage space.

In order to establish that these requirements have been fulfilled, a very careful physical examination must be done, and at least three radiographic views of the hip joint are required pre-operatively. This includes (1) a true anteroposterior view of the pelvis or hip with the thigh (hip) in neutral rotation; (2) an anteroposterior view of the pelvis or hip with the thigh (hip) held in abduction and inward rotation (*not* a 'frogleg' view); and (3) a groin or crosstable *lateral* view of the *acetabulum* with the thigh in neutral rotation. These combined views give a three-dimensional picture of the femoral head-acetabular relationships. The abduction and inward rotation view is especially valuable because if the femoral head seats *concentrically* into the acetabulum in this projection, then one of the prime prerequisites has been met for performing a reconstructive pelvic osteotomy.

The need for, and the place of, arthrography is a highly individualized issue. My indications for performing hip joint arthrography are very limited, and include those instances where I am in doubt about concentricity of reduction or congruency of the acetabular-femoral head relationships, as seen on the plain X-ray films noted above.

26 RECENT ADVANCES IN ORTHOPAEDICS

(A)

a

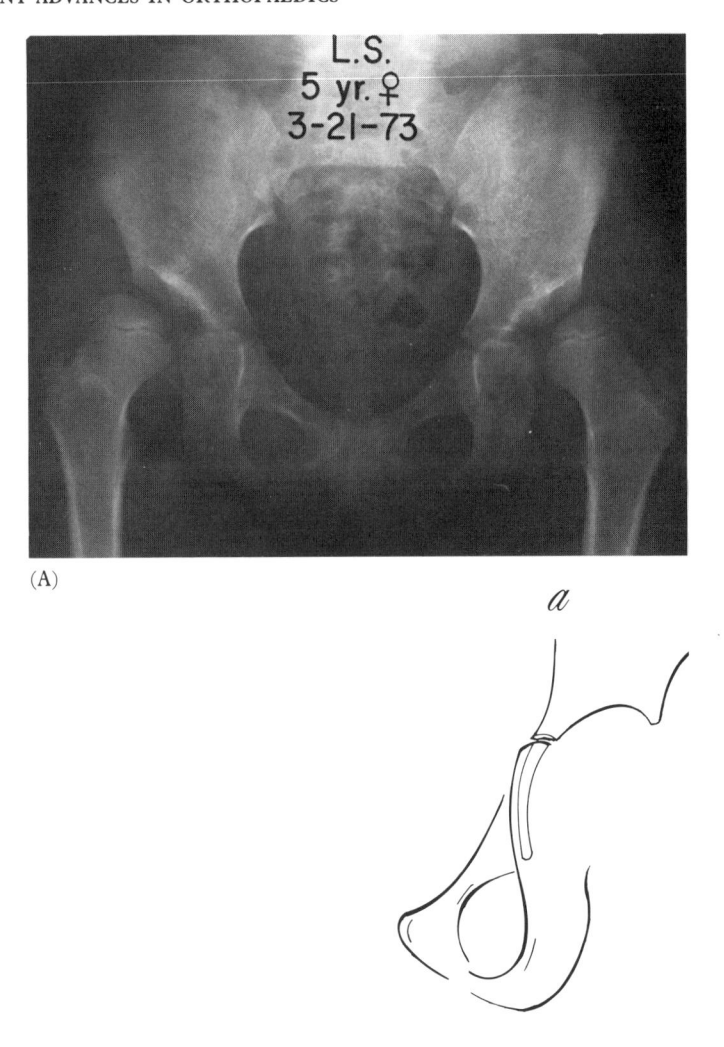

Fig. 2.1 Examples to show the variations in the configuration of the 'teardrop' on the medial wall of the acetabulum. Failure of the teardrop to appear at all in children over 18 months of age (A) means that the femoral head has never been properly reduced into the acetabulum. The normal teardrop is seen in the right hip in the roentgenogram (B) and the artist's depiction (a). Late reduction, but satisfactory, stable reduction of the hip is often accompanied by a teardrop of greater thickness as seen in the left hip in this roentgenogram (B) and the artist's depiction (b). Incomplete reduction, subluxation of the hip, or an unstable, subluxating hip usually is reflected by a 'V' or wedge shaped teardrop, as seen in the left hip in this roentgenogram (C) and the artist's interpretation (c). The right hip has a normal tear drop. (Roentgenograms A–B from Coleman S S, 1978 Congenital dysplasia and dislocation of the hip. C V Mosby, St Louis.)

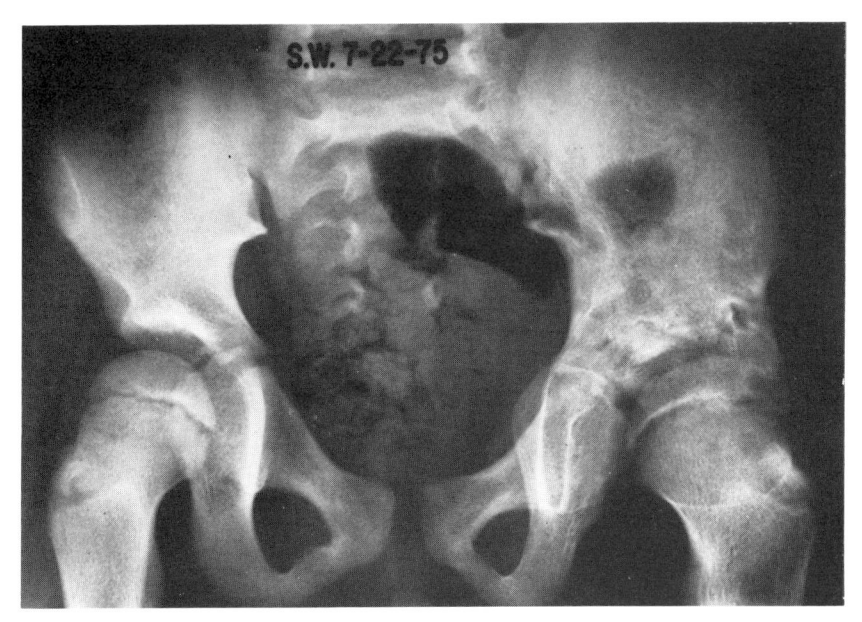

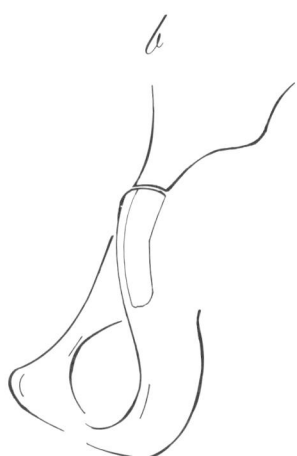

Fig. 2.1 (B)

In the large majority of instances, careful scrutiny of the plain films will be adequate to make the determinations. However, whenever there is doubt, arthrography may be helpful.

The place of CAT scans in establishing the acetabular-femoral head relationships has about the same position as arthrography. In other words, when in doubt one should use all *appropriate* ancillary studies that are available in an effort to define the acetabular-femoral head relationships accurately. The routine use of these invasive (arthrography) and expensive (CAT scan) techniques is, however, not warranted. Careful analysis of the three X-ray views listed earlier should, with rare exceptions, provide sufficient information in order to establish the presence or absence of a concentric reduction.

28 RECENT ADVANCES IN ORTHOPAEDICS

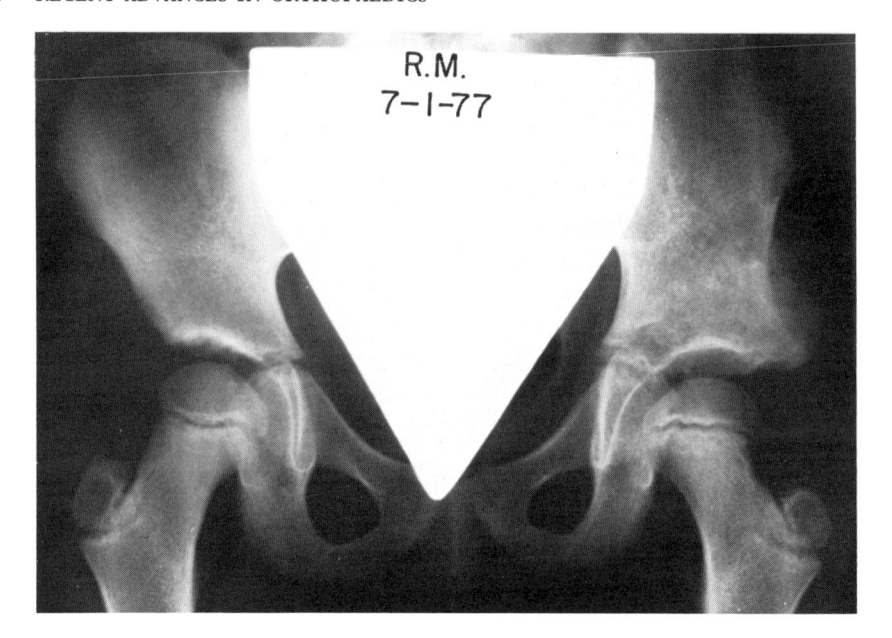

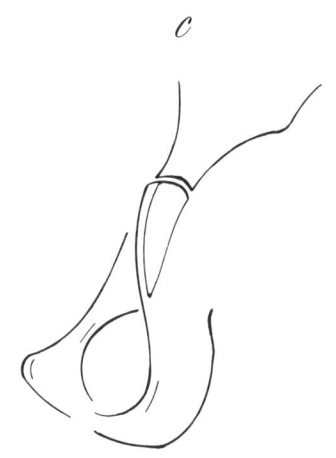

Fig. 2.1 (C)

I have utilized one radiographic determination that has been extremely helpful in establishing these femoral head-acetabular relationships. This consists of the configuration and thickness of the 'tear drop', which represents the response in development of the medial acetabular wall to femoral head articulation. In the normal development of the hip, the 'tear drop' eventually assumes a biconcave configuration. When the femoral head has not been or is not articulating in a normal concentric fashion, the medial wall (tear drop) will be either of greater thickness than normal, or it will assume a 'V' shape, reflecting either chronic subluxation, or failure of concentricity of reduction (Fig. 2.1). In young children, these abnormal findings on the medial acetabular wall can be reversed to some degree following pelvic (stabilizing) osteotomy. However, in older children and adolescents it is rare to see substantial alteration in either the thickness or the shape of the tear drop after pelvic osteotomy. The important thing to emphasize, however, is the value of scrutinizing carefully the medial acetabular wall, the rest of the acetabulum, and other aspects of the film in order to gain some valid impression of the functional relationships of the femoral head to the acetabulum. A weight-bearing AP view of the pelvis may be of special value in detecting instability, and it should be done in all cases when in doubt, and especially in those instances of a 'V' shaped teardrop.

Indications: The factors governing the need for reconstructive pelvic osteotomy are not easy to establish. The principal reasons for this difficulty consist of the following: (1) there is currently a substantial frailty in our ability to define the true configuration of the acetabulum, especially in the younger child; (2) the ability for the acetabulum to remodel and respond to a concentrically reduced femoral head is not well established, and it may vary substantially from one patient to another, especially in different age groups; (3) greater evidence is available to indicate that acetabular remodelling in response to a well reduced femoral head can continue through the entire growth of the pelvis and surely through the ages of eight or nine years and (4) the *long term* results of reconstructive pelvic osteotomy are still not known, specifically as they relate to the prevention or to the delay in onset of degenerative hip joint disease.

Nevertheless, from an intuitive point of view, and from the studies of Wiberg (1939), it seems justifiable to assume that in the presence of a persistently defective or inadequate acetabulum, wherein the femoral head is poorly covered, that some form of pelvic reconstructive osteotomy is justified. The problem arises when one is required to specify exactly what is a defective or inadequate acetabulum. The ability to establish this issue with confidence poses greater difficulty in younger age groups, but in late childhood and adolescence a reasonably accurate and defensible definition of the acetabular configuration can be synthesized. It is important, therefore, to establish the radiographic determinants for each age group; and to outline the method by which these criteria are established. Because reconstructive pelvic osteotomies are somewhat age-related, according to my own current concept of the indications, the osteotomies will be discussed separately from the standpoint of the indications.

Because the pelvis and upper femur of the growing patient exercise substantially different physical characteristics throughout growth; and because there is substantial variation in the ability of the acetabulum and hip joint to respond to corrective operative procedures at different skeletal ages, it becomes apparent that there is no single, exclusive reconstructive operation on either the acetabulum or the proximal femur that can be expected to solve all of the problems that are unique to the wide variation in pathology that can exist in congenital dislocation of the hip. Thus, it is essential that the problem and the pathology of the hip joint be clearly defined, so that the appropriate procedure is utilized in effecting a solution. The remainder of this chapter will deal with the indications and contraindications for each of the currently accepted technical *reconstructive* operations being utilized for the treatment of congenital dislocation of the hip and its sequelae. The technical details of the operative procedures will not be described or illustrated, except when considered necessary to clarify specific issues.

PEMBERTON 'PERICAPSULAR' OSTEOTOMY

Technique and indications: Pemberton (1965) designed this operation in order to achieve correction of an acetabulum that is deficient anteriorly and laterally. Within the limitations of our abilities to define this deficiency, this still remains the prime indication for the procedure (or *any* other reconstructive acetabular operation). Because of the unique technical characteristics of the operation, it is possible to execute only in children who have a flexible triradiate cartilage. The procedure also should be done only when there is clear cut evidence of a deficient acetabulum (instability) at the time of open reduction, or when the acetabulum fails to develop and improve over a substantial period of observation after successful closed or *stable* open reduction (Fig. 2.2).

It is technically a rather difficult operation to do because it requires a precisely placed pericapsular cut in the outer table of the ilium, extending from just above the anterior-inferior spine anteriorly to the posterior arm of the triradiate cartilage. A companion cut is then made in the inner table of the ilium, parallel to but somewhat lower (more distal) than the outer cut. The difference in the locations of these two cuts in the ilium governs the direction of rotation that can be achieved in the inferior fragment, i.e., the higher the outer cut with respect to the inner cut, the greater will be the degree of outward rotation of the distal fragment. Conversely, the closer these cuts are made parallel to each other, the lesser will be the degree of outward rotation. This technical detail, therefore, provides a substantial degree of versatility to the procedure.

Advantages: The versatility alluded to above is one of the prime advantages of the pericapsular osteotomy over other osteotomies of the ilium. Another advantage is that the posterior aspect of the acetabulum is not disturbed; therefore it can be used effectively in acetabular deficiencies associated with paralytic dislocation and subluxation of the hip (Coleman, 1981) (Fig. 2.3). An additional advantage of this operation is the fact that the osteotomy is incomplete and it is therefore inherently stable; thus, no internal fixation is required and therefore the possibility of penetrating the joint with pins is obviated. Also, a second procedure to remove internal fixation is unnecessary. Finally, a greater degree of acetabular roof rotation can be achieved with a lesser degree of opening of the osteotomy. This is because the fulcrum of rotation of the osteotomy is so close to the joint (triradiate cartilage).

Disadvantages: These consist of the following: (1) It is technically a more difficult procedure to learn to accomplish properly and the danger of entering the hip joint with an improperly done osteotomy is substantial; (2) It definitely changes the configuration of the acetabulum. This is a disadvantage only if done in older children who have little remodelling capacity of their acetabulum. In younger children, if done with proper indications, I have not found this to be a problem; and (3) Finally, it is restricted only to those children whose pelves have flexible triradiate cartilages. In other words, the operation cannot be done very effectively in children over six or

CONGENITAL DISLOCATION OF THE HIP 31

(A)

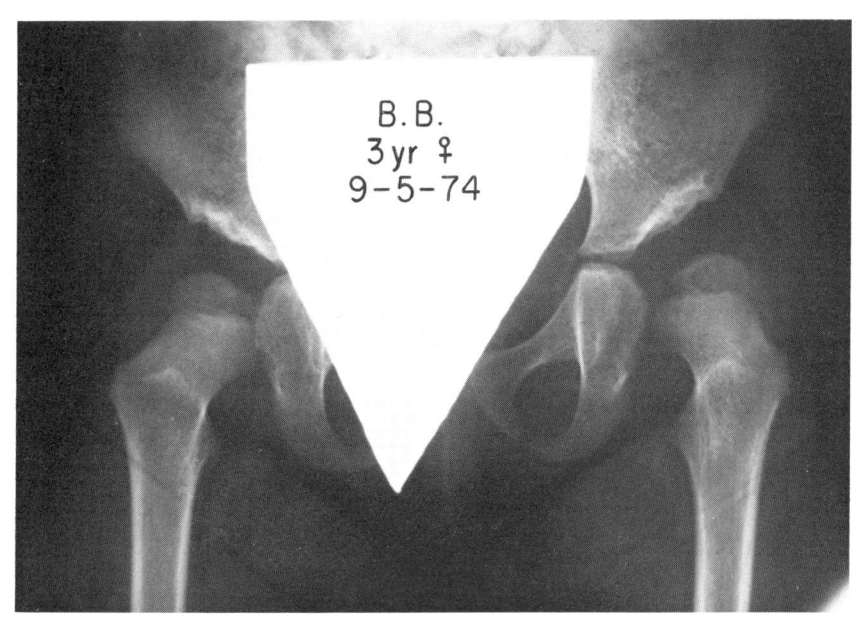

(B)

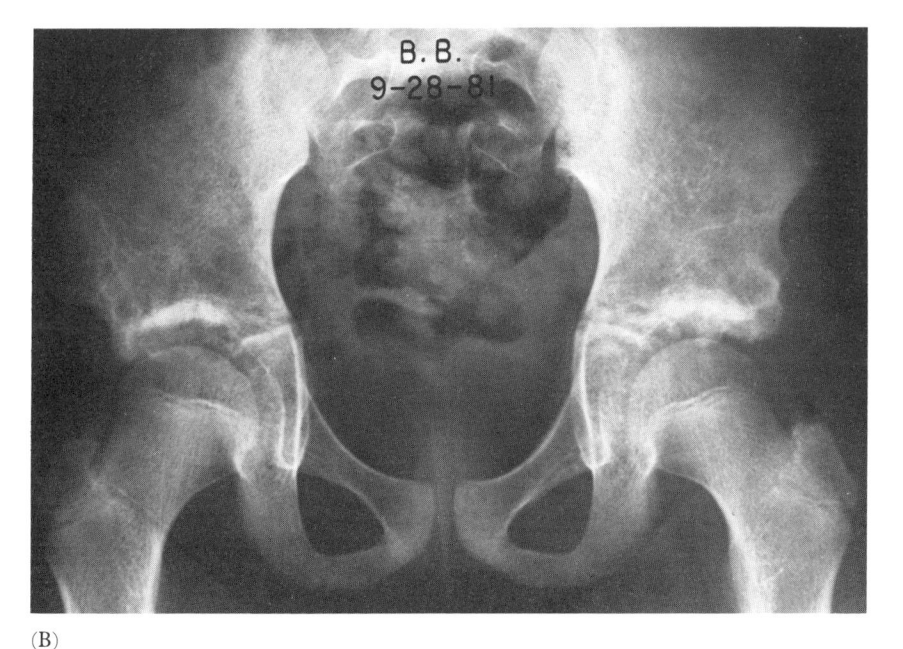

Fig. 2.2 Roentgenogram of the pelvis of a three year old female who had previously undergone an open reduction of both hips at age 18 months by means of the medial adductor approach (A). Because of failure of the acetabular roof to improve, because of the lack of definition of the teardrop, and because of the break in Shenton's line, a pericapsular Pemberton pelvic osteotomy was accomplished bilaterally. The result seven years later is seen in B. Note improved (almost normal) appearance of the medial teardrop, and the concentric and congruent relationship of the femoral head to the acetabulum.

32 RECENT ADVANCES IN ORTHOPAEDICS

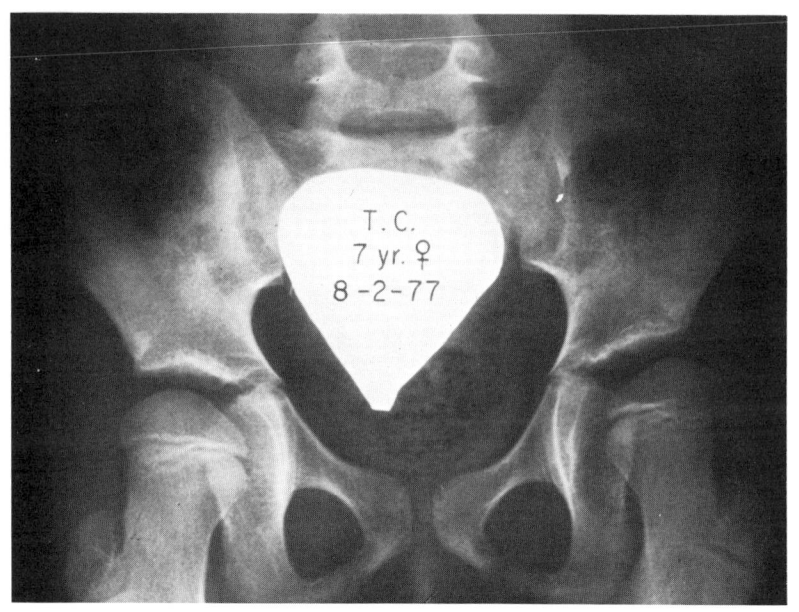

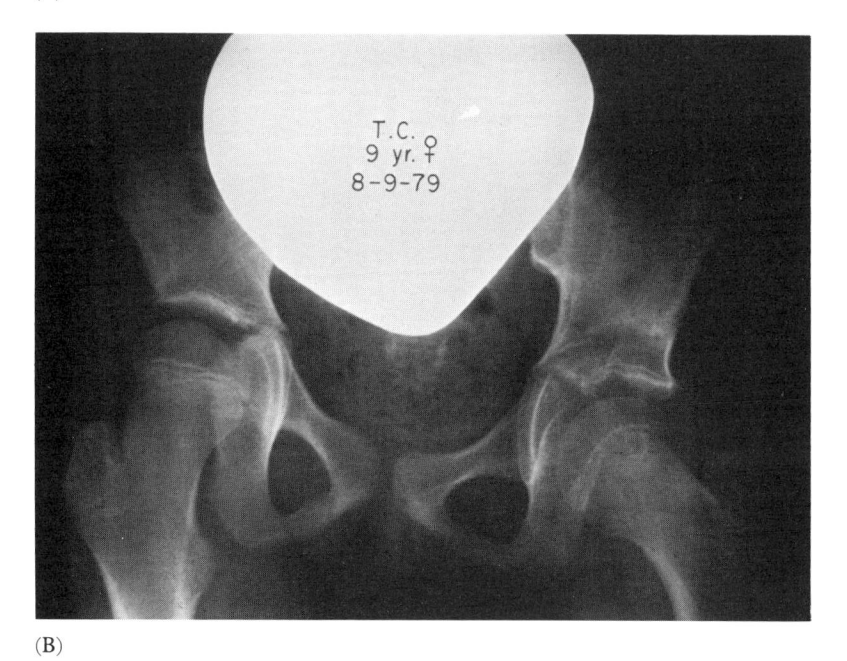

Fig. 2.3 An example of the value of the Pemberton osteotomy in paralytic hip disorders is seen in the pelvic roentgenogram of this seven year old female with cerebral palsy (A). Note the obliquity of the acetabulum, the increased valgus deformity of the proximal femur, the extrapelvic protrusion, and the 'V' shaped medial teardrop. Two years later, following a simultaneous pericapsular osteotomy and varus osteotomy of the proximal femur, substantially improved hip joint relationships are seen (B). Note the well-covered femoral head, but also observe that the configuration of the teardrop remains unchanged.

seven years of age. A conceptual disadvantage that rarely surfaces is the potential possibility of closing the triradiate cartilage. It has been reported by McKay, but I have not encountered it in my personal experience.

THE SALTER (REDIRECTIONAL) OSTEOTOMY

Technique and indications: Based upon the concept that the major problem of the deficient acetabulum is one of maldirection, resulting in deficient anterior and lateral femoral head coverage, Salter (1961) devised the redirectional pelvic osteotomy. It employs a complete osteotomy performed across the superior aspect of the acetabulum, extending from the sciatic notch to just above the anterior-inferior iliac spine. The inferior fragment is then rotated forward and somewhat outward and downward, thus correcting the maldirection. Because it is a complete osteotomy, there is need for internal fixation of the fragments in order to hold the fragments in their corrected position. Usually at least two threaded Steinmann pins (or hexhead screws) are necessary in order to stabilize the fragment satisfactorily. The indications are identical with those for the Pemberton osteotomy; namely, a deficient acetabulum demonstrable either at the time of open reduction (instability of reduction) or by virtue of a proven failure of the acetabulum to develop and remodel over a period of observation *following* either closed or *stable* open reduction (Fig. 2.4).

Advantages: These are best related to the operation of Pemberton: (1) the operation can be accomplished with greater simplicity (a single, straight pelvic osteotomy); (2) it produces no change in the acetabular configuration; and (3) it can be done in children through age 12 or 15 years of age (or even older than this according to Salter, 1981).

Disadvantages: These consist of the following: (1) The osteotomy is unstable; thus, internal fixation is necessary; (2) the possibility of penetrating the joint by the pins is very real; (3) removal of the pins necessitates a second (minor) operation; (4) there is less versatility in the direction that the lower (acetabular) fragment can be placed; and, (5) the posterior aspect of the femoral head is uncovered to the same extent that the anterior and lateral aspects of the head are covered. Thus, it cannot be employed effectively in paralytic dislocations, wherein the acetabular defect most often is posterior-superior.

SUTHERLAND 'DOUBLE' OSTEOTOMY

Technique and indications: This osteotomy was developed much later than the redirectional osteotomy. The reasons for its creation were based upon two concepts; namely, (1) that rotation of the inferior fragment, when performing the Salter osteotomy, became difficult to achieve in older children, and (2) that the redirectional osteotomy displaced the acetabulum laterally thus preventing medialization of the socket towards the centre of gravity of the body (Sutherland & Greenfield, 1977).

Therefore, the superior and inferior pubic rami are divided each by means of a single cut just lateral to the pubic symphysis, and the ilium is osteotomized in the same manner as that developed earlier by Salter. In order to achieve medial displacement of the acetabulum, a segment (about 1 cm) of the two pubic rami is

34   RECENT ADVANCES IN ORTHOPAEDICS

(A)

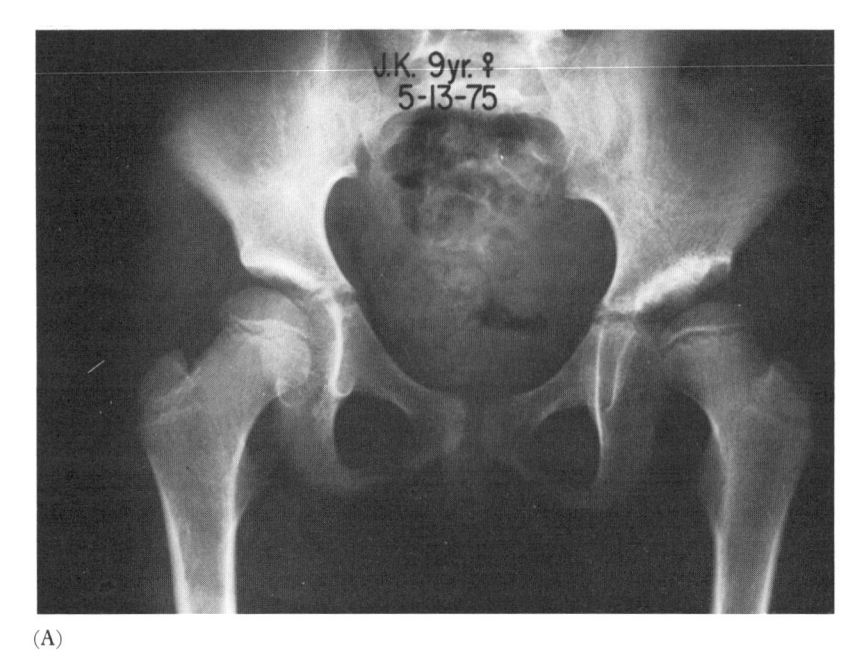

(B)

Fig. 2.4 Pelvic roentgenogram (A) of a nine year old female who developed a limp over the previous two years. There was no prior history of hip abnormality. Note the oblique, sloping acetabulum, the extrapelvic femoral head protrusion and the thickened and 'V' shaped teardrop, suggesting a long-standing subluxating hip. A Salter (redirectional) osteotomy was accomplished and the appearance nearly six years later is seen in B. Note the improved teardrop configuration, and the concentric, congruent relationship of the femoral head and acetabulum.

resected. As one might surmise, this results in a rather unstable acetabular fragment that necessitates internal fixation, not only in the area of the pubic rami, but also in the iliac osteotomy, exactly the same as that necessitated by the redirectional procedure of Salter. The indications for performing the operation are the same as for the pericapsular and the redirectional osteotomies. The major difference, as compared to the pericapsular osteotomy, is that the double osteotomy can be done (and is therefore indicated) in older, even skeletally immature adolescents.

The two *advantages* of the double osteotomy are those that prompted its conception; namely, it can accomplish rotation of the inferior (acetabular) fragment in older adolescents, at an age when most surgeons find it difficult to accomplish a simple redirectional (Salter, 1961) osteotomy; and (2) it is possible to medialize the rotated acetabulum towards the centre of gravity of the body.

The perceived *disadvantages* of the procedure have discouraged me from performing it; and therefore, I have never attempted this operation. This may not be a fair appraisal of the procedure, but there must be some significance in the fact that the operation is uncommonly done in the United States (Staheli, 1982; Tachdjian, 1982). These disadvantages consist of the following: (1) the osteotomy that is accomplished through the pubic rami requires internal fixation in a location uncomfortably close to many vital components of the urogenital system; (2) the axis of rotation of the inferior fragment (near the symphysis) is rather distant from the major site requiring correction (the acetabulum). Thus, any substantial anterior and lateral rotation of the acetabulum requires some degree of elevation of the superior pubic ramus at the site of the osteotomy. Sutherland claims that this has not been a problem; but Tachdjian (1982) has encountered unattractive superior and anterior prominence of the pubic ramus at the site of the pubic osteotomy. Finally, (3) the versatility of correction of the acetabular defect (whether abnormal direction or abnormal configuration) is less than that with a Pemberton (pericapsular) or the Steel (triple) innominate osteotomy (see below).

STEEL (TRIPLE) INNOMINATE OSTEOTOMY

Technique and indications: Steel (1973) observed the same difficulties that were discussed earlier when attempting to rotate the inferior fragment by means of the Salter redirectional osteotomy in adolescents and young adults. He, therefore, performed osteotomies of the ischium (through a separate buttock incision) and the pubis and ilium. This rendered the inferior fragment much more mobile, and permitted greater freedom of rotation of the acetabulum. Because the osteotomies are made closer to the acetabulum, there is a greater degree of versatility granted the surgeon in attempting to 'cover' the femoral head. Also, it can be done at any age through and well beyond skeletal maturity (Fig. 2.5). The indications are the same as for the pelvic osteotomies discussed previously, but the ability to mobilize the acetabular fragment makes it possible to accomplish coverage of the femoral head in almost any direction, thus it *may* have a role in older children and young adults with paralytic acetabular dysplasias.

The *advantages* have been alluded to above; namely, (1) there is greater freedom of movement of the inferior (acetabular) fragment; (2) the procedure has no age

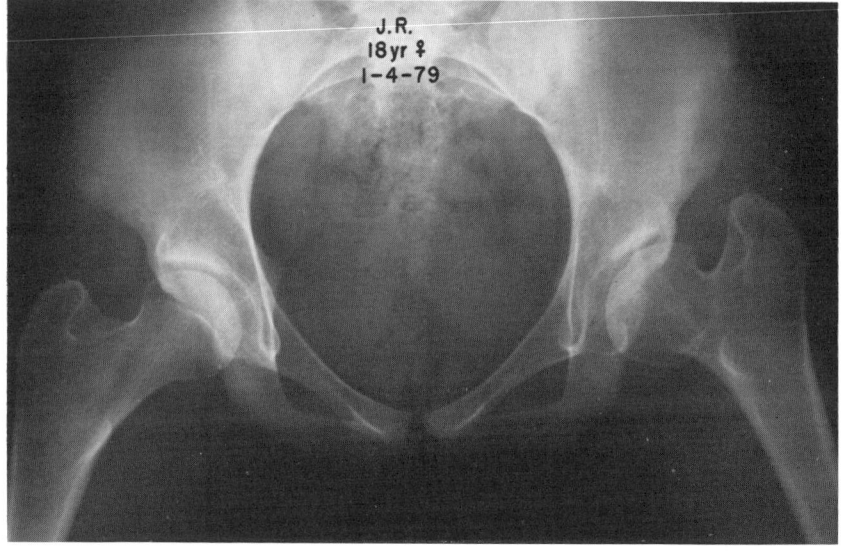

36   RECENT ADVANCES IN ORTHOPAEDICS

(A)

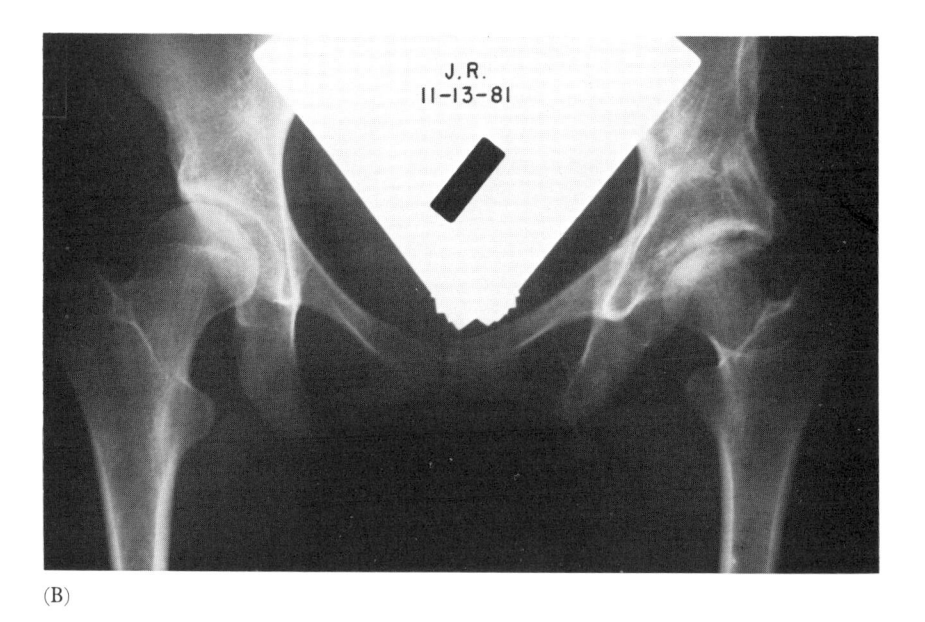

(B)

Fig. 2.5 Pelvic roentgenogram of an 18 year old female, with the femora held in abduction and inward rotation. She had hip pain with activities and had recently developed a substantial antalgic limp. Note the oblique, sloping acetabulum, the slightly narrowed cartilage space, and the narrow zone of articular cortex on the acetabular side, representing a substantially reduced weight-bearing area. Following a triple innominate osteotomy (Steel, 1973) the improved femoral head coverage, the increased weight-bearing area, and the more horizontal acetabular roof is seen three years later in B.

limitations; and (3) it has a potential advantage in treatment of paralytic acetabular dysplasias in older children.

The *disadvantages* are essentially the same as for the redirectional osteotomy of Salter. These are: (1) the inferior fragment is unstable and therefore, internal fixation is mandatory (my current preference is for large bicortical and cancellous screws with hex-heads); (2) penetration of the joint with the internal fixation is a major concern; (3) the operation is much more difficult to perform than a single redirectional osteotomy; and (4) a second (minor) operation is necessary in order to remove the internal fixation.

THE 'DIAL' (EPPRIGHT) AND 'SPHERICAL' (WAGNER) OSTEOTOMIES

Techniques and indications: Although these two procedures differ slightly in technique, the concept employed in their execution is so similar that it is appropriate to deal with them in the same section. Basically, each is designed to accomplish rotation of the subchondral bone and hyaline cartilage of the acetabulum by means of a spherical osteotomy made throughout the entire circumference of the socket. The desired thickness of the subarticular bone is about 1 cm, and the osteotomy is made in a pericapsular and subchondral fashion by means of curved, spherical osteotomes (Wagner, 1979) or by means of a saw (Eppright, 1981). The acetabular fragment maintains nearly all of its capsular attachments, except perhaps at the most inferior portion of the osteotomy, near the transverse acetabular ligament, and, therefore, if properly done, there is no compromise to the blood supply of the fragment. The osteotomy is, however, a technically demanding procedure that should only be attempted by one with extensive experience in hip joint surgery in adolescents and young adults.

The prime indication for the operation is a deficient acetabulum that is more or less otherwise spherical. Because the acetabular fragment is very mobile, it can be utilized in all varieties of hip dysplasia; and given considerable surgical expertise, the fragment can be placed over the femoral head wherever the greatest coverage is desired or needed (Fig. 2.6).

In addition, Wagner has devised three variations of the spherical osteotomy which are designed to correct either limb length discrepancies or gross deficiencies in the stock of the ilium and acetabulum. These variations require great technical expertise, and I have had no personal experience with either of them.

The *advantages* of these two procedures (dial and spherical osteotomy) include the following: (1) there is great versatility, because the osteotomy is made very close to the site of deformity, and the axis of rotation is essentially *at* the acetabulum; (2) the method of rotation of the acetabular fragment makes the *properly* done osteotomy rather stable, and thus internal fixation is usually much simpler; and (3) because of this, the chances of penetrating the joint with internal fixation devices are much less.

The *disadvantages* of these procedures are found primarily in their demanding technical nature. First, the cut in the ilium must be made so precisely that there is very little room for error. If the joint is entered, there is substantial likelihood of chondrolysis, and also efforts at successful rotation of the acetabular fragment are compromised. Second, if the medial acetabular wall is unusually thin, then it is very difficult to accomplish the operation safely or effectively.

38   RECENT ADVANCES IN ORTHOPAEDICS

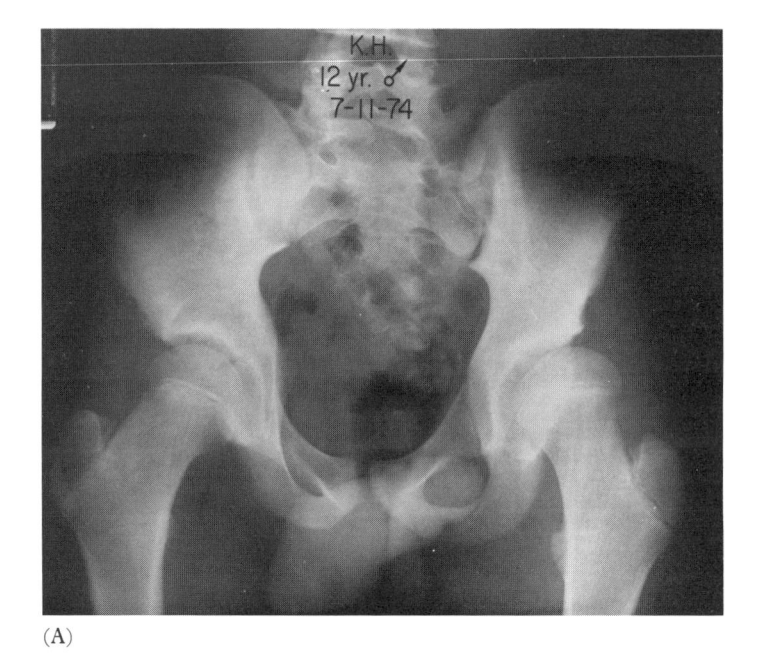

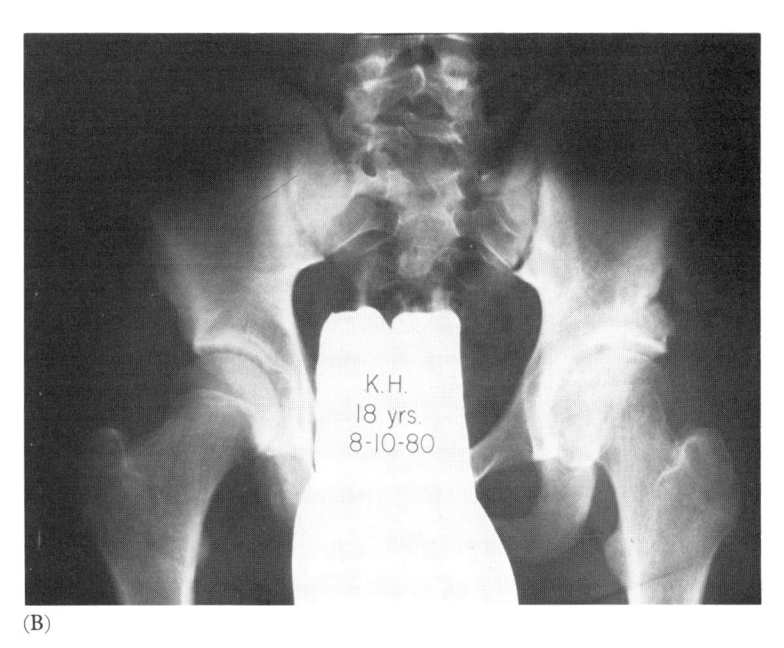

Fig. 2.6 Roentgenogram of the pelvis of a 12 year old male is seen in A. Note the shallow, dysplastic acetabulum, the extrapelvic femoral head protrusion, the congruency of the femoral head and the acetabulum, and the generous thickness of the medial acetabular wall in the left hip. Because the patient was painfully symptomatic in this hip, and because he fulfilled all of the prerequisites for a reconstructive procedure, a 'dial' acetabular rotation was accomplished. Six years later the patient had a normal range of hip motion and was asymptomatic. The greatly improved femoral head and acetabular relationships can be seen in B. (Courtesy Dr Richard H Eppright, Houston, Texas.)

Conclusions regarding reconstructive pelvic osteotomies
In review and analysis of the foregoing discussion I have come to the following programme in applying the various pelvic osteotomies to the treatment of the dysplastic acetabulum in Congenital Dislocation of the Hip. It is assumed, of course, that the prerequisites discussed earlier have been fulfilled in all instances, and that the indications have been satisfied. This means that the *need* for the osteotomy has been established by all of the available clinical and radiographic criteria. If the prerequisites or indications are *unmet*, then their performance is contraindicated.

For the young child ranging from 18 months of age through age seven or eight years, I prefer the Pemberton pericapsular osteotomy for correction of acetabular dysplasia. This dysplasia may be due either to congenital dislocation of the hip or paralytic dislocation and subluxation. Over age eight years and through age 12 or 15 years, I prefer the redirectional osteotomy of Salter. In older adolescents and adults, I prefer the triple innominate osteotomy of Steel. In that 'twilight' age group of 12 to 18 years, it has been my policy to attempt the simple, redirectional osteotomy, but to be prepared to carry out the triple osteotomy if it is found necessary. I have not utilized the double osteotomy, and I find the spherical or 'dial' osteotomy too difficult to accomplish on the 'occasional' basis.

Osteotomies on the femoral side of the hip joint

There is considerable controversy among orthopaedic surgeons in the United States, and between the American and Continental orthopaedic surgeons about the indications for and the expected results of performing a varus and/or rotational osteotomy of the femur in the treatment of congenital dislocation of the hip. It is difficult to rationalize these differences, because if the results of varus/rotational osteotomy were uniformly and eminently successful, and were predictable in producing improved acetabular development, it would be more universally used. Certainly it is a simpler procedure, with less likelihood of complications and problems than pelvic osteotomy.

It is established that a more varus configuration of the neck shaft angle is more stable than is a valgus configuration. This is one of the justifications for performing the operation. The same consideration applies to rotational attitudes of the femur. The greater the anteversion, the less stable the femoral head is within the acetabulum. Thus, reduction in anteversion of the femur is justifiably considered a means of enhancing stability. These two factors have been the principal arguments for performing varus rotational osteotomy of the proximal femur in treatment of congenital hip dislocation. These are appropriate operations, provided that they are done rather early in life when acetabular remodelling is so rapid (18 months to three years), and only when the prerequisites have been fulfilled. However, there is not a good *controlled* series that proves that there is any substantial effect upon the acetabular development when performing this operation (varus rotational osteotomy) in the femur that has a *normal configuration*. Thus, from my understanding, the prime indication for performing reconstructive osteotomies on the proximal femur is a proven deformity in either angulation or rotation, the correction of which will correct that deformity and consequently improve hip joint relationships.

As noted in a previous section, the ability to define the abnormality in the proximal femur, and therefore to determine the need for femoral corrective osteotomy, is much easier than it is on the pelvic side. If one assumes that the same prerequisites have been met as for pelvic osteotomy, and that there is a stable concentric reduction of the femoral head in the acetabulum in abduction and inward rotation, then correction of any *substantial* rotational and/or angular deformity of the proximal femur can be justified.

The biggest problem facing the orthopaedic surgeon in making a decision to perform this procedure is to establish the criteria that truly identify a *substantial* deformity. There are no hard and fast figures that can accurately establish the degree of deformity that unequivocally justifies surgical correction. Clearly, major deformities are rather easy to define, but the borderline abnormalities require considerable judgment, based upon a careful review of the X-ray films, and a substantial degree of intuition based upon clinical experience, in order that one may arrive at the proper decision. My own indications for utilizing the procedure or combinations of procedures are more or less implicit in the foregoing discussions; namely, when a clearly defined deformity of the proximal femur exists, and when this deformity is sufficiently great that it contributes to pelvi-femoral instability, or when it is a major cause of gait abnormalities, then correction of that deformity is justified (Fig. 2.7). Again, it is essential to emphasize that before any reconstructive proximal femoral osteotomy is accomplished, that the prerequisites are fulfilled; namely, that there is a concentric, congruent, reduction of the hip, a normal or near-normal range of hip

(A)

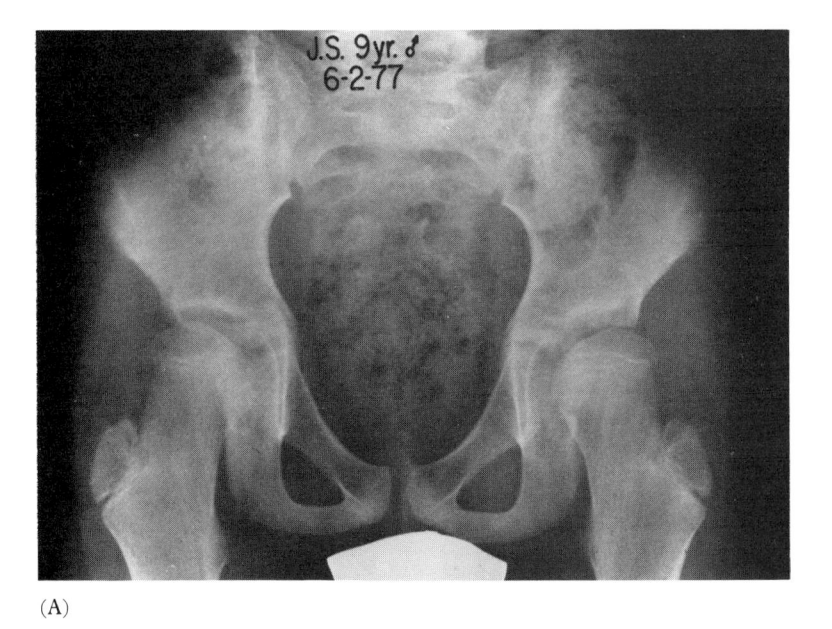

Fig. 2.7 An example of a deformity of the proximal femur that justified varus rotational osteotomy for correction. This nine year old male underwent treatment of bilateral congenital dislocation of the hip at age 18 months. At age nine years, the parents complained that he had developed a waddling gait. The roentgenogram (A) shows a well developed acetabulum bilaterally, but there is substantial valgus deformity of the femoral neck shaft angle. An abduction-inward rotation film (B) further confirms the valgus deformity and shows the femoral head to be well seated in this position. Therefore a biplane varus-rotational osteotomy was accomplished (C) resulting in substantial improvement in gait. (From Coleman S S, 1978 Congenital dysplasia and dislocation of the hip, C V Mosby, St Louis.)

CONGENITAL DISLOCATION OF THE HIP 41

(B)

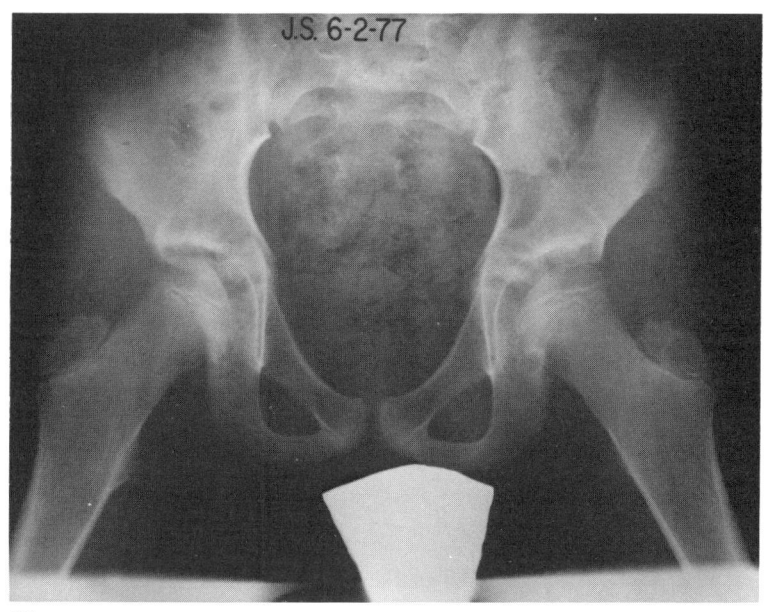

(C)

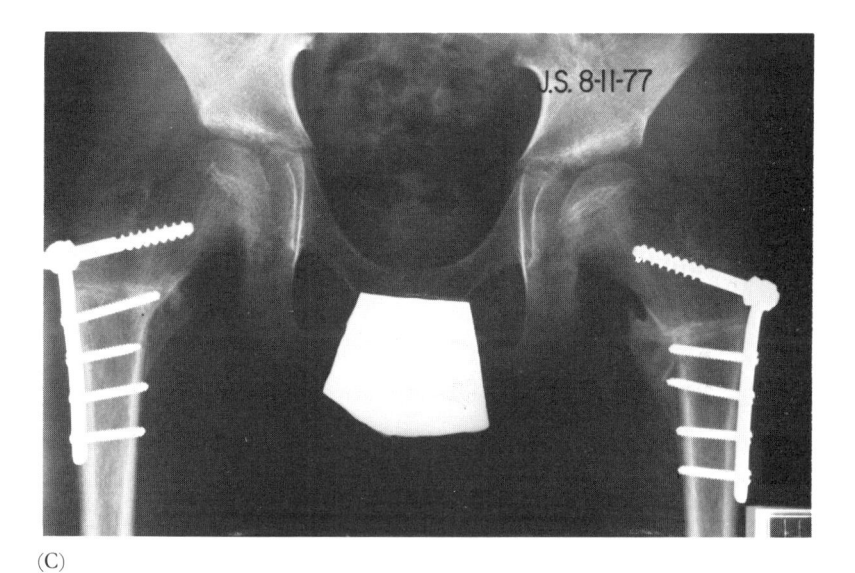

motion, and a normal or near-normal cartilage space. Failure to insist upon fulfilling these criteria will surely result in failure of the operation.

One final procedure that qualifies as a modified reconstructive operation on the proximal femur is transfer of the greater trochanter. The reason why one may challenge the inclusion of this procedure in such a discussion is because the operation is accomplished as treatment of a major complication; namely, physeal arrest of the femoral head due to aseptic necrosis. In this circumstance, the usually undamaged

42 RECENT ADVANCES IN ORTHOPAEDICS

(A)

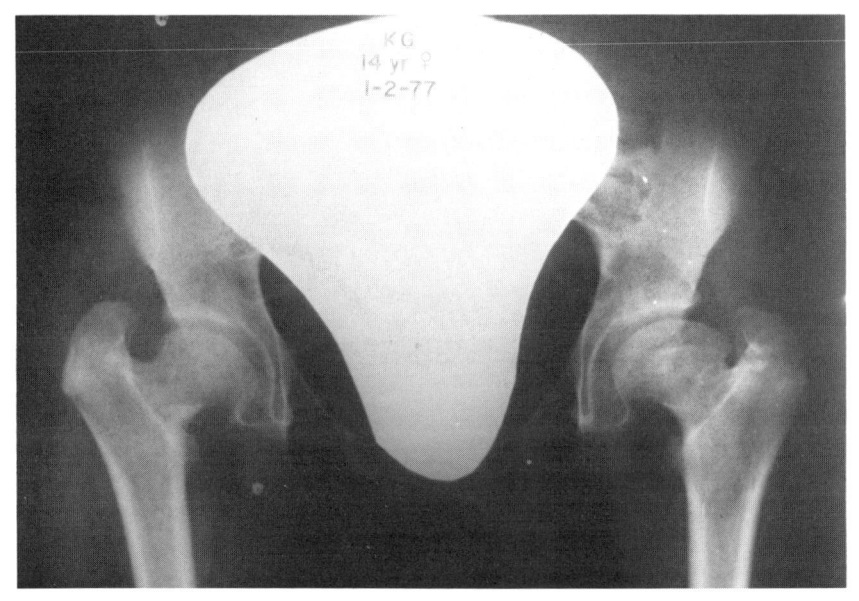

(B)

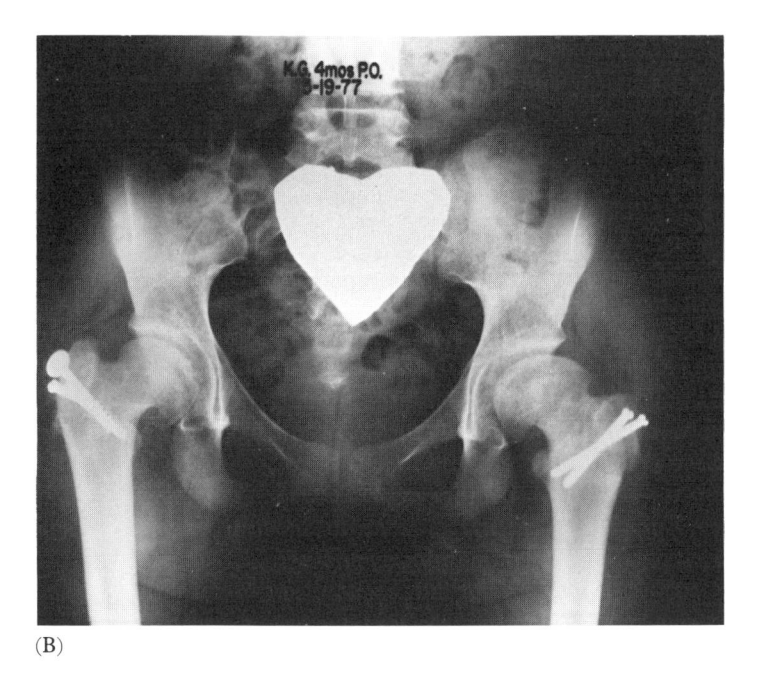

Fig. 2.8 An example of upward displacement of the greater trochanter due to its relative overgrowth resulting from growth arrest of the femoral head physis is seen in A. This 14 year old girl had a decidedly positive Trendelenburg gait. Distal transfer resulted in reversal of the Trendelenburg gait, as a result of improved hip mechanics (B). (From Coleman S S (1978) Congenital Dysplasia and dislocation of the hip, C V Mosby, St Louis.)

greater trochanteric physis continues to grow, leading to an upwardly displaced (relatively speaking) greater trochanter. The functional effectiveness of the abductors becomes compromised, resulting in a progressively worsening Trendelenburg gait. Distal transfer of the trochanter, so that the uppermost tip comes to lie directly opposite the centre of the femoral head will restore a more normal biomechanical relationship and often will reverse the previously positive Trendelenburg sign (Fig. 2.8). In some situations it may be necessary to *lateralize* the greater trochanter (Wagner, 1978). When this is done, iliac bone grafts are required in order to serve as a spacer that can displace the transplanted trochanter laterally.

REFERENCES

Eppright R 1981 'Dial' osteotomy. Presented at AAOS Inst. Course, Marco Island, Florida

Coleman SS 1981 Pemberton osteotomy in paralytic dislocations. Presented at AAOS Inst. Course. Marco Island, Florida

Jackson R T, Coleman S S 1981 The teardrop in congenital dislocation of the hip. Presented at Annual Scientific Meeting, Shriners Hospital for Crippled Children, Chicago

McKay D 1980 Personal communication

Pemberton P A 1965 Pericapsular osteotomy for congenital dislocation of the hip: indications and techniques. Some long-term results, Journal of Bone & Joint Surgery, 47A: 437

Ponseti I V, Lindstrom J, Wenger D R 1976 Acetabular development afer reduction in congenital dislocation of the hip. Journal of Bone & Joint Surgery, 58A: 725

Salter R B 1961 Innominate osteotomy in the treatment of congenital dislocation and subluxation of the hip. Journal of Bone & Joint Surgery 43B: 518

Salter R B 1981 Personal communication

Staheli L T 1982 Personal communication

Steel H H 1973 Triple osteotomy of the innominate bone, Journal of Bone & Joint Surgery 55A: 343

Sutherland D H, Greenfield R 1977 Double innominate osteotomy. Journal Bone & Joint Surgery 59A: 1082

Tachdjian M O 1982 Personal communication

Wagner H 1979 Personal communication

Wagner H 1978 Proximal femoral osteotomies. Int Ped Ortho Seminar, San Francisco

Wiberg G 1939 Relation between congenital subluxation of the hip and arthritis deformans (roentgenological study). Acta Orthopaedica Scandinavica 10: 351

3. Knee replacements
W. Waugh

KNEE REPLACEMENT OPERATIONS

Introduction
There have been many developments in knee replacement operations over the last decade, so that by 1980 a wide range of prostheses had become available. The aim of this chapter will be to consider the broad principles on which the changes have been based: it will not be possible to describe every new knee joint and it seems preferable to deal mainly with those which are within the experience of the author. Nevertheless, other models will be introduced when they have a direct bearing on any argument being followed. It is regretted that many implants, some no doubt excellent, will receive no mention. Although the theme must be 'advances', it will be necessary to look back from time to time to try to understand on what grounds the advances have been made, but the chapter will not aim to be a complete historical review. Knee replacements will be considered from the viewpoint of the practising surgeon who has to treat patients with chronic arthritis of the knee joint. Advances in bioengineering and material sciences in relation to the design of prostheses will not be discussed in any detail.

Experience at Harlow Wood Orthopaedic Hospital
The changing pattern in the use of prostheses is illustrated by our experience at Harlow Wood Orthopaedic Hospital. The type and number of primary knee replacement operations done or supervised by the author and his colleague, Mr J P Jackson, is shown in Figure 3.1.

	1966-71	1972	1973	1974	1975	1976	1977	1978	1979	1980	1981	Total
Walldius	24	9	9	12	11	1	9	7				82
MacIntosh	18	11	18	4	2				1			54
Freeman		8	16	33	29	16	33	32	21	12	15	215
Sheehan				4	25	15	26	20	18	2	5	115
Manchester					18	26	14	6	1			65
Stanmore								1	5	4	9	19
Oxford										15	18	33
Total	42	28	43	53	85	58	82	66	46	33	47	583

Fig. 3.1 This shows the changing pattern in the number and type of knee replacements carried out at Harlow Wood Orthopaedic Hospital each year between 1971 and 1981.

In 1972 we established special knee clinics for assessment of patients before operation (in collaboration with rheumatologists) and at regular intervals afterwards. As the interval from the early operations lengthened and the number of unsuccessful replacements increased, we stopped using the MacIntosh hemiarthroplasty, the Walldius and the Manchester prostheses. We progressively changed to more recently developed types which appeared to overcome the deficiencies of the earlier models. But we cannot yet know whether the prostheses we use now will last for longer and therefore will represent true advances.

From the outset, pain has been our main indication for operation and we have selected patients who have widespread joint disease or who are elderly. The basic principle which we adopted was to attempt to conserve bone stock as far as possible whilst using a prosthesis which would allow correction of deformity and restoration of stability. This led us to use a small bicompartmental implant where there was loss of articular cartilage but little or no bony collapse and where the ligaments were preserved; a condylar replacement in knees with a fixed deformity and a semiconstrained prosthesis in knees with more bony destruction and subluxation.

Evaluation and the presentation of results

There is as yet no general agreement about the information which needs to be collected for proper evaluation to be carried out; the Research Sub-Committee of the British Orthopaedic Association proposed an assessment form (Aichroth et al, 978) which, however, had some shortcomings (Tew & Waugh, 1979).

Clinical assessment
In Nottingham we have developed a method which depends on using non-medical personnel to ask questions about pain and then to carry out simple functional tests designed to assess the contribution which the affected knee makes towards the patient's total disability. The surgeon next examines the patient and records the minimum basic data which we believe to be necessary. The methods of assessment and our form have been published (Waugh, 1982) and a manual is available which gives precise instructions for recording the data in a uniform manner. This information enables the surgeon to assess an individual patient's progress, but it also allows the experience of patients as a whole to be studied, so that the possible advantages and disadvantages of different kinds of operations can be compared.

We also use a sophisticated technique which makes it possible to measure knee function in the patient's home throughout the day. The early results of this project have been reported (Johnson et al, 1982) and a review of our methods has been outlined in a paper by Waugh et al (1981).

Measurement of coronal knee angles
There is little disagreement about the need to achieve correct alignment at operation (Hood et al, 1981; Freeman et al, 1978 and Lotke et al, 1977), but a detailed discussion of the intricacies of measuring the coronal knee angles is beyond the scope of this chapter. It is, however, important to define which angle is being measured and to state the method used, if useful comparisons are to be made. There are two angles to be considered:

1. *The coronal tibiofemoral angle (CTF)* which is the acute angle made by the axis of the tibial shaft to the axis of the femoral shaft (normal range: 5° to 10° valgus).
2. *The angle of deviation of the mechanical axis (DMA)* which is made by the line joining the centre of the femoral head to the centre of the knee with the line joining the centre of the knee to the centre of the ankle (normally 0°).

Some authors prefer to express their 'neutral angle' as 180° instead of 0°. This avoids having to add the suffix 'valgus' or 'varus' to the number of degrees, so that 185° is varus and 175° is valgus.

Standing radiographs have been used for many years and the value of having a film which includes the hip, knee and ankle has been emphasised (Maquet et al, 1967). However, standardisation can be difficult and minor degrees of rotation of the whole leg will introduce errors, particularly when there is a flexion contracture, a problem which can only be overcome by the use of a complicated method such as that described by Hagstedt et al (1980). The necessary equipment is not widely available and even at the Hospital for Special Surgey, New York, 'logistical and technical' reasons have precluded the routine use of standing films which include the whole leg (Hood et al, 1981).

Clinical measurement of the CTF, using a long-armed goniometer, may have an interobserver error of only ±1.5° in normal subjects (Lawrence, 1980); but as is the case with radiographic measurements, obesity and deformity of the knee will introduce inaccuracies.

Until international (or even, national) standards are recognised, each surgeon must choose his method and use it consistently. Measurements are needed to record changes in alignment of an individual knee and to provide data from groups of patients which will allow a general conclusion to be drawn.

In our knee clinic we measure the CTF clinically, with the tibia stressed laterally and medially, and in lying and standing radiographs taken on a 43 cm film.

The value of radiographs

Radiographs provide the best evidence for predicting the final outcome of knee replacements which may initially appear satisfactory. The attitude of each component to the femur or tibia can be measured in both planes. The significance of translucent lines of less than 1 mm is uncertain, but their presence should be observed and recorded at regular intervals if loosening is to be recognised early.

Analysis of results

The results of knee replacement operations can be classified by grades of success, and success and failure rates calculated. Ultimate failure is the removal of the prosthesis, but reoperation does not encompass all failure; a more complete definition would include patients who have severe pain but in whom, for various reasons, revision or arthrodesis has not yet been carried out. Using the wider as well as the narrower criteria, we have adapted the statistical model of survivorship tables (Armitage, 1971) to calculate for our own series of 365 knee replacements the annual failure rate in relation to the number of knees at risk throughout each year after operation and, hence, the proportion of implants which survive successfully for any given period.

Our findings are that the failure rate on both criteria is very low in the first two years after operation, but rises significantly in the third. Since the number at risk necessarily diminishes as the period since operation lengthens, the confidence with which subsequent trends can be identified is eventually limited by small numbers, but the incidence of severe pain seems to increase rapidly from the sixth year. The passage of time was found to be a far more important factor determining the result than the type of prosthesis used, diagnosis, the age of the patient or the preoperative deformity of the knee. It follows that the larger the proportion of recent implants in any series, the smaller will be the proportion of failures. Thus comparisons of failure rate, measured in the conventional way, in series with different follow-up periods could be completely invalid. This illustrates the necessity of developing appropriate statistical techniques if the surgical advances are to be accurately evaluated.

The indications for knee replacement
Knee replacement must not be regarded as the only possible operation for knees with chronic arthritis which are causing increasing pain and disability. Tibial osteotomy is the best treatment for medial compartment osteoarthritis in younger patients, particularly if the changes are not too advanced (bony collapse of less than 0.5 cm, may be taken as the limit). Similarly, supracondylar osteotomy is indicated for lateral compartment osteoarthritis. If the disease is more advanced and there is lateral subluxation of the tibia, arthrodesis may be the wisest choice when only one knee is affected and where the patient is under 60 years old. However, the success of hip replacement operations has led many patients to believe that a similar procedure on their knee would be equally successful and they are consequently unwilling even to consider an arthrodesis. It is important that the surgeon concerned should describe in what he believes to be realistic terms the possible outcome of a knee replacement. There are, however, a number of factors which will determine the decision and which are relevant to the choice of operation.

1. *Age* It is generally agreed that in patients over the age of 65 years recovery is easier and quicker after a replacement operation than an osteotomy. Life expectancy is obviously shorter and the level of active use of the knee is likely to get less year by year.

2. *Involvement of other joints* Operation may be justifiable at a younger age in patients with rheumatoid arthritis when hips, knees and both feet may be, or may be going to be, affected. This implies that the patient's activities will always be restricted and it may be hoped that this will mean that the life of the replacement will be longer than it would be in a normally active person. Certainly a woman of 30 years with flexion contractures of both knees may be so grossly disabled that bilateral replacement can be justified. The early result may be spectacularly successful, but it really is impossible to predict the outcome in 10, let alone 15 or 20, years.

3. *The state of the affected knee* This does not in itself determine the need for operation, but it may affect the choice of prosthesis. The more deformity is present (whether valgus, varus, flexion or rotational), the greater will be the amount of bony collapse and the more likely it will be that the ligaments will be either shortened or stretched. These factors may determine the extent of the operation in terms of bone resection and soft tissue release. The rest of this chapter will be concerned with

different types of replacement and it should be clear that the smaller prostheses will be indicated in the earlier stages of rheumatoid or osteoarthritis and that the larger types (which may be semiconstrained or constrained), may be needed if there is very severe deformity, bony collapse or subluxation.

Types of knee replacements

The large number of prostheses available for total replacement of the knee joint can be grouped together in various ways, and it is helpful to do this in order to be able to make general observations about each type.

In the following sections replacements are considered under four main headings:

1. *Compartmental replacements* (Manchester, Marmor and Oxford) These are small implants which depend on the integrity of intact ligaments. Unicompartmental replacement will also be considered in this section.

2. *Condylar replacements* (Freeman, Insall) These prostheses are inserted after resection of the condylar surfaces and depend, to a greater or lesser degree, on correct ligament balance for stability.

3. *Semiconstrained linked replacements* (Sheehan, Attenborough, Spherocentric) These types of replacement have more inherent stability and need considerable excavation of bone from femur and tibia for their insertion. They have intramedullary stems of varying lengths.

4. *Constrained hinges* (Stanmore) Bone has to be resected from the length of the femur and tibia to accommodate the hinge and fixation is obtained with long intramedullary stems. This type of implant, and the semiconstrained linked prosthesis, can be regarded as large replacements in relation to the amount of bone removed and invaded.

Compartmental replacements

These are small prostheses which replace the damaged articular surface and preserve the cruciate ligaments. The amount of bone to be resected is minimised and, in general, the bone is not invaded deeply for fixation. The surfaces of both femoral and tibial condyles are replaced using four separate components and this type of design was first developed by Gunston (1971). The aim was to simulate normal knee movement, but there were technical difficulties and complications (Gunston & Mackenzie, 1976; Skolnick et al, 1976). Other surgeons then sought to simplify the design and technique.

The Manchester replacement

This four-part compartmental replacement was designed by Newton & Shaw and was described by Shaw & Chatterjee (1978). Excellent and good results were reported in 84.5% of a series of 51 knees followed up for from 23 months to 5 years. We began to do this operation at Harlow Wood in 1975 and by 1979 had used it in 65 knees. Early results were excellent, but when reviewed in 1980, 17 knees had failed and had been converted to another prosthesis: 8 were unsatisfactory in that patients complained of moderate to severe pain (7 patients had died). The average time between the original operation and the second intervention was only 33 months. Williams et al (1979) reported 31 Manchester operations, 15 of which, were carried out for osteoarthritis; of these, 8 failed for mechanical reasons often with considerable wear of the tibial components. There were, however, no failures in their 16 patients who had rheumatoid arthritis.

Certainly our results in both osteoarthritic and rheumatoid knees were not satisfactory and we gave up the procedure as Figure 3.1 indicates. There may be a number of explanations for our lack of success. First, it was not easy to insert all four components correctly and to achieve correct alignment; there were no alignment jigs and the operation had to be done 'by eye'. Lack of technical skill may explain some of our early failures and we also operated on a few knees with more deformity than is possible to correct with this type of operation. Second, it seems likely that point-loading, followed by tracking, could occur and this was followed by excessive wear of the polyethylene. Third, loosening was accompanied by considerable bone destruction so that, for example, the slots made for the femoral components became large cavities. Reconstruction was consequently difficult and it was nearly always necessary to use a large constrained hinge for conversion.

Other compartmental replacements
Favourable results from somewhat similar types of implant have been reported by Marmor (1976), Laskin (1976) and Engelbrecht et al (1976), but the average follow-up was less than 3 years in each series. Marmor (1982) has now published the results of 147 bicompartmental knees with a follow-up of between 5 and 8 years. Seventy-two per cent were rated as excellent or good.

The Oxford knee replacement
The principles, on which the design of this new prosthesis is based, have been described by Goodfellow & O'Connor (1978) and Goodfellow et al (1980). The theoretical concept was skilfully argued, but it was possible to express some doubts of a practical nature. First, the operation seemed more complicated than most since six components are inserted: a metal runner on to each femoral condyle and a flat metal plate on to each tibial condyle; finally, high-density polyethylene meniscal bearings were placed between the metal components on each side of the new joint (Fig. 3.2). Second, success seemed to depend on restoring the correct tension in the ligaments, both cruciate and collateral, and it remained to be seen whether this could be done in knees badly damaged by arthritis. Although jigs were designed to allow the correct resection of bone from the femur and tibia; tension was determined using graded spacers and trial menisci, but the choice of size was a matter of 'feel'.

The author was fortunate enough to be invited to take part in the clinical trial after we had given up the Manchester operation, and so reasons need to be given as to why it was hoped that the Oxford knee would be better. First, the concept of biomechanical design was more soundly based and the advantages of the flat tibial component in reducing shear forces exerted by the femur on the tibia have been demonstrated (O'Connor et al, 1982). Second, the possibility of point-loading and tracking is almost certainly eliminated. Third, the joint surfaces are conforming so that fragments of acrylic cement are less likely to produce abrasive wear of the plastic meniscal bearing.

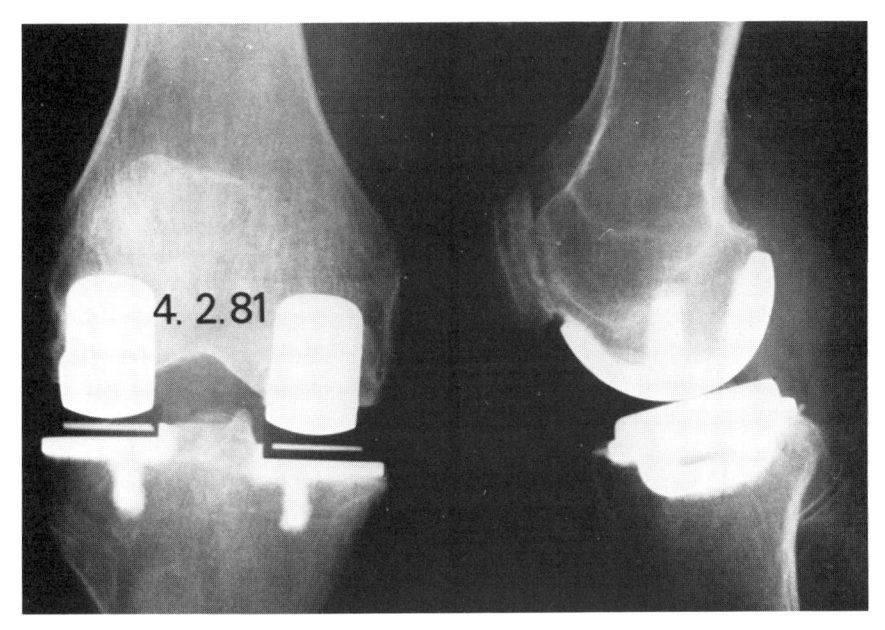

Fig. 3.2 This radiograph shows an Oxford replacement. In the anteroposterior view wire markers show the position of the polyethylene meniscal bearing.

Fourth, the insertion of the bearing between metal femoral and tibial components makes it easier to adjust tension in the ligaments, and thus correct deformity and achieve stability, than was the case in the Manchester replacement. The amount of bone sacrificed is less; in the Oxford operation, very thin slices are removed from the surface of each femoral condyle, but the inside of the bone is only encroached by a drill hole (6.5 mm × 22 mm) to receive a stud.

There is, however, one very important and entirely new idea which concerns the state of the ligaments. Freeman et al (1978) argued that fixed varus or valgus deformity is due to 'bone loss followed by soft tissue contracture which fixes the deformity'. This leads to the need for release of the shortened soft tissues to realign the knee (stability being achieved by 'blocking open the knee' with the prosthesis). Insall et al (1979) also emphasised that there was shortening of the capsule and ligaments on the concave side of the deformity and a soft tissue release was considered necessary in a great many knees to restore 'ligamentous balance'. Goodfellow (1981), on the other hand, considers that the collateral ligaments maintain their normal length (except perhaps in the most severely damaged knees) and the only soft tissue structure to shorten is the posterior capsule. The theory can be confirmed, not only by observation at operation, but by stress radiographs before operation. Varus or valgus deformities can almost always be corrected to 'neutral' if the correcting force is applied with the joint sufficiently flexed to relax the posterior capsule. In this way 'fixed' deformities can often be demonstrated to be correctable. In a fixed valgus knee without a flexion deformity, coronal alignment can be corrected by inserting spacers of the correct height, and this produces a flexion deformity in place of the valgus. The other important implication is that the normal coronal tibiofemoral angle is achieved by restoring the proper tension in the collateral ligaments and the essential alignment of the limb is independent of the alignment of the femoral or tibial components.

The role of the cruciate ligaments now needs to be considered. Theoretically, they would seem to be essential to the proposed function of the Oxford knee. Freeman et al (1977) pointed out the reasons for removing these ligaments in his type of operation, but their arguments do not necessarily apply to the Oxford knee because of the freedom allowed by the movement of the menisci. The posterior cruciate ligament is likely to be normal except where there is lateral subluxation, but the anterior cruciate is sometimes destroyed, or at least attenuated. In a prospective observation of 86 knees (41 osteoarthritis, 45 rheumatoid arthritis) Goodfellow found at operation that the anterior cruciate was intact in 44, 'damaged' in 18 and absent in 24. Although it is theoretically desirable that the ligament should be present, its absence does not seem to affect the clinical result.

The first operation was carried out in Oxford in 1976 and the prototype components were implanted in 31 knees during the following 2 years. The meniscal bearing displaced on six occasions and accordingly its shape was modified to minimise this complication. By December, 1980, 67 knees had been replaced by the new design. In general the outcome was very satisfactory in most patients, pain being relieved and stability restored. Dislocation of the new design of meniscal bearings occurred only once. But in the total series of 92 knees reviewed, 20 had a flexion contracture of 15 degrees or more after operation.

The author has inserted 33 Oxford knees between March 1980 and October 1981, and it is too soon to give the detailed results. Although the operation takes more time than some of the 'simpler' replacements, it is not technically difficult. Restoration of alignment and stability has been satisfactorily achieved in most knees, but the persistence of a flexion contracture in some has been of concern. It is true that the degree of contracture left at the end of operation decreases over subsequent weeks, but full extension is sometimes not regained. This may be related to the degree of deformity (in both planes) before operation, so that the surgeon may be advised to choose knees with a flexion contracture of less than 15° and a CTF angle in the range of 0° varus to 10° valgus until wider experience shows that these limitations are unnecessarily narrow.

The Oxford replacement seems to represent a true advance, both in its concept and design. Time will tell how successful it proves in practice.

Unicompartmental replacement
Satisfactory results have been reported with the use of a unicompartmental replacement in knees where osteoarthritis is largely confined to the medial or lateral compartment (Marmor, 1979; Scott & Santori, 1981 and Jones et al, 1981). On the other hand, Laskin (1978) reported a 20% failure rate and considered that the operation should only be used for posttraumatic osteoarthritis of the lateral compartment. Insall & Aglietti (1980) agreed that the early results were satisfactory, but there was marked deterioration at between 5 and 7 years. These authors no longer use unicompartmental replacement for medial compartment osteoarthritis, but consider that in lateral compartment disease the operation is a 'viable alternative to the total condylar prosthesis and is preferable to osteotomy'.

Surgeons must make their own decisions in the light of these reports, but we have

icompartmental replacements at Harlow Wood. The knees of our
:ither to be suitable for tibial osteotomy or else so severely involved to
acement.

acements

lacements which resurface the femoral and tibial condyles with two
onents. There are a number of variants, but this section will consider
:nt and principles of only two designs.

of the Freeman knee replacement

;wanson (1972) reported a completely original knee arthroplasty: the
:he femur was replaced with a metal component and the upper end of the
dished high density polyethylene component. The two parts were not
y way and, since the cruciate ligaments were removed, stability was
the geometry of the articulating surfaces and by the capsule, extensor
mechanism and the collateral ligaments.

The Freeman-Swanson arthroplasty was first carried out at Harlow Wood in 1972 and, as with so many operations of this kind, the early results seemed encouraging. However, as time passed, failures began to occur. Of the first 24 operations done in 1972 and 1973, only 8 were satisfactory in 1980. Four patients had died and one was lost to follow-up; and 10 knees had been converted to another prosthesis or had been arthrodesed. A further two knees were unsatisfactory, but had not had a further operation. The average time between the first and second operation was from 4 to 5 years. Other surgeons had had a similar experience: Goldberg & Henderson (1980) reported an overall reoperation rate of 28.5% in a series of 70 replacements carried out between 1973 and 1975.

Some of the deficiencies of the earliest model were described by Freeman et al in 1978, by which time various modifications had already been made. Sinkage of the small tibial component of the first model was a major problem and this was overcome by designing a component which completely overlapped the cut surface of the bone. The introduction of the tensor and an awareness of the importance of releasing the tight soft tissue on the concave side of the joint made it possible to achieve correct tibiofemoral alignment. Our experience at Harlow Wood is shown in Figure 3.3 which compares the alignment in two groups of operations: the first between 1972 and 1974 and the second between 1977 and 1979. In the early period most knees were aligned in some degree of varus, whereas in the recent group the aim of between 5° and 10° of valgus was more often achieved. Failure to obtain correct alignment occurred more frequently in knees with the most severe deformities before operation, probably because an adequate soft tissue release had not been carried out. The balancing of the collateral ligaments can be crudely assessed by comparing the coronal tibiofemoral angle when the tibia is stressed laterally and medially. For example, when examined in 1980, lateral mobility of more than 5° was seen in 4 out of 10 knees operated on in 1973, but in only six out of 26 knees operated on in 1978. When the tensor is used much less bone is removed from the femur than was the case in the original technique.

Other innovations were the high anterior flange to the femoral component

54   RECENT ADVANCES IN ORTHOPAEDICS

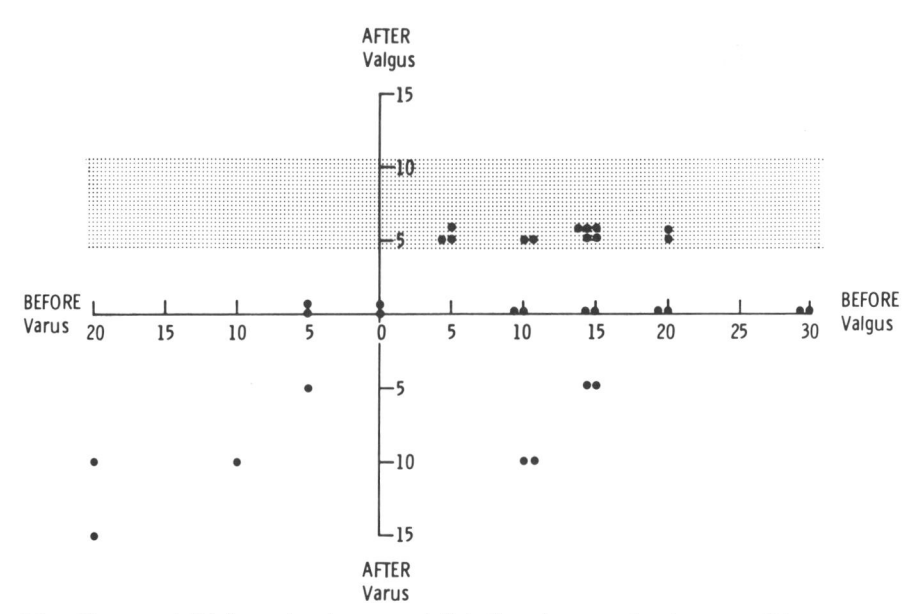

Fig. 3.3a   The coronal tibiofemoral angle measured clinically and expressed to the nearest 5° in a consecutive series of 32 Freeman replacement operations between 1972 and 1974. This method of demonstrating this aspect of the results relates the angle before to the angle after operation in each individual knee. In 20 knees the angle after operation was outside the 5°–10° valgus range and many knees were left in an unacceptable degree of varus.

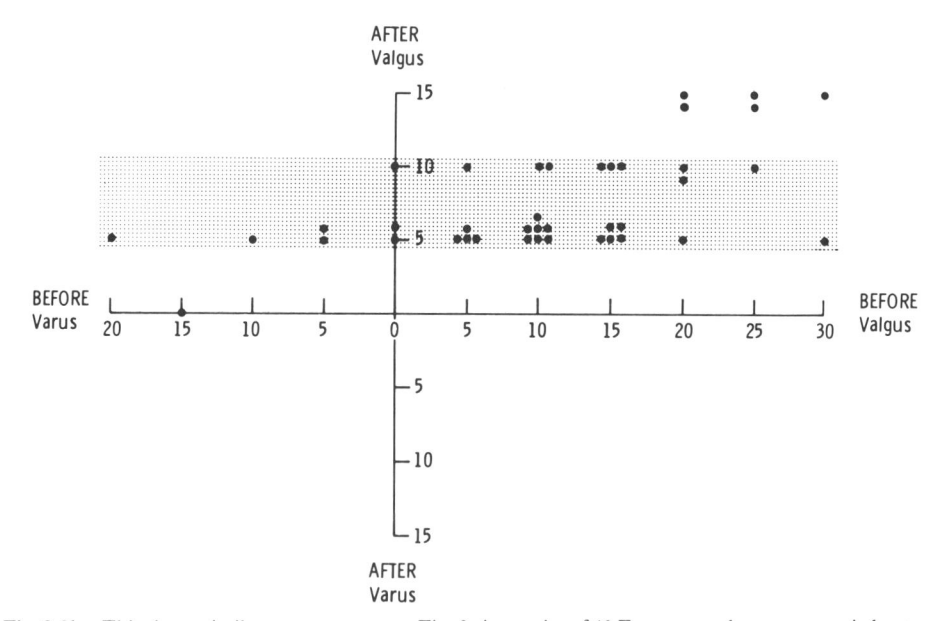

Fig. 3.3b   This shows similar measurements to Fig. 3a in a series of 40 Freeman replacements carried out between 1977 and 1979. In the majority the coronal tibiofemoral angle after operation fell within the range of 5°–10° of valgus. No knees were left in varus, but correction of severe valgus (20°–30°) in 5 patients was not satisfactorily achieved.

(cemented in position after the tibial component) and the allows redundant cement to be removed from the back of t

Freeman's next development was the introduction in 1977 the tibial component (Freeman et al, 1978). Fixation dep pegs with flanges which provide an immediate interlock (Fig. 3.4). Satisfactory results were reported by Morel follow-up was three years or less. A similar technique was 1977 and to the femur in 1979 (Freeman, 1980).

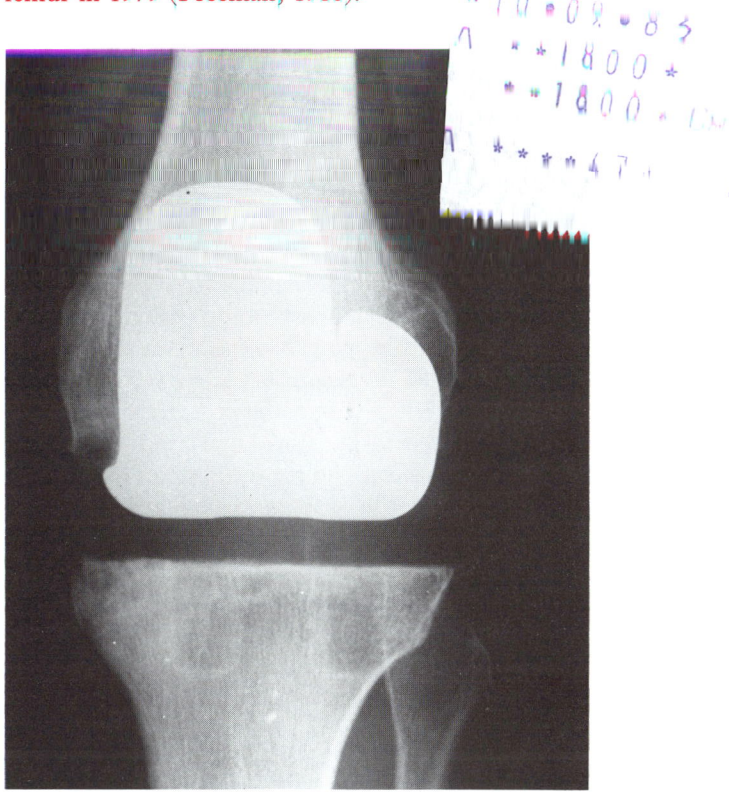

Fig. 3.4 An anteroposterior radiograph of a Freeman replacement showing the high anterior flange and two studs in the tibial component which provide fixation without the use of cement.

Up to the present the tibial component has provided no constraint to lateral subluxation, but division of the popliteus tendon is an important step which helps to prevent this complication, particularly in knees with a flexion–valgus–external rotation deformity.

The new Freeman-Samuelson knee, which became available in 1981, has a central eminence on the tibial component. There are also side walls on the patellar surface of the femoral component to protect the suture line in the medial capsule during the first few weeks after operation. Lateral patellar dislocation had been a complication (Freeman et al, 1981); it may be necessary to carry out lateral retinacular release and to confirm that the patella moves in the mid-line during flexion and extension at the end of the operation. Correction of rotational deformity is essential and the tibial tuberosity must be lined up with the centre of the tibial component.

Although the initial fundamental concept was sound, numerous elements in its application have needed to be improved. The ability to achieve correct alignment and ligament balance has been demonstrated and these factors, together with a better understanding of the principles involved and improvements in design, give grounds for hoping there will not be a deterioration in the quality of the results after another 4 or 5 years.

Insall's total condylar prosthesis

The practice some years ago at the Hospital for Special Surgery in New York was to use four different prostheses (unicondylar, duocondylar, geometric and the Guépar) which were selected according to the degree of pathological damage in the knee being operated on. Results of 198 operations (of the 4 types), followed-up from 2 to 3½ years, were reported (Insall et al, 1976). Although 'a significant improvement from the preoperative state' was achieved, the results were considered to be 'far from ideal'. Their dissatisfaction was such that Insall and his colleagues designed a new prosthesis (called the total condylar) and a preliminary report (Insall et al, 1976) was made in the same year as they published their comparison of the four models.

In 1979, Insall et al reported the results of 220 total condylar arthroplasties which had been followed for from 3 to 5 years. The prosthesis could be used whatever the pathological state of the knee before operation and this had the advantage of eliminating what can be a difficult choice; furthermore, only one technique had to be learnt. Considerable optimism was expressed and the results were claimed to approach the excellence achieved by replacement of the hip joint (Insall et al, 1979).

Modifications, however, have subsequently been introduced and there are now two types of Insall-Burstein replacement. The first, the total condylar, consists of a single bicondylar metallic femoral component and single bicondylar polyethylene tibial component with a central intramedullary stem; the patella is replaced by a convex polyethylene button. A metal-retained base is available in an attempt to prevent plastic deformation. All components are fixed with cement. The second type is the posterior stabilised knee which is described as a 'semiconstrained' nonlinked condylar system. The tibial component has a central eminence which is accommodated within an enlarged intercondylar box in the femoral component. This is intended to 'ensure a more natural path of motion and to prevent subluxation in flexion'. At the present time, Insall (1981) uses the posterior stabilised knee exclusively. An account of the short term results using this prosthesis has been published by Scott & Schoscheim (1982).

A detailed comparison between the Freeman and the Insall knees is difficult, particularly in view of changes which are currently being introduced. It is important to appreciate that there are wide areas of agreement and this can be seen in a chapter written by Freeman & Insall (Freeman, 1980). The need to correct all elements of the deformity by adequate soft tissue release is, for example, an essential requirement for both operations. Both authors agree on the various reasons for sacrificing cruciate ligaments (Freeman et al, 1977) and on achieving stability by obtaining a correct balance of the collateral ligaments and to a greater or lesser degree by the geometry of the surface of their components. It seems likely that the basic designs and instrumentation will draw closer together in the future.

Semiconstrained linked knee replacements

The Sheehan knee replacement

Sheehan (1974) described his new prosthesis at the International Knee Meeting in Rotterdam and in the same year we began using it at Harlow Wood Orthopaedic Hospital. At the time we felt it would be useful to have a prosthesis which was inherently more stable than the Freeman knee replacement and which could be used to replace severely damaged knee joints, particularly when there was lateral subluxation of the tibia. Sheehan (1978a) reported his results and has also given an account of the development of the operation and his experience with it in his Manual of Knee Arthroplasty (Sheehan, 1978b).

We carried out 90 Sheehan arthroplasties in the 5 years up till 1978 and 72 of them were available for review at the end of 1980. Only 2 knees at that time were considered total failures. A further 17 were not satisfactory in that the patients were complaining of pain, though there was no evidence at that time of mechanical failure. It also seemed as though the results did not deteriorate with time: 16 out of 22 (73%) of operations carried out in 1974 and 1975 were satisfactory, as were 71% of operations in 1978.

Nevertheless, there were some knees in which we did not achieve adequate correction of deformity; in particular, it proved difficult to reduce a coronal tibiofemoral angle of, say, 30 degrees of valgus, to within the 5–10° range (Fig. 3.5). It seemed that these knees, even if not painful, must be at risk from either breaking the stud or excessive plastic wear on one side of the articulation. This has proved to be the

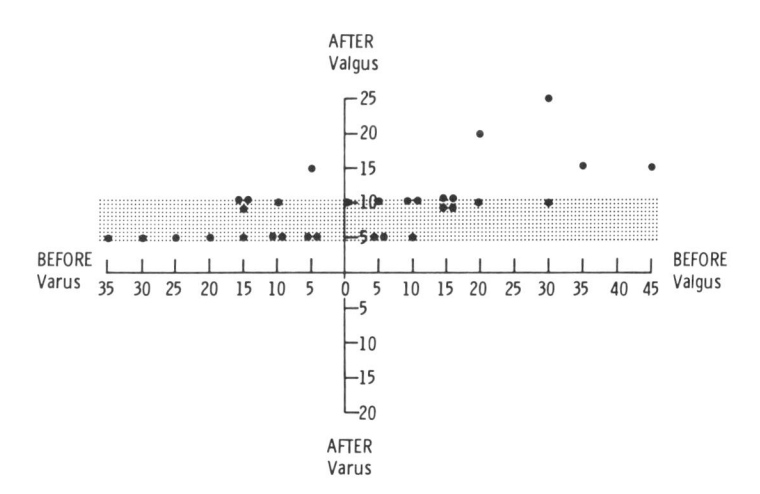

Fig. 3.5 This demonstrates the coronal tibiofemoral angle measured before and after operation in 33 consecutive Sheehan replacements. Satisfactory correction to within 5°–10° of valgus was achieved in 28. Severe varus deformities were well corrected, but there was failure in severe valgus deformities (from 20°–45°). The cause in the latter group was probably an inadequate soft tissue release, but it does indicate that intramedullary stems cannot always guarantee correct alignment.

case, and during 1981 we have operated on 4 knees with this complication. Chen & Helal (1980) reported similar, or rather worse, failures in 50 Sheehan replacements, 8 of which required further operations. It seems clear that intramedullary stems cannot, by themselves, ensure correct alignment.

Sheehan (1978b) recognised the difficulty of correcting severe deformities. He emphasised the need for soft tissue release and also the correction of the external rotation deformity in a valgus knee. During the past 2 years, Sheehan (1981) has been using a modification of the original design with broader condyles in order to increase the area of load transmission. There is also a revision tibial component with a bigger and stronger stud. A femoral component is also being designed which will provide an articulating surface for a patellar replacement.

Other semiconstrained linked knee replacements
Attenborough (1974) also presented his new design at the Rotterdam Meeting. Although quite different from the Sheehan prosthesis, it can be regarded as a semiconstrained linked replacement. Both operations, whilst conserving length, demand considerable excavation of intramedullary bone to insert the components. Vanhegan et al (1979) reviewed 100 Attenborough replacements followed from 1 to 4 years. There were only two knees with loosening and three deep infections. It seems possible that severe bone destruction can be associated with loosening and that fractures may occur above and below the rather short stems of the prosthesis.

The spherocentric arthroplasty is in this category and was first used in 1973 (Sonstegard et al, 1977). Kaufer & Matthews (1981) reported 82 consecutive operations with an average follow-up of 4 years (range 2–6 years). The overall reoperation rate was 9%. Convery et al (1980) had rather less satisfactory results with 11 complications (loosening 5; supracondylar fracture 2; infection 1 and suspected loosening 3) in a series of 36 operations. They modified the design with the aim of improving alignment.

The case of linked, but not totally constrained, replacements can be well argued, but the complicated design of the implants and the amount of bone which has to be removed for their insertion may create difficulties if failure does occur.

Constrained hinges
In the 1950s considerable interest was aroused by the possibility of replacing a severely damaged knee with a hinge which had intramedullary stems for fixation (Shiers, 1954). This appeared to be a straightforward solution to a difficult problem and early results were satisfactory. But later a relatively high incidence of complications was reported (Arden & Kamdar, 1974). Young (1971) reported the results achieved using a vitallium hinged prosthesis of his own design in 38 patients with rheumatoid arthritis. At a 5-year follow-up 65% were considered satisfactory; but at 10 years, the 'failures were 100%' (mostly due to late infection). It is difficult to ignore the high incidence of late infection when large hinges are used (whether or not they are cemented in position). At Harlow Wood in a series of 111 uncemented Walldius replacements the incidence of early and late deep infection was 8.5% (an incidence which will no doubt increase further as time passes) whereas there has been no infection in 65 Manchester replacements.

The arguments advanced against the use of a constrained hinge are well recognised;

in particular, the high forces generated at the bone-cement interface are likely to lead to loosening. In June 1980, the American Journal of Bone and Joint Surgery published three papers (Wilson et al, 1980; Bargar et al, 1980 and Hui et al, 1980) on hinged replacements and the editorial (Murray, 1980) expressed a firm view that surgeons should become 'unhinged'.

Has the case against the constrained hinge really been proved? Even though acceptable results have been reported with the Walldius prosthesis (Phillips & Taylor, 1975) it is difficult to justify a hinge with a metal-on-metal bearing. The Stanmore hinge with its metal-on-plastic bearing has its enthusiastic advocates. Lettin et al (1978) reported on 100 prostheses which were inserted between March 1969 and December 1976. The functional results were good with some exceptions: there were three deep infections and two patients had an above-knee amputation. The early results are excellent in our experience and it may be that better techniques for cement insertion will decrease the possibility of loosening. There have also been improvements in design (Scales, 1981) and titanium plateau plates are available which effecively increase the surface area in contact with bone. As with the Sheehan arthroplasty it is best to cement each component separately with the knee in flexion in order to avoid angulation of the intramedullary stems in the coronal or sagittal planes. There will inevitably be cases of late infection when the amount of bone removed and the mass of intramedullary cement will make salvage difficult. There are thus theoretical reasons for limiting this operation to the old and to those knees in which severe bone loss makes any other procedure unlikely to succeed.

Although this chapter is concerned with the treatment of chronic arthritis of the knee, it should be pointed out that the Stanmore prosthesis was first introduced in 1952 for replacement after excision of tumours around the knee: when used for this purpose, in relatively young patients, there has been no evidence of loosening (Scales, 1981).

The management of failed replacements

Most surgeons have to admit to an increasing experience of failed knee replacements. The size of the problem is indicated by the increase of secondary operations (revision, conversion or arthrodesis) at Harlow Wood. During the past 4 years, an average of 48 primary replacements have been carried out each year and each year there has been an average of 14 secondary operations. The average time between the first operation and the salvage procedure was 50 months. Ahlberg & Linden (1981) described their experiences in a series which included the Geometric, the St Georg sledge prosthesis and two types of constrained hinge. The authors point out that failure is most likely to occur in knees where there has been a previous operation (for example, synovectomy, tibial osteotomy or patellectomy).

Most prostheses have been designed in the knowledge that arthrodesis is a possible outcome. It is, however, a delusion to think that the amount of bone left at the end of the first operation will be available for reconstruction if failure occurs. Loosening and infection produce extensive destruction of the bone ends and this may be made worse by a polyethylene synovitis when wear has been a factor. Consequently, arthrodesis may be difficult to achieve. The situation will be worse when a hinge replacement has been used (Brodersen et al, 1979).

It is easiest to deal with a failed Manchester or Freeman knee replacement by substituting a Stanmore hinge. It is, in fact, tempting to do so since patients are unwilling to accept a stiff knee. The Freeman-Samuelson revision knee may provide an acceptable solution. This prosthesis is similar in design to their primary replacement, but the femoral component has a stem and there is a metal-stemmed tibial component on which the conventional polyethylene component is fitted.

In facing up to the problems of failure, the surgeon should try to diagnose loosening before extensive bony destruction occurs. This is not to suggest that painless knees with translucent lines at the bone-cement interface should be operated on. Nevertheless, it is wrong to watch progressive destruction occur (Fig. 3.6) before intervening.

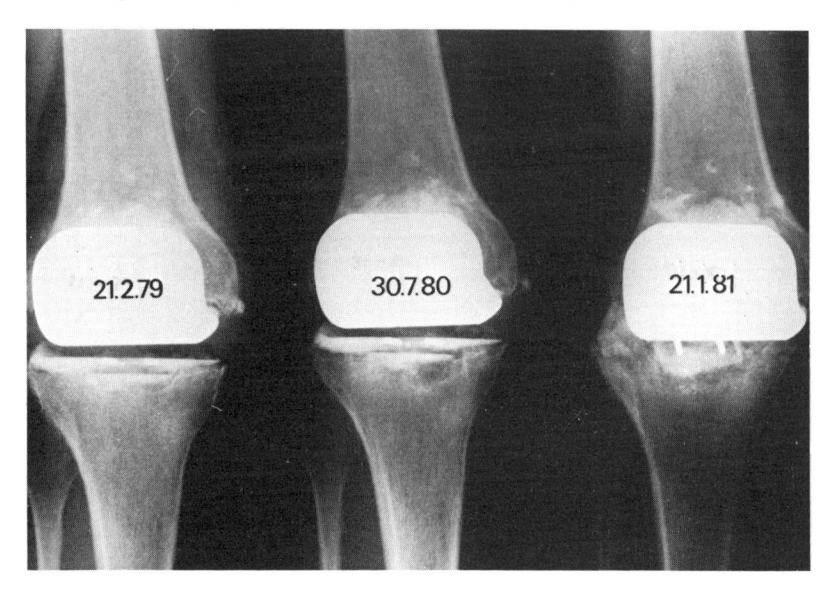

Fig. 3.6 Serial radiographs of a patient's knee with an early type of Freeman replacement showing progressive loosening and bony destruction. It would have been theoretically desirable to carry out an arthrodesis or revision between February 1979 and July 1980 before the bony damage became so far advanced.

It had been hoped that gait analysis might give objective evidence of abnormal loading so that failure could be more certainly predicted (Waugh, 1980). This, however, is not the case since at present our method is not sufficiently accurate (Johnson et al, 1981) to allow such individual predictions. At present, it is best to rely on clinical assessment and regular radiographic examination of every patient to be at risk from progressive loosening. Earlier operation will increase the prospect of a successful arthrodesis or conversion.

Discussion

Concepts and techniques of knee replacement operations continue to change, but it is possible to recognise some emerging patterns.

At present many surgeons appear to favour a condylar type of replacement with some in-built constraint. Deformity can be corrected (by appropriate soft tissue release) and stability restored in most knees. The basic concept was introduced by Freeman & Swanson (1972) and has proved to be fundamentally sound. Nevertheless,

Freeman has made many changes in the design and other surgeons and bioengineers have produced their own modifications. The Freeman-Samuelson prosthesis offers a little more constraint than was present in the earlier models: the new technique of fixation without cement may well prove to be a major advance. The Insall-Burstein posterior stabilised prosthesis provides more constraint with its intercondylar cam, the advantages of which have to be balanced against the theoretical risk of an increased incidence of loosening at the bone-cement interface.

Fixation of the tibial component (rather than the femoral) continues to provide a challenge and Walker (1981) has produced and tested in vitro a variety of different designs. His evidence suggests it is best to use a one-piece metal-tray plastic component with one or two posts or a one-piece component with a post on each side.

Wear of polyethylene certainly occurs, but it has not yet become a common cause of failure unless it is associated with malalignment or instability. In the long-term this factor may well become important, and new materials (such as carbon-fibre impregnated polyethylene, new plastics or ceramics) are likely to be tested.

Patellar replacement has now become an integral part of most modern replacements and when it is done, it is essential to ensure normal tracking by soft tissue release, if necessary, and to correct any external rotation deformity of the tibia.

Is it then likely that only one replacement will ever be needed to deal with every knee from the earliest to the most advanced stages of destruction? In the recent report from New York (Hood et al, 1981), the posterior stabilised total condylar knee was almost exclusively used, but it was also occasionally necessary to implant a 'custom metal-backed tibial component' where there was a deep bony defect and also to use titanium mesh to contain and re-enforce unsupported cement. Furthermore, in three revision operations 'a constrained total condylar III prosthesis' was needed.

This might seem to indicate the need for a linked prosthesis with a greater element of constraint, particularly when there is severe bone loss or subluxation. The Sheehan prosthesis has a good record in this class, but reviews with a longer follow-up are needed.

Some surgeons may still feel that there is a place for a totally constrained hinge; recent modifications to the Stanmore knee and better cementing technique may decrease the risk of loosening. It is probably correct to restrict its use to problems which cannot be easily solved by a less radical operation. Late infection is always likely to present a serious hazard particularly in rheumatoid patients.

If it is agreed that more than one type of replacement is needed, is there a place for having a system like the recently introduced Kinematic series? This should provide for all eventualities and has the advantage of using the same basic instrumentation for each of four different prostheses. The designs are based on sound bioengineering studies (Walker, 1981), but the results of clinical evaluation over a sufficiently long period are not yet available.

Finally, is there an indication for the 'small' compartmental implant? This type of replacement is only likely to be successful in knees where the destructive changes are not too advanced. Our own experience with the Manchester replacement led us to abandon this operation. It certainly appears to be more difficult to insert small implants correctly, although in some techniques alignment jigs are available (Cavendish et al, 1978). The advantage of conserving stock is balanced by the severe destruction which can be associated with loosening. The Oxford replacement may offer a solution, but it is too early to determine the precise place for this ingenious design.

Surgical and technological advances have produced very rapid changes in the development of knee replacement operations. It is to be hoped that we may now have a period of relative stability and, although improvements will inevitably be made, designs will not alter as frequently as they have in the past. Then we may look forward to reports of longer reviews presented in a way which will make possible comparison between different implants. Meanwhile it is still right to be cautious about the future of the great variety of operations that are available. If efforts are directed to look for the common ground, rather than exaggerating minor differences, we may reach a position where fewer implants are available and instrumentation becomes more standardised. Old designs should be discarded when they are shown to have an unacceptably high failure rate, but they should not be over-criticised because each has made a contribution in a difficult field. New designs must represent significant advances and be underwritten by sound bioengineering, appropriate physical tests and clinical experience.

The author appreciates the co-operation of those orthopaedic surgeons and bioengineers who have discussed their own designs of replacement with him, either by the spoken or written word: these are acknowledged in the list of references as personal communications. He is also very grateful to Mr John Goodfellow and Mr Michael Freeman for reading the sections describing their operations and for making helpful comments.

REFERENCES

Ahlberg A, Lunden A 1981 Secondary operations after knee joint replacement. Clinical Orthopaedics 156: 170–174

Aichroth P, Freeman M A R, Smillie I S, Souter W A 1978 Knee function assessment chart. Journal of Bone and Joint Surgery 60B: 308–309

Armitage P 1971 Statistical methods in medical research. Blackwell, Oxford, 408–414

Attenborough C G 1974 Stabilised gliding total knee replacement. The Knee Joint, Proceedings of the International Congress 1973. Excerpta Medica, Amsterdam

Attenborough C G 1978 The Attenborough total replacement. Journal of Bone and Joint Surgery 60B: 320–327

Arden G P, Kamdar B A 1975 Complications of arthroplasty of the knee. Total Knee Replacement. Institute of Mechanical Engineers, London, 118–122

Barbar L, Cracchiolo A, Amstutz H C 1980 Results with the constrained total knee prosthesis in treating severely disabled patients with failed total knee replacements. Journal of Bone and Joint Surgery 62A: 405–511

Broderson M P, Fitzgerald R H, Peterson L S A, Coventry M B, Bryan R S 1979 Arthrodesis of the knee following failed total knee arthroplasty. Journal of Bone & Joint Surgery 61A: p 181–185

Cavendish M E, Wright, J T M 1978 The Liverpool Mark II prosthesis. Journal of Bone and Joint Surgery 60B: 358–370

Chen S C, Helal B 1980 Preliminary results of Sheehan total knee prosthesis. International Orthopaedics 4: 67–71

Convery F R, Minteer-Convery M, Macolm L L 1980 The spherocentric knee: a revaluation and modification. Journal of Bone and Joint Surgery 62A: 320–327

Engelbrecht E, Siegel A, Rottger J, Bucholz H W 1976 Statistics of total knee replacement: partial and total knee replacement, design St Georg. Clinical Orthopaedics 120: 54–64

Freeman M A R, Swanson S A V 1972 Total prosthetic replacement of the knee. Journal of Bone and Joint Surgery 54B: 170

Freeman M A R, Insall J N, Besser W, Walker P S, Hallel T 1977 Excision of the cruciate ligaments in total knee replacement. Clinical Orthopaedics 126: 209–212

Freeman M A R, Todd R C, Bamert P, Day W H 1978 ICLH arthroplasty of the knee: 1968–1977. Journal of Bone and Joint Surgery 60B: 339–344

Freeman M A R, Insall J N 1980 Tibiofemoral replacement using two unlinked components and cruciate resection (The ICLH and total condylar prostheses). Arthritis of the Knee, Springer-Verlag, Berlin, Heidelberg and New York, ch 13, p 254
Freeman M A R, Blaha J D, Insler H 1981 Replacement of the knee in rheumatoid arthritis using the ICLH prosthesis. Reconstruction Surgery and Traumatology 18: 147–174
Goldberg V M, Henderson B T 1980 The Freeman-Swanson ICLH total knee arthroplasty. Journal of Bone and Joint Surgery 62A: 1338–1344
Goodfellow J W, O'Connor J 1978 The mechanics of the knee and prosthesis design. Journal of Bone and Joint Surgery 60B: 358–370
Goodfellow J W, O'Connor J, Biden E 1981 Designing the human knee. In: Stokes I A (ed) Mechanical factors and the skeleton, John Libbey, London, ch 9, p 52–64
Goodfellow J W 1981 Personal communication
Gunston F H 1971 Polycentric knee arthroplasty: prosthetic simulation of normal knee movement. Journal of Bone and Joint Surgery 53B: 272–277
Gunston F H, Mackenzie R I 1976 Complications of polycentric knee arthroplasty. Clinical Orthopaedics 120: 11–17
Hagstedt B, Norman O, Olsson T H, Tjornstrand B 1980 Technical accuracy in high tibial osteotomy for gonarthrosis. Acta Orthopaedica Scandinavica 51: 963–970
Hood R W, Vanni M, Insall J M 1981 The correction of knee alignment in 225 consecutive knee replacements. Clinical Orthopaedics 160: 94–108
Hui F C, Fitzgerald R H 1980 Hinged total knee arthroplasty. Journal of Bone and Joint Surgery 62A: 513–519
Insall J N, Ranawat C S, Aglietti P, Shine J 1976a A comparison of 4 models of total knee replacement prostheses. Journal of Bone and Joint Surgery 58A: 754–765
Insall J N, Ranawat C S, Scott W N, Walker P 1976b Total condylar replacement. Clinical Orthopaedics 120: 149–154
Insall J N, Scott W N, Ranawat C S 1979 The total condylar prosthesis. Journal of Bone and Joint Surgery 61A: 173–180
Insall J N, Aglietti P 1980 A five to seven year follow-up of unicondylar arthroplasty. Journal of Bone and Joint Surgery 62A: 1329–1337
Insall J N 1981 Personal communication
Jones W T, Bryan R S, Lowell F A, Peterson M D, Ilstrup D M 1981 Unicompartmental knee arthroplasty using polycentric and geometric hemicomponents. Journal of Bone and Joint Surgery 63A: 946–954
Johnson F, Leitl S, Waugh W 1980 Assessments of load across the knee — a comparison of static and dynamic measurement. Journal of Bone and Joint Surgery 62B: 346–349
Johnson F, Scarrow P, Waugh W 1981 Assessments of loads in the knee joint. Medical and Biological Engineering and Computing 19: 237–243
Johnson F, Oborne J, Allen M, Waugh W 1982 Continuous assessment of knee function and patient mobility. Journal of Biomedical Engineering, 4: 2–8
Kaufer H B, Matthews L S 1981 Spherocentric arthroplasty of the knee. Journal of Bone and Joint Surgery 63A: 545–559
Laskin R S 1976 Modular total knee replacement. Journal of Bone and Joint Surgery 58A: 766–773
Lawrence M R 1980 The role of goniometry and radiography in the assessment of tibiofemoral alignment and knee joint mobility. B Med Sci Thesis, University of Nottingham
Le Nobel J, Patterson F P 1981 Guépar total knee prosthesis. Journal of Bone and Joint Surgery 63B: 257–260
Lettin A W F, Deliss L J, Blackburne J S, Scales J T 1978 The Stanmore hinged knee arthroplasty. Journal of Bone and Joint Surgery 60B: 327–332
Lotke P A, Ecker M L 1977 Influence of positioning of prosthesis in total knee replacement. Journal of Bone and Joint Surgery 59A: 77–79
Maquet P, Simonet J, Marchin P 1967 Biomechanique du genou et gonarthrose. Rheumatologie 19: 51–70
Marmor L 1976 The modular Marmor knee: case report with minimum follow-up of two years. Clinical Orthopaedics 120: 86–94
Marmor L 1979 Marmor modular knee in unicompartmental disease. Journal of Bone and Joint Surgery 61A: 347–353
Marmor L 1982 The Marmor knee replacement. The Orthopedic Clinics of North America 13: 55–64
Moreland J R, Thomas R J, Freeman M A R 1980 ICLH replacement of the knee 1977 and 1978. Clinical Orthopaedics 145: 47–59
Murray D G 1980 In defence of becoming unhinged. Journal of Bone and Joint Surgery 62A: 495–496
O'Connor J, Goodfellow J W, Perry N 1982 Fixation of the Oxford knee. The Orthopedic Clinics of North America 13: 65–87

Phillips H, Taylor J G 1975 The Walldius hinge arthroplasty. Journal of Bone and Joint Surgery 57B: 59–62
Scales J T 1981 Personal communication
Scott R S, Santore R F 1981 Unicondylar unicompartmental replacement for osteoarthritis of the knee. Journal of Bone and Joint Surgery 63A: 536–544
Scott W N, Schoscheim P 1982 Posterior stabilised knee arthroplasty. Orthopedic Clinics of North America 13: 131–139
Shaw N E, Chatterjee R K 1978 Manchester knee arthroplasty. Journal of Bone and Joint Survery 60B: 310–313
Sheehan J M 1974 Arthroplasty of the knee. The Knee Joint, Proceedings of the International Congress 1973. Excerpta Medica Amsterdam
Sheehan J M 1978a Arthroplasty of the knee. Journal of Bone and Joint Surgery 60B: 333–338
Sheehan J M 1978b Manual of Knee Arthroplasty. Deloro Surgical, Swindon
Sheehan J M 1981 Personal communication
Shiers L G P 1954 Arthroplasty of the knee. Journal of Bone and Joint Surgery 36B: 553–560
Skolnick M D, Bryan R S, Peterson L F A, Combs J J, Ilstrup D M 1976 Polycentric total knee arthroplasty: a two-year follow-up study. Journal of Bone and Joint Surgery 58A: 749–753
Sonstegard D A, Kaufer H, Matthews L S 1977 Spherocentric knee: biomechanical testing and clinical trial. Journal of Bone and Joint Surgery 59A: 602–616
Tew M, Waugh W 1979 Total replacement of the knee. Journal of Bone and Joint Surgery 61B: 225–228
Vanhegan J A D, Dabrowski W, Arden G P 1979 A review of 100 Attenborough stabilised gliding knee prostheses. Journal of Bone and Joint Surgery 61B: 445–450
Walker P S, Greene R D, Thatcher J, Ben-Dor M, Rutherford M S, Ewald F C 1981 Fixation of tibial components of knee prostheses. Journal of Bone and Joint Surgery 63A: 258–267
Walker P S 1981 Personal communication
Waugh W, Tew M, Johnson F 1981 Methods of evaluating results for chronic arthritis of the knee. Journal of the Royal Society of Medicine 74: 343–347
Waugh W 1982 Assessment of knee function. Acta Orthopaedica Belgica 48: 36–44
Williams E A, Hargadon E J, Davies D R A 1978 Late failure of the Manchester prosthesis. Journal of Bone and Joint Surgery 61B: 451–454
Wilson F C, Fajgenbaum D M, Venters G C 1980 Results of knee replacement with the Walldius and geometric prosthesis. Journal of Bone and Joint Surgery 62A: 497–503
Young H H 1971 Use of a hinged vitallium prosthesis (Young type) for arthroplasty of the knee. Journal of Bone and Joint Surgery 53A: 1658–1659

4. The surgical treatment of osteoarthritis of the hip by reduction of articular pressure

P. Maquet

INTRODUCTION

Different conservative operations have been proposed in the past for treating osteoarthritis of the hip. Some aimed at modifying the blood circulation in the femoral head by drilling the bone (Duvernay cited by Herbert, 1950) or at stimulating the cartilaginous cells of the joint by dividing the bone (Nissen, 1960). However, no series of lasting good results of these operations has ever been published to our knowledge. Other procedures have been aimed at reducing the load on the joint: Voss (1956) divided the adductor and the abductor muscles; McMurray (1935, 1939) claimed to bypass the hip by transmitting part of the load directly from the pelvis to the shaft of the femur. However, although we can put forward a rationale for McMurray's osteotomy, our explanation is radically different from that suggested by McMurray himself (Maquet, 1966). Pauwels (1959 and 1973) was the first to analyse thoroughly the mechanics of the hip. He devised operations, the aim of which consisted of decreasing the joint pressure by diminishing the load to be transmitted and by enlarging the load bearing surface of the joint. We have proposed other procedures with the same aim (Maquet 1971b, 1976).

RATIONALE

During gait each hip alternately supports the mass of the body minus the loaded leg (Fig. 4.1). This mass acts on the hip with force K. Force K is exerted eccentrically on the joint. Equilibrium requires a force M which is provided by the abductor muscles. The hip joint thus transmits the resultant R of the two forces K and M. Force R normally attains more than four times body weight during the single limb support period of gait and acts on the joint like a hammer. Its line of action oscillates back and forth in the sagittal plane to a small degree but remains close to the coronal plane. Therefore, the analysis of the mechanical equilibrium of the hip can be restricted to the projection of the forces in this latter.

The magnitude of the resultant R depends on the distance from the centre of the femoral head to the line of action of force K, exerted by the partial body mass, and to that of force M exerted by the abductor muscles. In a normal hip force K acts with a lever arm h' which is approximately three times longer than h of force M.

If force K acts closer to the joint, the force M necessary for equilibrium will be smaller as will be the resultant R. This is what happens in limping. On the other hand, if they act with a longer lever arm, the abductor muscles will counterbalance the force K with a smaller force M and the resultant R will also be smaller. Therefore, for the same length of femoral neck, the resultant R is greater in coxa valga than in a

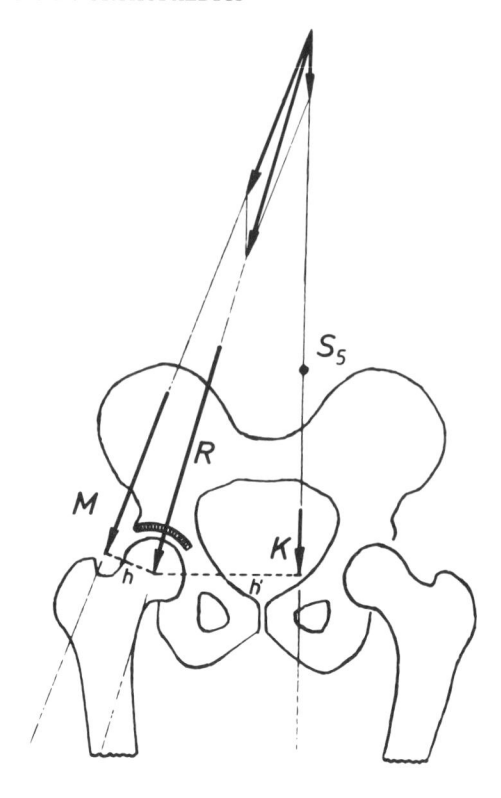

Fig. 4.1 Mechanical stresses on the hip joint during the single limb support period of gait
S_5, centre of gravity of the body minus the supporting leg
K, force exerted by the mass of the body minus the supporting leg
h', lever arm of force K
M, force exerted by the abductor muscles
h, lever arm of force M
R, resultant of forces K and M
(Redrawn after Pauwels)

normal hip because the lever arm of the abductors is shorter. It is smaller in a coxa vara than in a normal hip because the lever arm of the abductors is longer (Pauwels, 1973).

The force R evokes compressive stresses in the joint. In a normal hip the stresses are evenly distributed over the weight bearing surface of the joint. This even distribution is suggested by the subchondral sclerosis of even thickness throughout, in the roof of the acetabulum. As shown by Pauwels, the quantity of bone depends on the magnitude of the stresses. Therefore, the subchondral sclerosis presents the same shape as the stress diagram (Fig. 4.2a).

If one of the layers of cartilage has been removed, as in the replacement of the femoral head by a prosthesis, or if the cartilage no longer distributes the articular stresses evenly, a cup shaped sclerosis develops in the roof of the socket (Fig. 4.2b). This cup shaped sclerosis indicates an uneven distribution of joint stresses, although symmetrical on both sides of the line of action of the resultant force R. This constitutes the first sign of primary osteoarthritis the cause of which is to be sought for in a disturbance of the tissues rather than in the mechanical conditions.

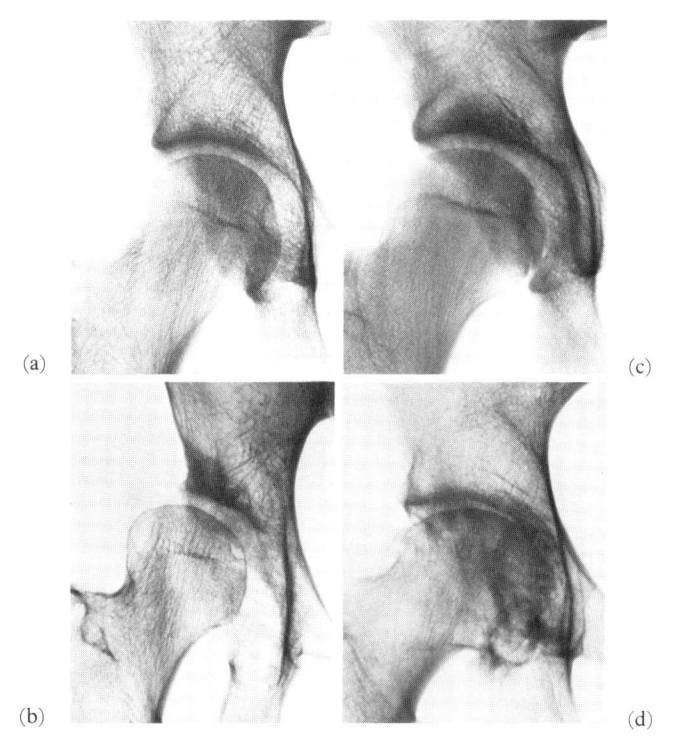

Fig. 4.2 (a) Subchondral sclerosis of uniform thickness in the roof of the acetabulum in a normal hip.
(b) Cup shaped subchondral sclerosis: the first sign of primary osteoarthritis.
(c) Sclerotic triangle at the edge of the acetabulum in osteoarthritis with subluxation.
(d) Sclerotic traingle in the depths of the acetabulum in osteoarthritis with protrusio (Maquet, 1975)
(Courtesy of Expansion Scientifique Française)

In a subluxated hip the resultant R acts closer to the edge of the socket than in a normal hip and part of the articular contact surface no longer bears weight. The stresses are then asymmetrically distributed over a smaller weight bearing area. They are at their greatest at the edge of the acetabulum and their distribution diagram is now triangular as is the subchondral sclerosis (Fig. 4.2c).

While the subluxation of an osteoarthritic hip progresses, the contact surface of the joint may increase considerably as a result of the alterations in shape of the socket and of the femoral head. However the line of action of the force R continues to pass through the centre of the femoral head. Since the latter is more and more extruded laterally by a medial osteophyte, the resultant force R is brought closer to the edge of the acetabulum. Thereby the weight bearing surface of the joint is decreased despite the increase of its contact surface (Pauwels, 1973). This is very important for the understanding of the mechanics of subluxating osteoarthritis of the hip.

In osteoarthritis with protrusio acetabuli the resultant force R acts more deeply in the socket. A dense triangle can now be observed in the depths of the acetabulum (Fig. 4.2d). It demonstrates an uneven distribution of the articular compressive stresses with a maximum medially. The transverse component Q of the resultant R — or rather of its reaction R_1 — appears too great for the resistance of the tissues (Fig. 4.11). This transverse component Q pushes the femoral head into the acetabulum.

Osteoarthritis thus appears as the result of a breakdown of a physiological equilibrium which exists between the resistance and the stressing of articular tissues. Either pathological tissues cannot withstand normal stresses or increased stresses overwhelm the resistance of normal tissues. The biological factors which determine the resistance of the tissues can be little influenced. Furthermore, bringing this resistance up to normal again would not be sufficient if the mechanical stressing is further increased, as it soon becomes, in the course of the disease. This is illustrated by the progressive subluxation of the femoral head. The only sensible mechanical approach to the condition thus consists of decreasing the compressive stresses in the joint sufficiently to make them tolerable.

There are two ways of decreasing the articular compressive stresses: (1) to decrease the force R transmitted; (2) to enlarge the load bearing surface of the joint.

The best solution, whenever possible, would be to combine these two possibilities.

HANGING-HIP (Voss-Pauwels)

The hanging hip operation combines a division of the tendons of the adductors and abductors of the hip (Voss, 1956) with a tenotomy of the ilio-psoas (Pauwels, 1959) (Fig. 4.3). The adductors and the ilio-psoas are divided through a 5 cm longitudinal

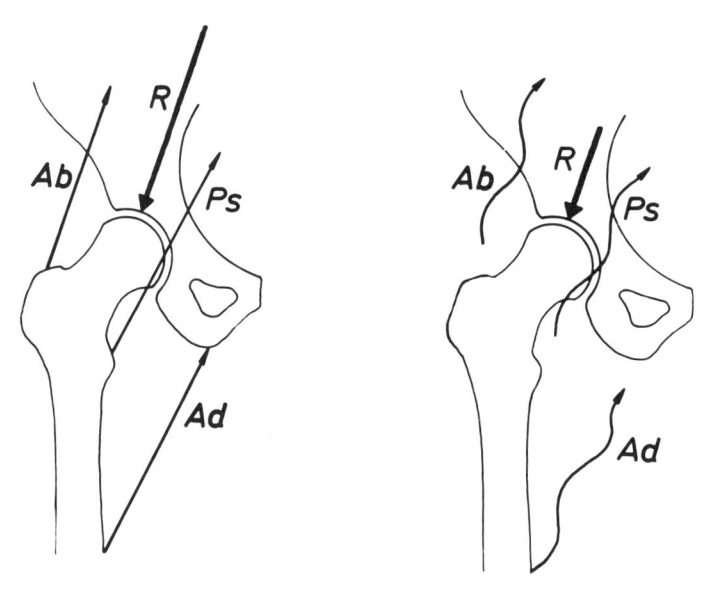

Fig. 4.3 Hangling hip. Division of the abductor-, adductor- and ilio-psoas muscles and of the fascia lata (Voss-Pauwels)
(Redrawn after Pauwels)

incision along the tendon of adductor longus, the fascia lata and abductors through a lateral longitudinal incision. The patient can walk immediately. He is asked to use two crutches for at least three months, one crutch for three additional months. Any active exercise is avoided so as not to strengthen the muscles.

In all cases the operation decreases the load transmitted by the joint, particularly if the divided muscles were contracted. Two requirements must be fulfilled before considering this operation: good congruence of the articular surfaces and the absence of a triangle of subchondral sclerosis which would correspond to a reduced weight bearing area. Provided that these requirements are met, the procedure can give spectacular results. The 78-year-old female patient (Fig. 4.4a) complained of a painful hip with a restricted range of movement (fl. 75°; ext. 0°; add. 5°; abd. −5°; int.rot. −5°; ext.rot. 10°). The joint surfaces were congruent but there was no joint space. There was no triangular increase in density but rather a cup shaped subchondral sclerosis in the roof of the acetabulum. Nine years after a hanging hip operation (Fig. 4.4b), the patient remains painfree, the range of movement has improved (flex. 100°; ext. 10°; add. 35°; abd. 5°; int. rot. 45°; ext.rot. 55°) and a joint space has reappeared. The subchondral sclerosis has evolved for the better, and now approaches the same thickness throughout.

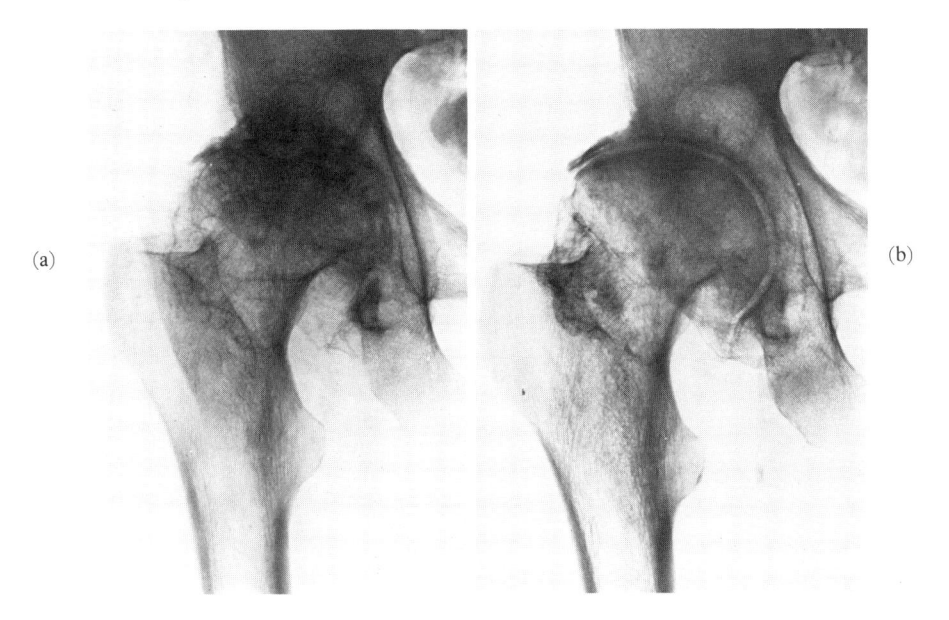

Fig. 4.4 78-year-old female patient before (a) and nine years after a hanging hip (b)

Fifty-two hips considered to be good candidates for this procedure were reviewed with a follow-up between 1 and 14 years. Forty-four (85%) were relieved of pain, 32 (62%) had a good or better gait with little need for a walking stick. In 23 (44%) the radiological signs of osteoarthritis had regressed, in 20 (38%) they had not evolved further and only in nine (17%) were they aggravated (Radin et al, 1975).

However, the hanging hip procedure is doomed to fail if carried out in the presence of a dense subchondral triangle, indicating a decrease in the weight bearing area. This happened in a 64-year-old female patient (Fig. 4.5a). Four years after the operation the situation has become worse than before (Fig. 4.5b). This results from an error of indications! The patient then underwent an intertrochanteric osteotomy which enlarged the weight bearing surface of the joint, with an excellent result at eight years follow-up (Fig. 4.5c). If the weight bearing area of the joint has become decreased, it

70 RECENT ADVANCES IN ORTHOPAEDICS

Fig. 4.5 Poor result of a hanging hip in a 67-year-old patient. The hip before (a) and four years after the operation (b). The indication was incorrect! The patient then underwent an osteotomy which enlarged the weight bearing surface of the hip with an excellent result at eight years follow-up (c) (Maquet, 1975) (Courtesy of Expansion Scientifique Française)

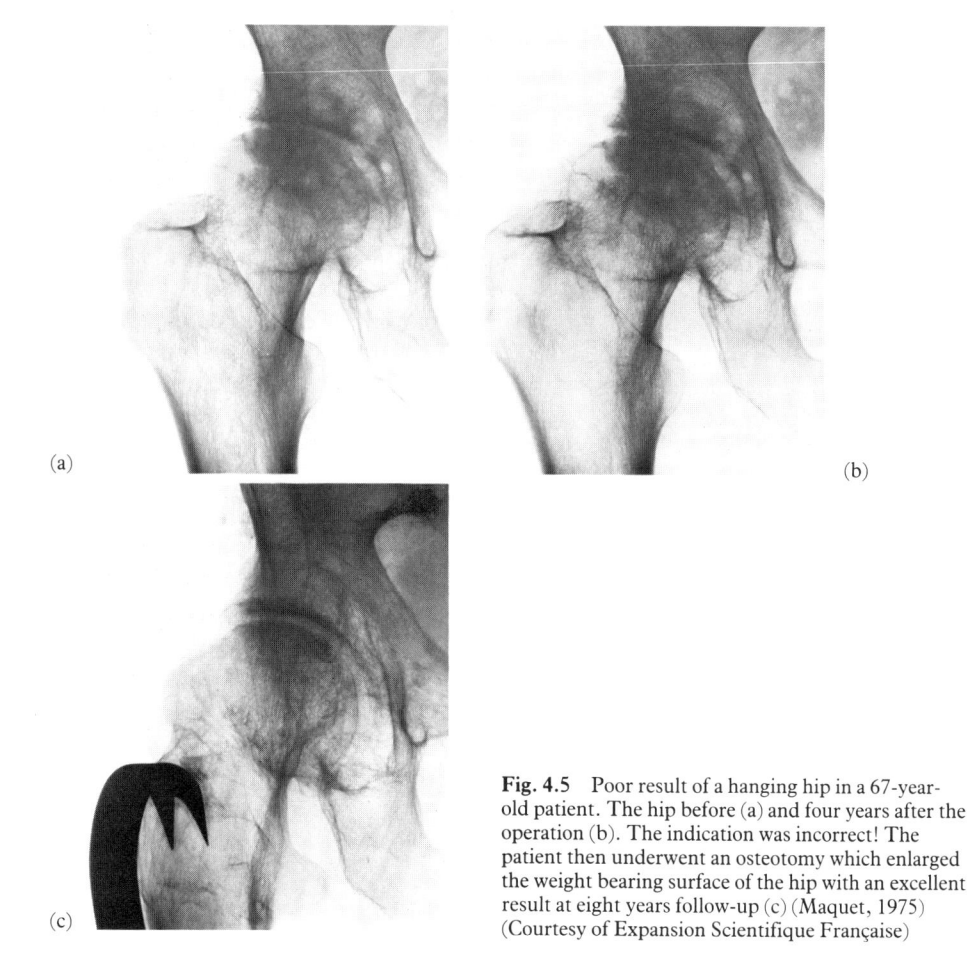

must be enlarged because in this situation, diminishing the load is not sufficient. Different ways of enlarging the weight bearing area of the hip joint exist, depending on the particular configuration of the articulation.

VARUS INTERTROCHANTERIC OSTEOTOMY (Pauwels I)

Varus intertrochanteric osteotomy (Pauwels, 1959) lengthens the leverarm and changes the direction of the abductor muscles M (Fig. 4.6). A longer lever arm allows the muscles to carry out their work with less force. Furthermore the osteotomy changes the direction of the force M. This brings downwards the intersection of the two forces K and M and thus displaces the resultant force R further into the socket which enlarges the weight bearing area of the joint. Both diminishing force M and opening the angle formed by the forces M and K (Fig. 4.1) decrease the load R. The operation therefore entails a decrease and a better distribution of the compressive stresses in the joint. This can only be achieved if the articular surfaces remain congruent when the leg is brought into full abduction preoperatively.

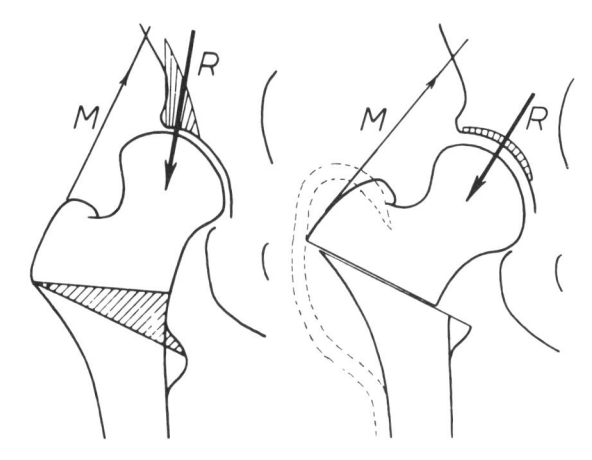

Fig. 4.6 Varus intertrochanteric osteotomy (Pauwels I): increase of the weight bearing joint surface and decrease of the load (Redrawn after Pauwels)

Triangular subchondral sclerosis illustrates the increased and asymmetrically distributed articular pressure in a 73-year-old female patient (Fig. 4.7a). Thirteen years after a varus osteotomy a thin ribbon of even thickness throughout has replaced the dense triangle and the pressure is now evenly distributed over a large weight bearing area (Fig. 4.7b). The clinical result was excellent.

If the varus osteotomy does not ensure congruity of the joint surfaces it may not change or it may even decrease the articular weight bearing area. It then leads to failure. This happened in this 31-year-old female patient (Fig. 4.8). This failure must not be attributed to the method but to the surgeon: the indication was wrong!

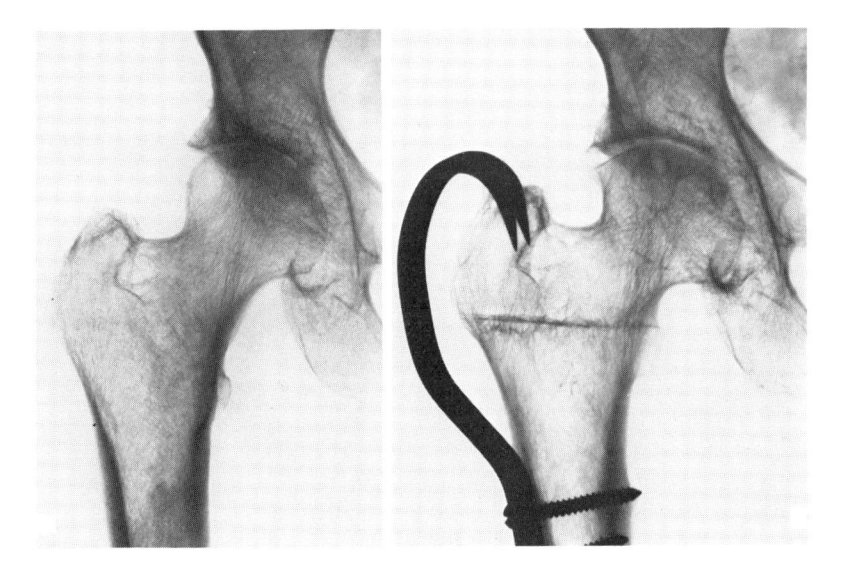

Fig. 4.7 73-year-old female patient before (a) and 13 years after a varus intertrochanteric osteotomy (b)

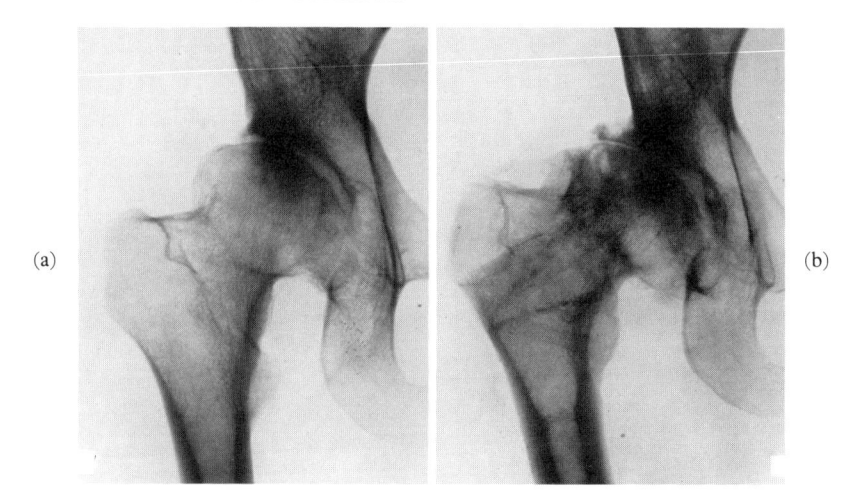

Fig. 4.8 Poor result after a varus intertrochanteric osteotomy which decreased the weight bearing surface of the joint. (Maquet, 1975)
(Courtesy of Expansion Scientifique Française)

VALGUS INTERTROCHANTERIC OSTEOTOMY + TENOTOMY
(Pauwels II)

In some cases it is often possible to enlarge the articular load bearing area by a valgus intertrochanteric osteotomy (Fig. 4.9). The osteotomy is combined with a tenotomy of the abductor-, adductor and ilio-psoas muscles (Pauwels, 1959) and makes the

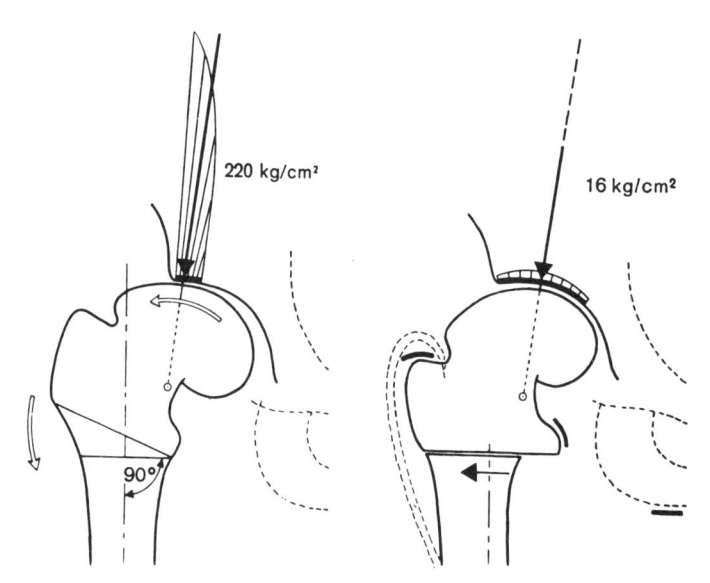

Fig. 4.9 Valgus intertrochanteric osteotomy combined with tenotomy of the abductor-, adductor- and ilio-psoas muscles (Pauwels II): increase of the weight bearing surface of the joint and decrease of the load (Redrawn after Pauwels)
(Courtesy of Expansion Scientifique Française)

osteophyte developed medially on the femoral head part of the weight bearing surface, thus increasing the latter, sometimes very considerably, while the tenotomy reduces the load transmitted. The operation results in a diminution and an even distribution of the compressive stresses in the joint.

A dense triangle at the edge of the socket betokens the increased pressure in the joint of a 55-year-old female patient (Fig. 4.10a). Eleven years after a valgus osteotomy combined with a multiple tenotomy, subchondral sclerosis of uniform thickness demonstrates a diminution and even distribution of the articular stresses over a large weight bearing area (Fig. 4.10b). The clinical result was excellent.

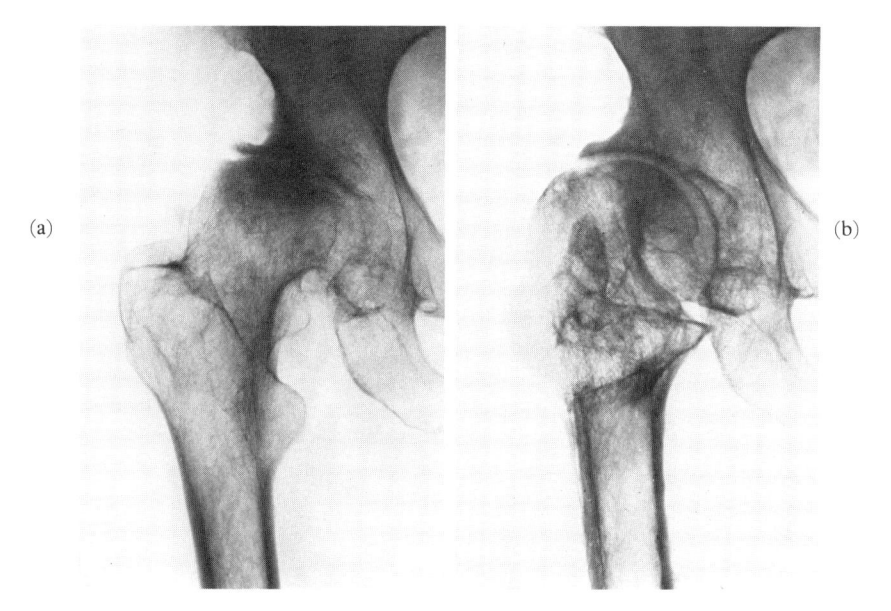

Fig. 4.10 55-year-old female patient before and 11 years after a valgus intertrochanteric osteotomy + tenotomy

Treatment of osteoarthritis with protrusio acetabuli

In osteoarthritis with protrusio acetabuli a valgus osteotomy combined with a tenotomy (Pauwels II) will reduce the pressure in the depth of the acetabulum by decreasing the force R supported by the hip and above all its transverse component Q which pushes the femoral head medially (Fig. 4.11). The operation enlarges the weight bearing surface of the joint by displacing the line of action of force R towards the upper part of the socket. A female patient underwent this procedure at age 48 on one side (Fig. 4.12a), at age 49 on the opposite side (Fig. 4.13a). At 10 and 9 years follow-up the result is excellent bilaterally. The signs of osteoarthritis have regressed and regular joint spaces have reappeared (Fig. 4.12b and 4.13b).

Progressive reappearance of the joint space

It should be emphasised that the Pauwels osteotomies do not replace, in the weight bearing area, a part of the femoral head from which the cartilage has been worn off by another part on which the cartilage has been preserved. This is demonstrated by the slow development of a new joint space in most patients.

74 RECENT ADVANCES IN ORTHOPAEDICS

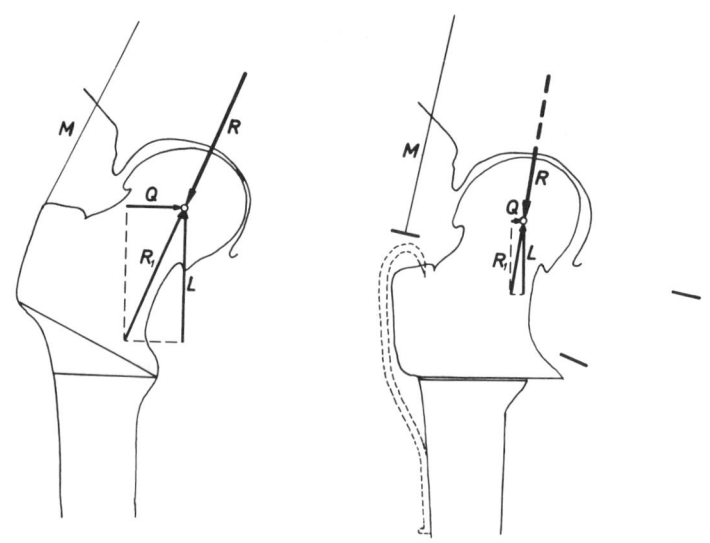

Fig. 4.11 In osteoarthritis with protrusio acetabuli, a valgus intertrochanteric osteotomy combined with a tenotomy of the abductor-, adductor- and ilio-psoas muscles will decrease the load R transmitted (= the reaction force R_1) and above all its transverse component Q (Redrawn after Pauwels) (Courtesy of Expansion Scientifique Français)

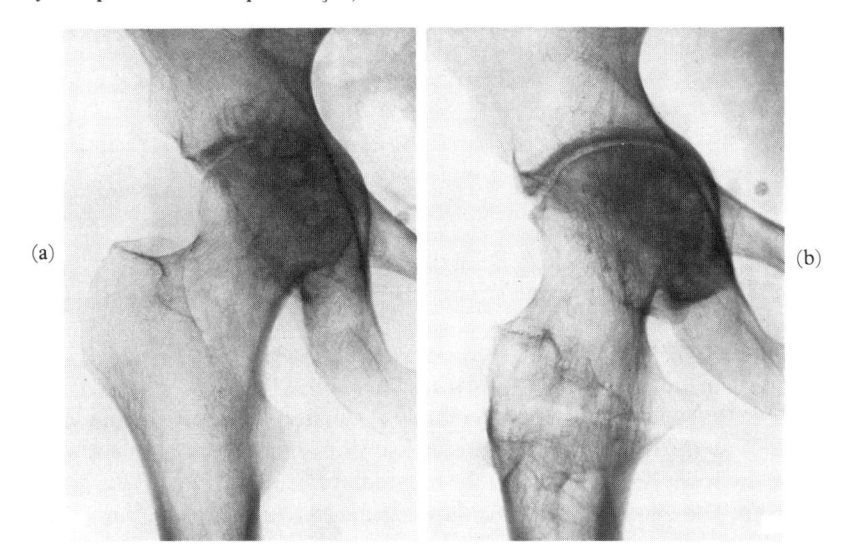

Fig. 4.12 48-year-old female patient before (a) and 10 years after a Pauwels II (b)

Preoperative X-rays, planning and surgical procedure

In order to choose the proper osteotomy, A.P. X-rays are taken with the beam centred on the femoral head, with the leg in internal rotation, in the neutral position, in full abduction and in full adduction. Congruence of the joint surfaces in abduction would tend to indicate a varus osteotomy (Fig. 4.14a). The operation must then be precisely planned on a tracing of the X-ray in the neutral position, with accurate measurement of the angle of the wedge to be resected (Fig. 4.14b). If the joint surfaces are

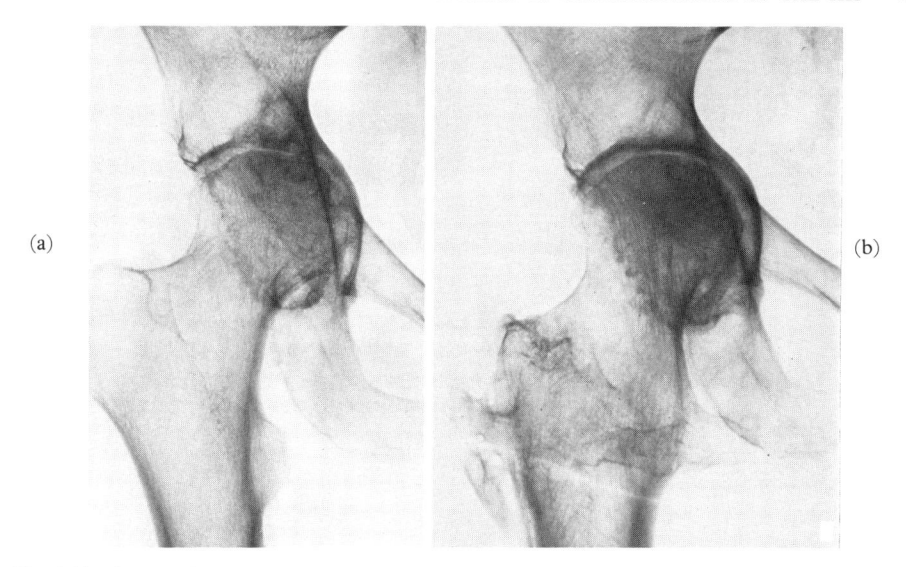

Fig. 4.13 Same patient as in Figure 4.12. Opposite hip before (a) and nine years after a Pauwels II (b)

incongruous in abduction and tend to be congruous in adduction, a valgus osteotomy must be considered (Fig. 4.15a). The valgus osteotomy is also planned graphically (Fig. 4.15b). It must ensure congruent articular surfaces with some opening of the joint space at the edge of the acetabulum. The wedge required to be resected may be greater than the range of adduction available but the subsequent abduction corrects itself spontaneously in the course of the first post-operative year.

The procedure has been described elsewhere (Maquet, 1977), but will be summarised briefly. Firstly, all the adductors are divided near their pubic attachment as is the ilio-psoas at its attachment to the lesser trochanter, through a 5 cm longitudinal incision over the tendon of adductor longus. (This tenotomy is not necessary if a varus osteotomy is planned.) Then the patient is placed in the prone position. A lateral approach to the upper end of the femoral shaft and greater trochanter is used. The skin incision is 12 to 15 cm long, distal to the greater trochanter. The fascia lata is split along its fibres. The vastus lateralis is disinserted from the greater trochanter and the linea aspera. The wedge to be resected is then marked by K-wires drilled into the bone and forming the desired angle. One of the two cuts must be perpendicular to the long axis of the femur, the proximal for a varus osteotomy, the distal for a valgus one. The wedge is resected accurately with a hand saw under the image intensifier. Pre-operative flexion contracture is corrected by cutting the wedge larger posteriorly than anteriorly. The knee is then flexed to a right angle and the lower leg kept vertical to ensure accurate rotational correction. The fragments are then brought close together by bringing the leg into as much adduction as possible for a varus osteotomy and into abduction for a valgus osteotomy. They are fixed under compression using a plate which is hooked into the greater trochanter by two spikes and screwed onto the lateral aspect of the shaft. *This plate (Maquet, 1971a) will act as a pre-stressed tension band.

* Manufactured by JRI, 104–112, Marylebone Lane, London W1.

76 RECENT ADVANCES IN ORTHOPAEDICS

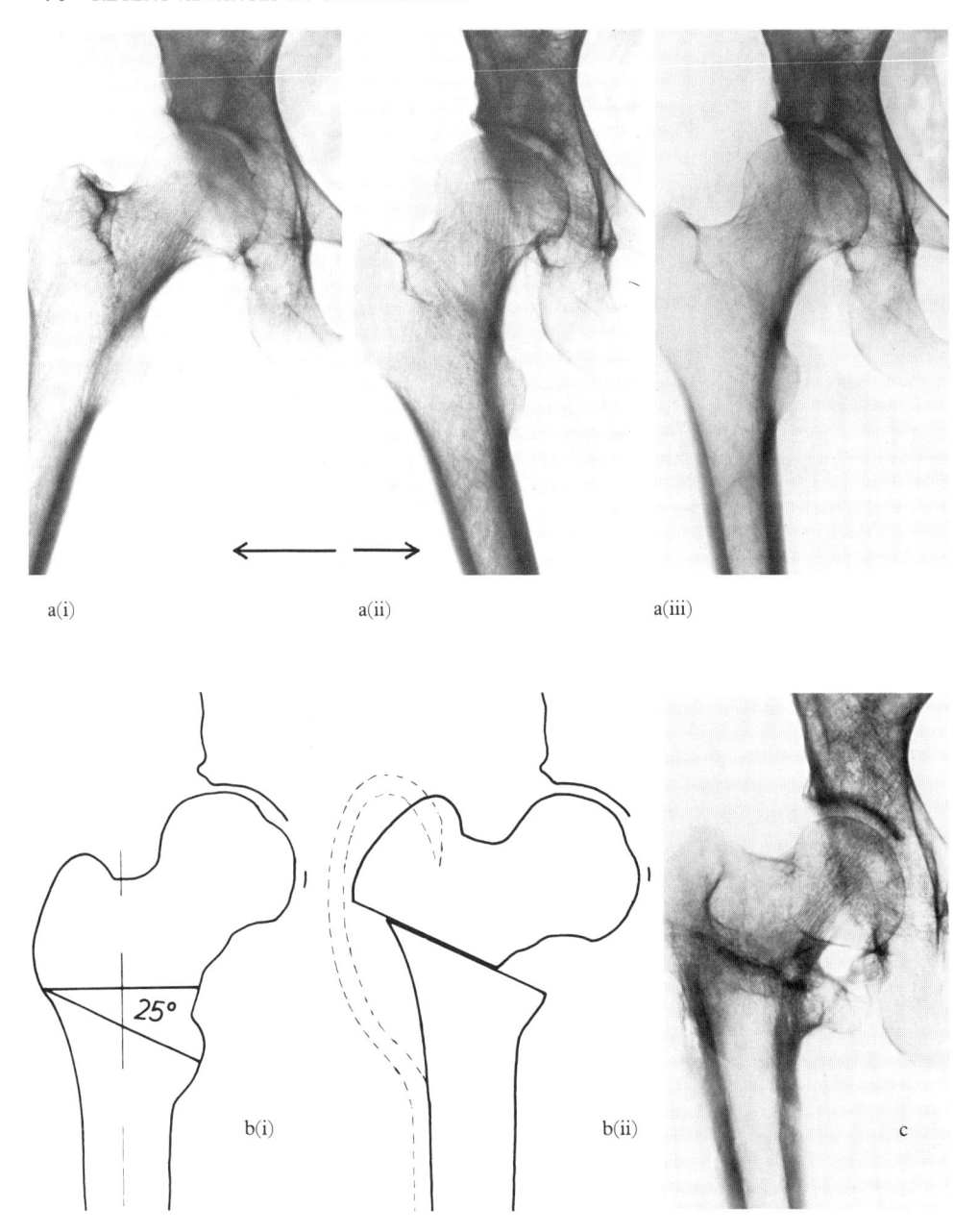

a(i) a(ii) a(iii)

b(i) b(ii) c

Fig. 4.14 Good congruence of the joint surfaces in full abduction (a). A varus osteotomy is indicated (b). 59-year-old patient. Result at five year follow-up (c)

The patient may be mobilised immediately after surgery. He stands up on the second day and starts to walk with two crutches, partially loading the operated leg (20% of body weight). In cases of severe osteoarthritis, two crutches are recommended for six months and then one crutch is used for six additional months. Any

TREATMENT OF OSTEOARTHRITIS OF THE HIP 77

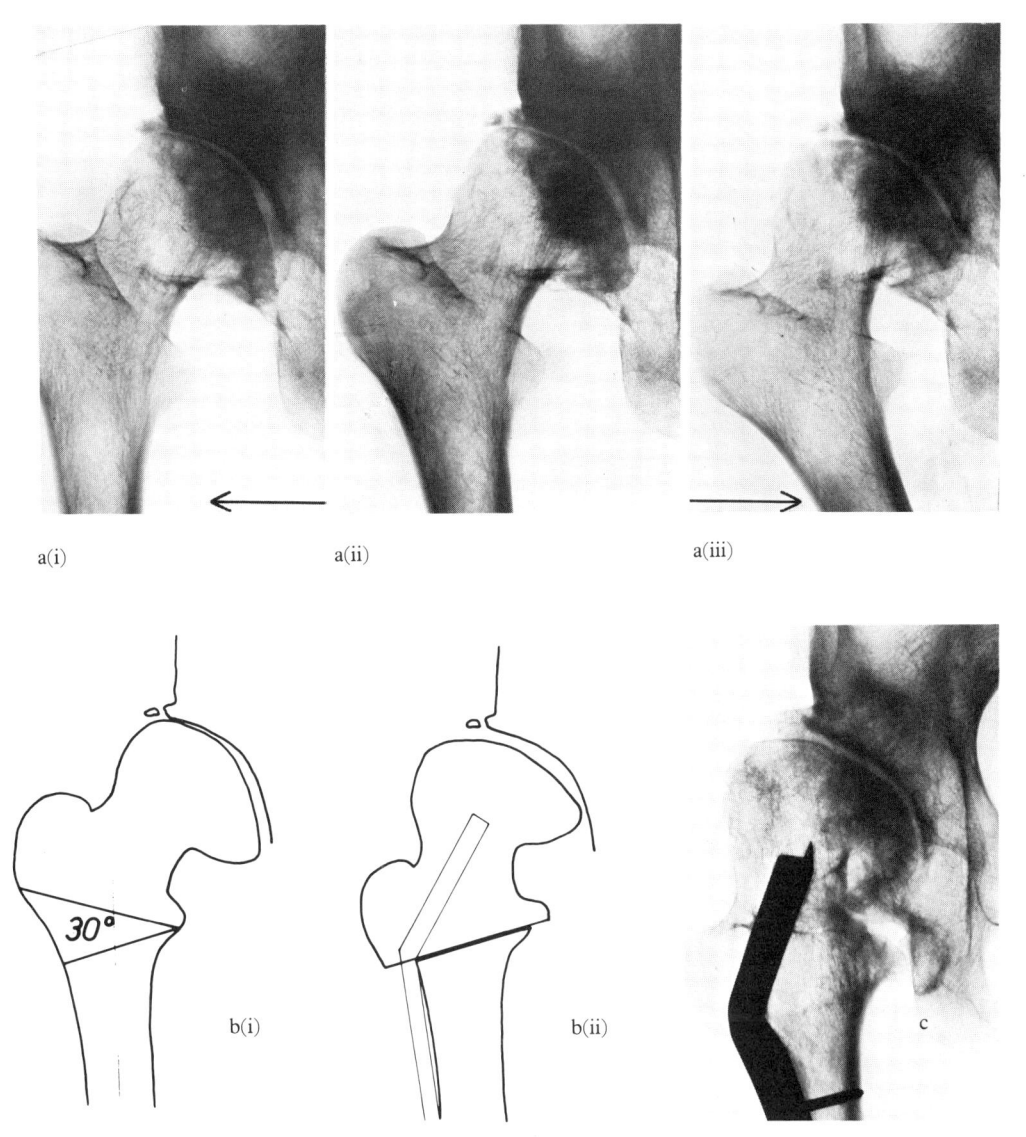

a(i) a(ii) a(iii)

b(i) b(ii) c

Fig. 4.15 Better congruence of the joint surface in full adduction (a) A valgus osteotomy seems appropriate. This must be confirmed by drawing (b) 42-year-old patient. Result at 16 year follow-up (c)

active exercise, except walking, is avoided. Strengthening the muscles would increase the articular pressure which is just the opposite of the aim pursued by the operation!

Usually the pain disappears immediately, the range of movement improves and the signs of osteoarthritis regress.

In some cases neither a varus nor a valgus osteotomy can enlarge the weight bearing surface of the joint. In neither abduction nor adduction can the femoral head re-enter the acetabulum, leading to satisfactory congruence of the articular surfaces. In such cases any osteotomy is doomed to failure. Further progress must be awaited or another solution sought.

78 RECENT ADVANCES IN ORTHOPAEDICS

Decreasing the compressive stresses rather than restoring normal anatomical shape

This approach to the problem does not aim at restoring anatomy but rather at decreasing the stresses in the joint. A 37-year-old female patient (Fig. 4.16a)

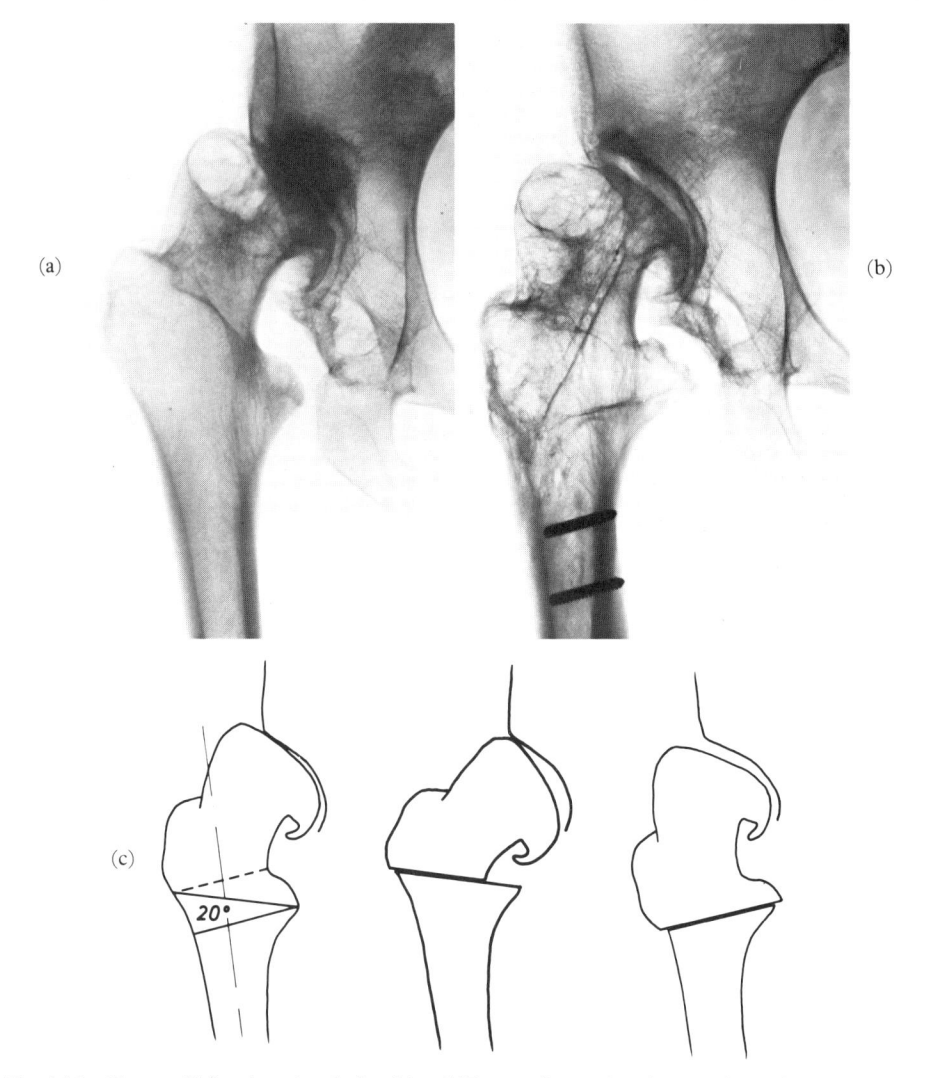

Fig. 4.16 37-year-old female patient before (a) and 17 years after a valgus intertrochanteric osteotomy + tenotomy (b) Valgus osteotomy is indicated rather than varus osteotomy even though the latter would tend to restore anatomy (c)

developed severe osteoarthritis in a subluxating dysplasic hip with coxa valga and a shallow acetabulum. A varus osteotomy would tend to restore anatomy but would certainly not ensure congruence of the articular surfaces (Fig. 4.16c). Therefore, it would not enlarge the weight bearing area of the joint. To achieve this, a valgus osteotomy appears to be necessary even though this increases the valgus deformity of the upper end of the femur and the subluxation. However, it was carried out with a multiple tenotomy and did indeed reduce considerably the compressive stresses in the joint, as shown by the regression of the dense triangle at the edge of the socket and its progressive replacement by subchondral sclerosis of even thickness throughout (Fig. 4.16b). The follow-up covers seventeen years and the clinical result remains excellent.

Old age does not constitute a contra-indication. It is amazing to observe that osteoarthritis can heal whatever the age. The patients, in Figure 4.4 and 4.7 represent good examples of this. Several of our patients were over 70 years of age when they were submitted to a tenotomy or an osteotomy and they reacted as well as younger patients.

Watillon et al (1978) have reviewed 804 cases of Pauwels' osteotomy for severe osteoarthritis in which the mechanical aim seemed to have been attained. The minimum follow-up was 3 years, the maximum 28 years. Not only did the pain relief appear very satisfactory but the range of movement and the gait improved considerably. The regression of the X-ray signs of osteoarthritis was also spectacular. Improvement of articular congruence was followed by excellent or good results in 79% of the cases. Conversely the cases in which incongruence of the joint surfaces had been aggravated gave mostly poor results. These results support Pauwels' rationale as do the following observations.

Reoperation after a poor result due to faulty case selection
A varus intertrochanteric osteotomy was carried out for severe osteoarthritis in a 61-year-old female patient (Fig. 4.17a). It could not enlarge the weight bearing area of the joint and presumably even decreased it. Aggravation of the clinical state was noted and the X-ray did not show any improvement (Fig. 4.17b). A valgus intertrochanteric osteotomy was then carried out. This second osteotomy achieved good congruence of the articular surfaces and thus enlarged the weight bearing area of the joint. Clinical improvement occurred. Eleven years later the result remains excellent (Fig. 4.17c).

SHORTENING OF THE OPPOSITE LEG (Maquet, 1976)

So far as the load bearing area of the hip is concerned, turning the socket around the femoral head (clockwise in the diagram Fig. 4.18c) must be equivalent to turning the femoral head in the socket as in a valgus osteotomy. A 57-year-old female patient (Fig. 4.18) presented a dysplasia of the right hip which articulated in a neo-acetabulum more proximal than normal. The patient developed bilateral severe osteoarthritis (Fig. 4.18a) with a tilt of the pelvis to the right such that the apparent discrepancy of leg length attained 4 cm. A left valgus osteotomy of 55° was carried out combined with a 4 cm shortening. The shortening of the left leg caused the pelvis to turn around the right femoral head as if a valgus osteotomy of 10° had been carried out on the right side (Fig. 4.18c). Both hips soon improved. Eleven years later the result remains excellent not only on the left side which has been operated on but also on the right side which did not undergo any surgery. On both sides a large joint space has reappeared and the signs of osteoarthritis have dramatically regressed (Fig. 4.18b). The clinical result is excellent.

Simple division of the bone with the changes in blood supply which this may entail

80 RECENT ADVANCES IN ORTHOPAEDICS

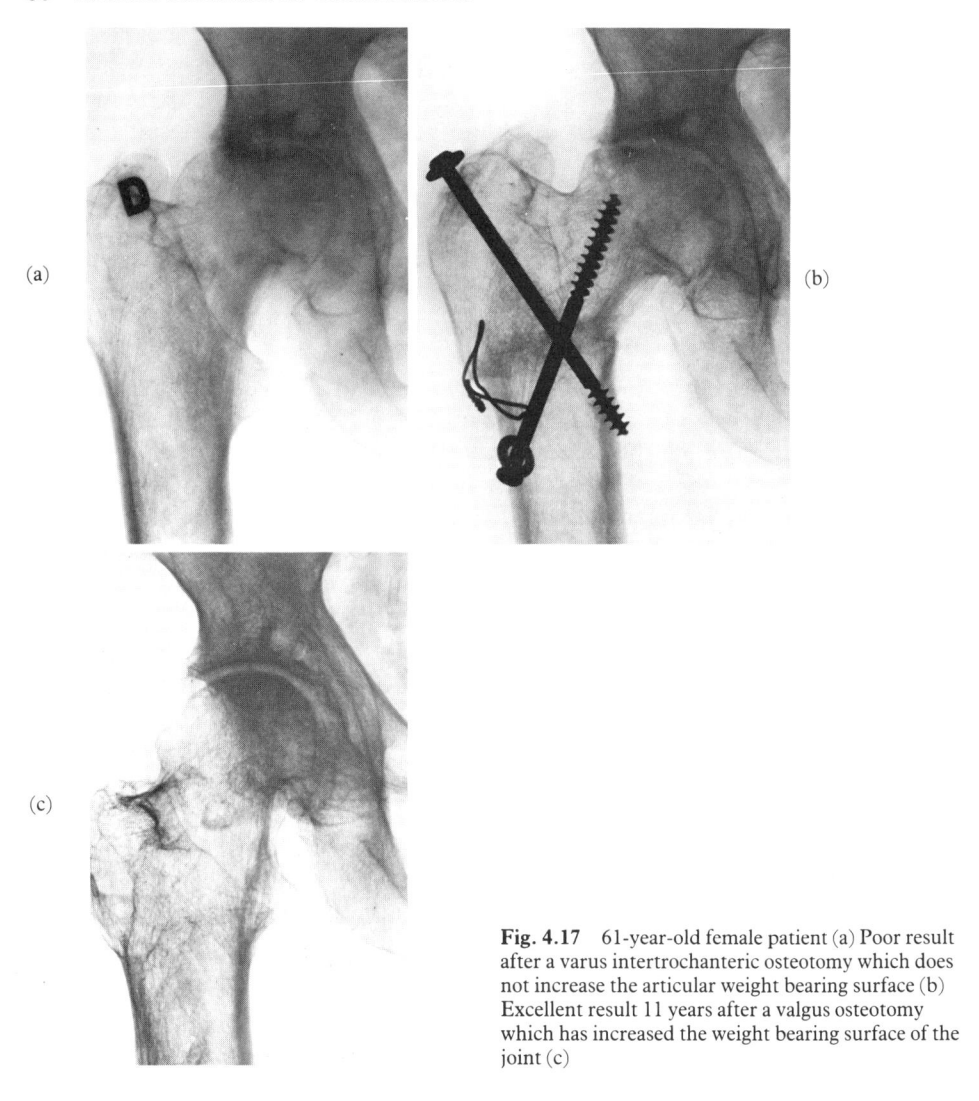

(a)

(b)

(c)

Fig. 4.17 61-year-old female patient (a) Poor result after a varus intertrochanteric osteotomy which does not increase the articular weight bearing surface (b) Excellent result 11 years after a valgus osteotomy which has increased the weight bearing surface of the joint (c)

cannot be invoked as causing the good result in the right hip. Here, only a change in mechanics with an increase of the weight bearing surface of the joint, can be implicated.

LATERAL DISPLACEMENT OF THE GREATER TROCHANTER (Maquet, 1976)

If the articular surfaces are congruent, lateral displacement of the greater trochanter will lengthen the lever arm h of the abductor muscles M and by changing the direction of force M, will displace the resultant R medially into the acetabulum (Fig. 19). The operation thus decreases the load R and distributes it over a larger weight bearing area as does a Pauwels I osteotomy. We combine it with a tenotomy of the adductors and

TREATMENT OF OSTEOARTHRITIS OF THE HIP   81

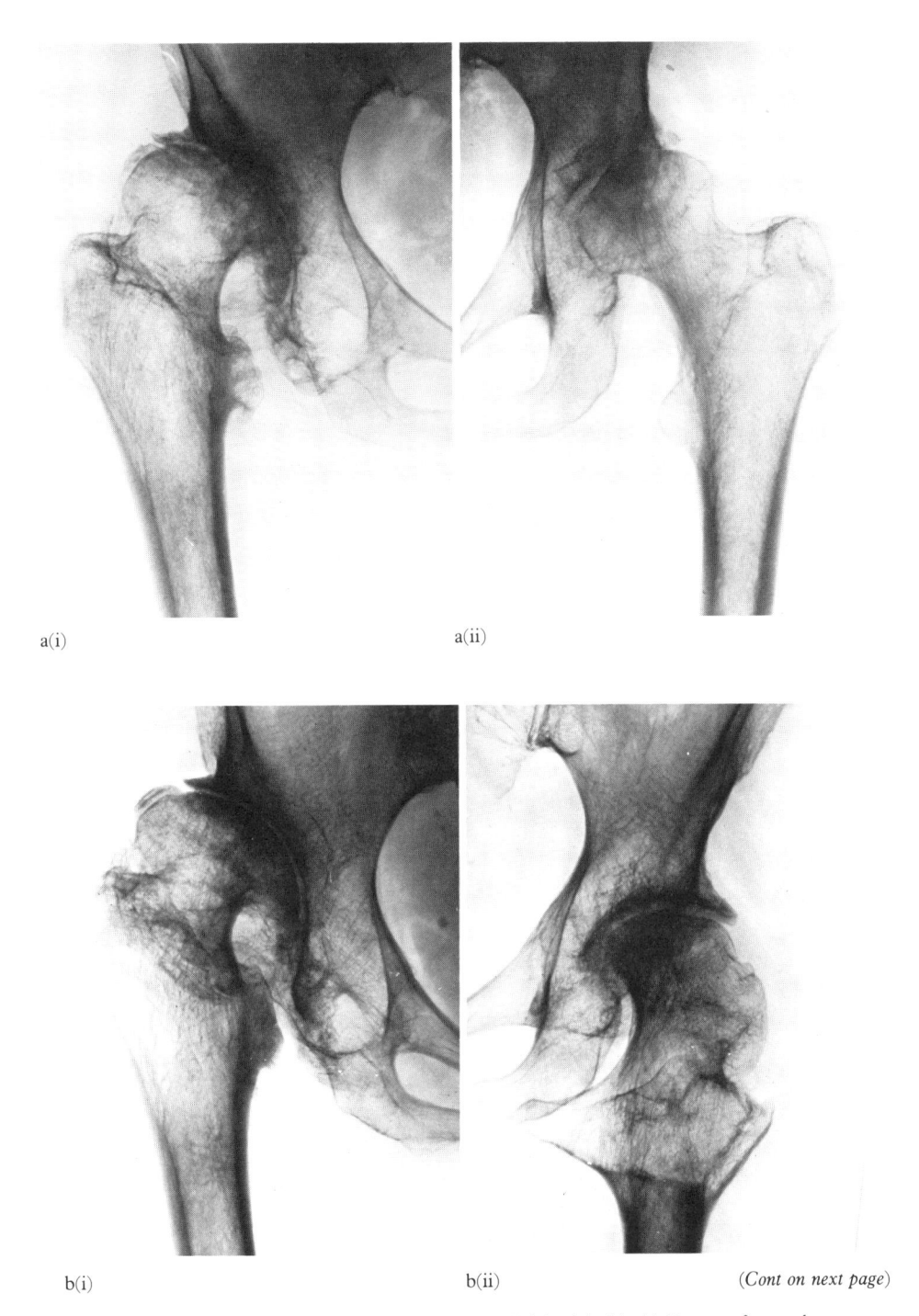

a(i)   a(ii)

b(i)   b(ii)   (Cont on next page)

Fig. 4.18 57-year-old female patient with bilateral osteoarthritis of the hip (a) 11 years after a valgus osteotomy and a shortening of the femur on the longer side (b) Turning the pelvis around the opposite femoral head is equivalent to a valgus osteotomy (c)

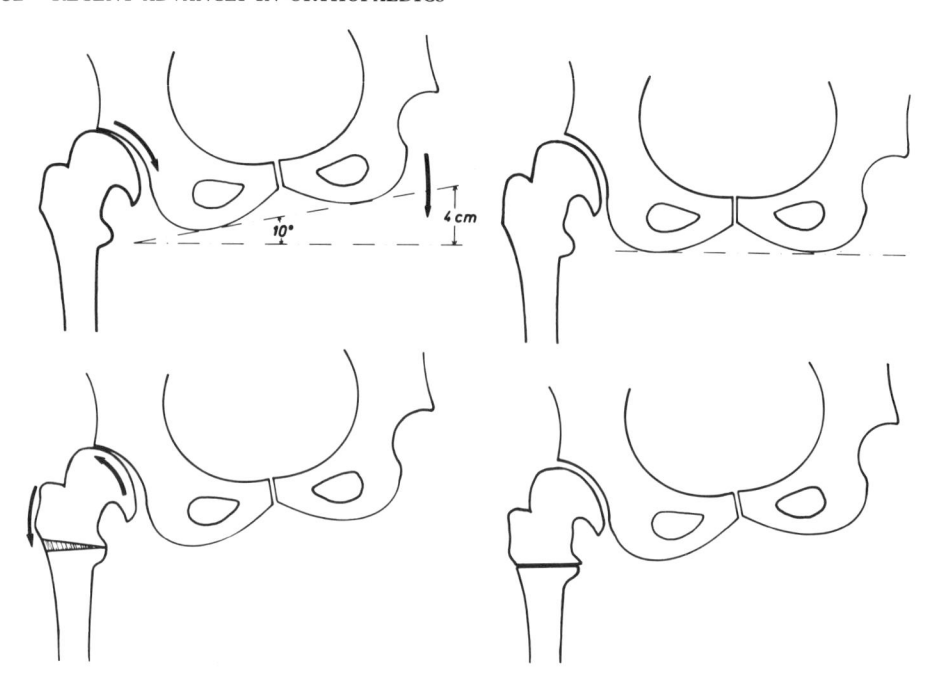

Fig. 4.18(c) (*cont*)

ilio-psoas. The tenotomy of the adductors and of the ilio-psoas is carried out through a 4 to 5 cm longitudinal incision along the tendon of adductor longus, the patient lying supine. The patient is then turned into the prone position. The upper end of the femur is approached, through a postero-lateral incision. The femoral shaft is split longitudinally for a distance of 12 cm from a distal postero-anterior drill hole at the junction of the lateral 1/4 and medial 3/4 of its transverse diameter, to the medial aspect of the greater trochanter. The split portion of the femur is displaced laterally and fixed in this position by inserting an iliac graft, on edge, between the greater trochanter and the neck of the femur. The junction of the split portion and the shaft of the femur usually breaks. A screw is used to fix the fragments. Two transverse K wires can be inserted through the two femoral fragments and the graft. The patient is encouraged and helped to get up and walk from the second day. Crutches are advised as after the Pauwels' osteotomies.

We would recommend this lateral displacement of the greater trochanter in congruent hips with a relatively high greater trochanter. A dense triangle at the edge of the socket does not constitute a contra-indication since the procedure is aimed at enlarging the weight bearing surface of the joint.

A 56-year-old female patient (Fig. 4.20) developed severe osteoarthritis. A dense triangle was present at the edge of the acetabulum and the joint space had disappeared (Fig. 4.20a). Six years after a 2.5 cm lateral displacement of the greater trochanter combined with a tenotomy of the adductors and ilio-psoas, the dense triangle is replaced by a thin ribbon of sclerotic bone of even thickness throughout and a wide joint space has developed (Fig. 4.20b). The clinical result is excellent.

Out of 23 hips which had undergone lateral displacement of the greater trochanter

TREATMENT OF OSTEOARTHRITIS OF THE HIP 83

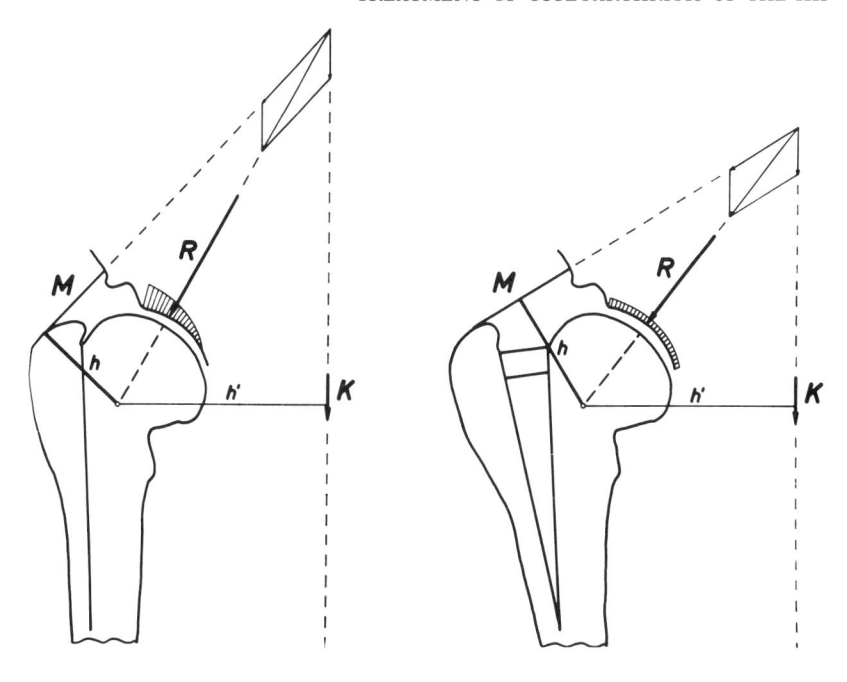

Fig. 4.19 Lateral displacement of the greater trochanter; if the joint surfaces are congruent, this reduces the load transmitted and increases the weight bearing surface of the joint. (Maquet, 1976)

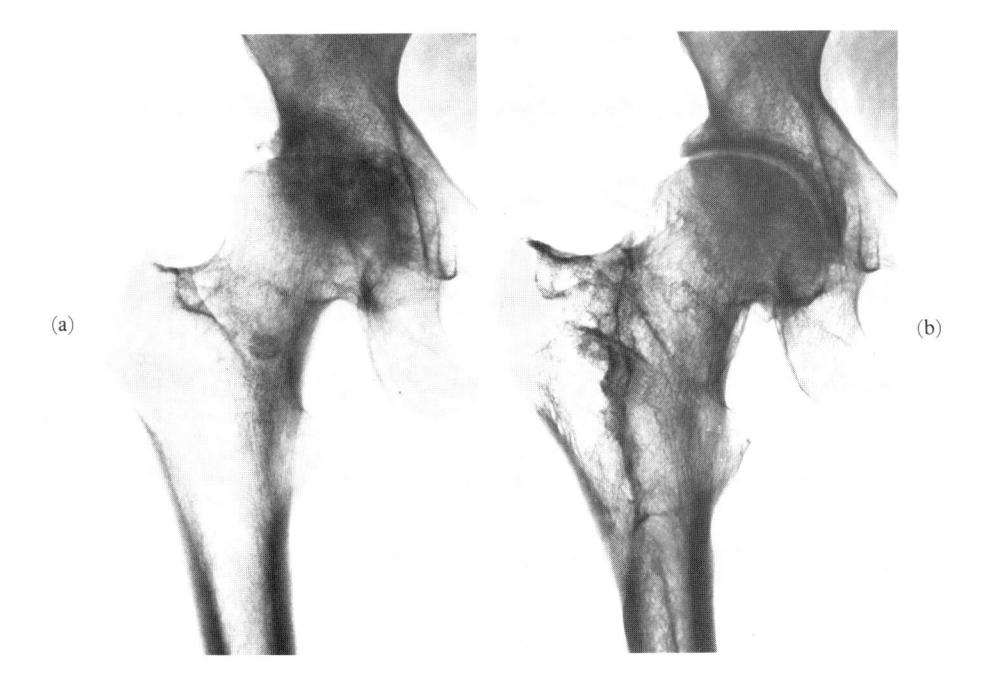

(a)

(b)

Fig. 4.20 56-year-old patient before (a) and six years after a lateral displacement of the greater trochanter + tenotomy (b)

21 have been reviewed with a minimum follow-up of one year and a maximum of six years. The pain relief was spectacular, the range of movement and the gait considerably improved. Three parameters were assessed according to Merle d'Aubigné (1970). Absence of pain, full range of movement and normal gait were each rated six. A normal hip is thus rated 6+6+6 or 18. At the other end, 0 means permanent pain, a stiff hip in bad position and inability to walk. The other figures describe intermediary states.

The average rating of the 21 hips was 10.1 before operation. It had become 17 at follow-up. The hips had improved by 2 to 10 points with an average improvement of 6.1 points. On the X-rays the subchondral sclerosis became normal in most patients and the joint space widened.

The same operation has also been carried out with success for hips in which a previous intertrochanteric osteotomy had provided congruence of the joint surfaces but an unsatisfactory overall result. Lateral displacement of the greater trochanter improved these hips dramatically.

CONCLUSION

All the aforementioned operations have one common denominator: they aim at decreasing the joint pressure sufficiently to make it tolerable for the tissues. They certainly do not constitute a standard method of treatment. They require careful thought on the part of the surgeon. Their results depend on:
1. a good appraisal of the mechanical situation of the affected hip. Special X-rays, with the beam centred on the joint, in different positions of the latter, are also necessary;
2. a precise pre-operative planning on paper, using an exact tracing of the X-rays;
3. an accurate operative procedure realising the preoperative drawing, considerably helped by adequate instruments and by an image intensifier. X-rays during the operation are required in order to check the accuracy of the procedure;
4. a careful postoperative follow-up avoiding overstressing of the joint.

However, if the indications are correct and if these prerequisites are met, the results, even in very severe cases, appear amazingly good and long lasting, equivalent to true biological healing.

REFERENCES

Herbert J J 1950 Chirurgie et orthopédie du rhumatisme. Masson, Paris
Maquet P 1966 Ostéotomie de McMurray. Etude biomécanique. Revue de chirurgie orthopédique 52: 525–532
Maquet P 1971a Le coapteur à griffes pour ostéotomie inter-trochantérienne. Acta orthopaedia belgica 37: 495–504
Maquet P 1971b Le principe de Pauwels dans le traitement de la coxarthrose. Congrès Franco- Hellénique d'orthopédie. 1970 Athènes p 365–368
Maquet P 1975 Biomécanique de la hanche et traitement chirurgical conservateur de la coxarthrose. Cahiers d'enseignement de la SOFCOT. Expansion Scientifique Française, Paris
Maquet P 1976 Réduction de la pression articulaire de la hanche par latéralisation chirurgicale du grand trochanter. Acta orthopaedica belgica 42: 266–271
Maquet P 1977 Ostéotomie intertrochantérienne valgisante (Pauwels II). Techniques orthopédiques. Fiche 11/1. Expansion Scientifique Française, Paris

Maquet P, Vu Anh T 1981 On the forces exerted on the hip during gait, Archives of Orthopaedic Traumatic Surgery 99: 53–58

Merle d'Aubigné R 1970 Cotation chiffrée de la fonction de la hanche, Revue de chirurgie orthopédique 56: 481–486

Mc Murray T P 1935 Osteoarthritis of the hip joint. British Journal of Surgery 22: 716–727

Mc Murray T P 1939 Osteoarthritis of the hip joint, Journal of Bone and Joint Surgery XXI: 1–11

Nissen K I 1960 The arrest of early primary osteoarthritis of the hip by osteotomy, Journal of Bone and Joint Surgery 42.B: 423–424

Pauwels F 1959 Directives nouvelles pour le traitement chirurgical de la coxarthrose, Revue de chirurgie orthopédique 45: 681–702

Pauwels F 1973 Atlas zur Biomechanik der gesunden und kranken Hüfte, Springer, Berlin, Heidelberg, New York

Radin E L, Maquet P, Parker H 1975 Rationale and indications for the 'Hanging hip' procedure, Clinical orthopaedics and related research, 112: 221–230

Voss C 1956 Die temporäne Hangenhüfte Münchener medizinische Wochenschrift 98: 1

Watillon M, Hoet F, Maquet P 1978 Analyse de 804 cas d'ostéotomies, Acta orthopaedica belgica 44: 248–279

PLATE SECTION

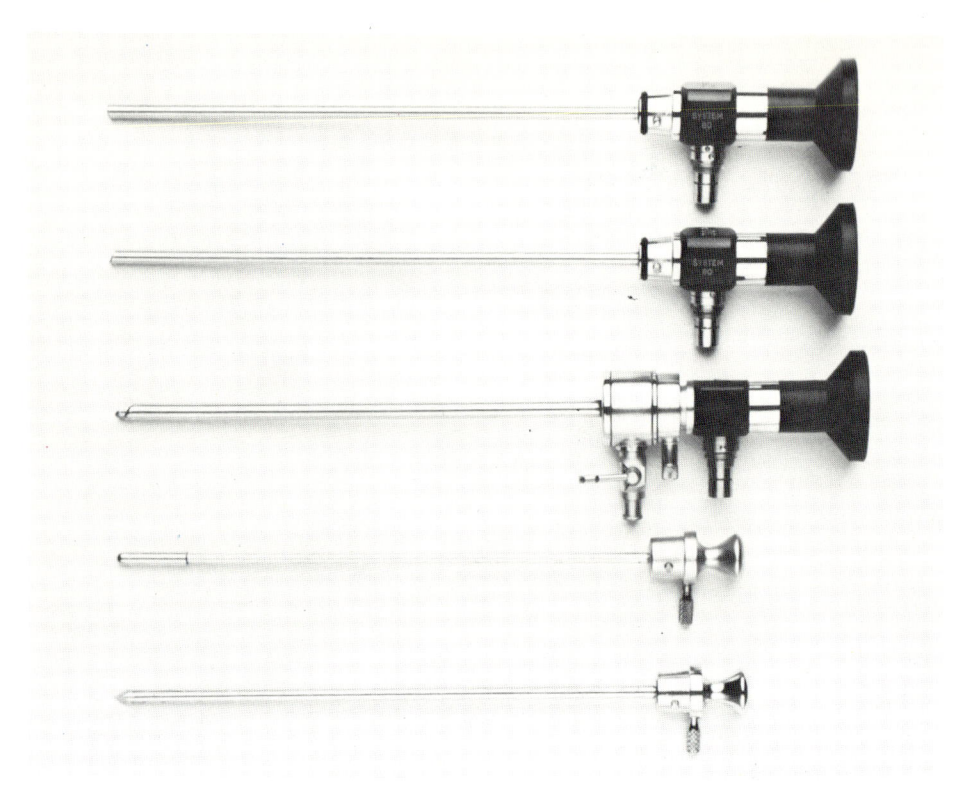

Plate 5.1 A set of arthroscopes. From above downwards; 0° telescope, 30° telescope, 70° telescope in sheath, blunt obturator and sharp trochar.

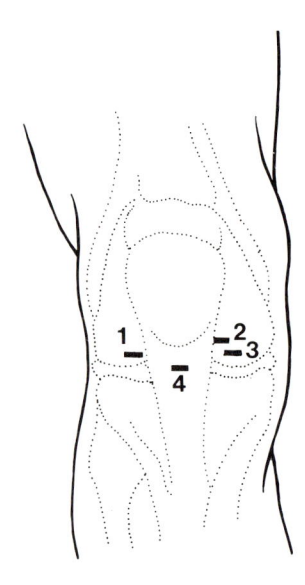

Plate 5.2 Site of insertion of the arthroscope. (1) Antero-lateral approach. (2) Antero-medial approach. (3) Lower and more medial point of insertion for approaching the posterior horn of the medial meniscus with operating instruments. (4) Central approach.

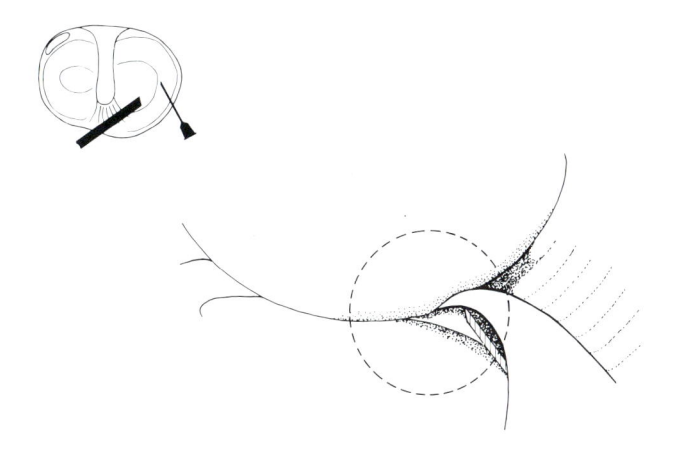

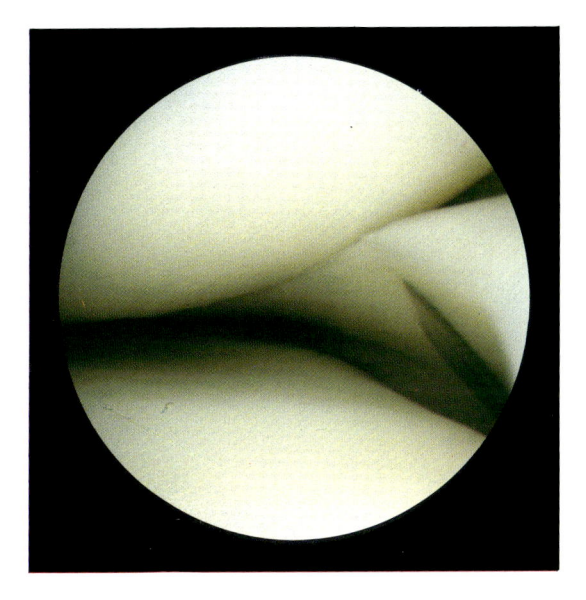

Plate 5.3 Lifting the medial meniscus with a percutaneous joint line needle to expose its under-surface and the inferior coronary ligament.

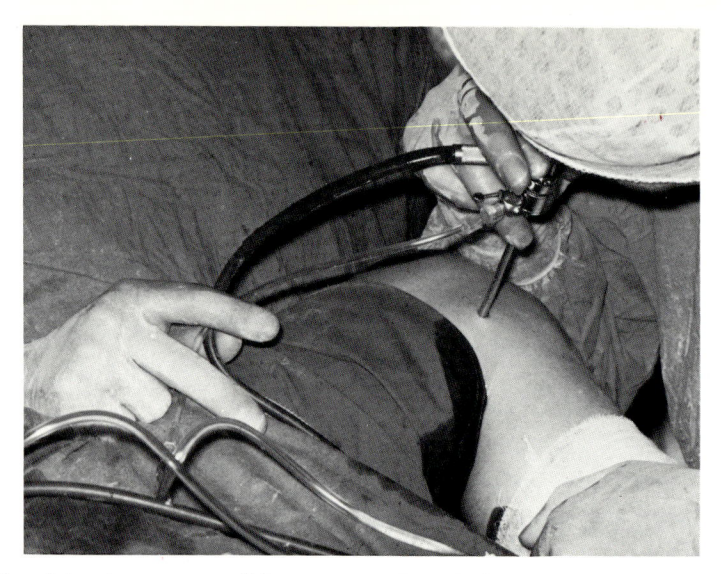

Plate 5.4 Examining the postero-medial compartment from the postero-medial approach.

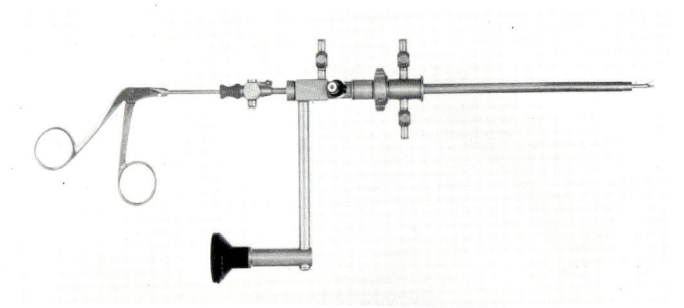

Plate 5.5 The Wolf operating arthroscope with the scissors in the instrument channel.

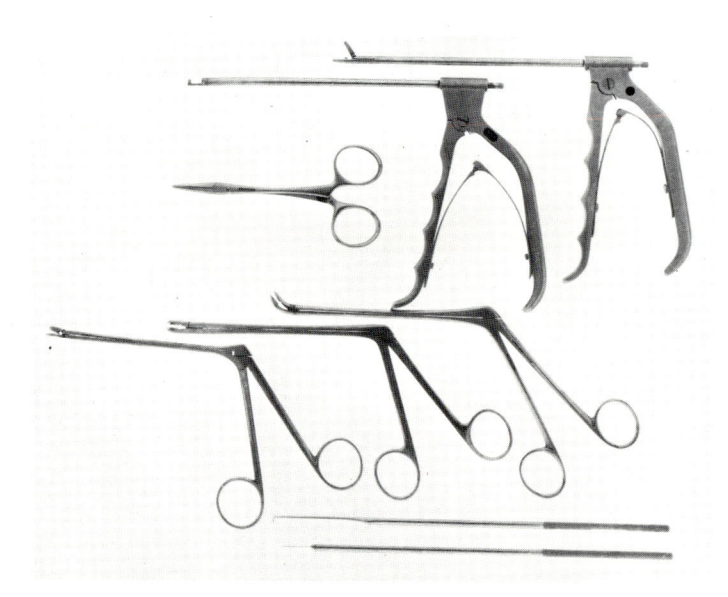

Plate 5.6 Basic set of simple instruments for the double puncture technique. From above downwards; arthroscopic scissors, guillotine, artery forceps with screw joint, Northfield's curved pituitary rongeurs, Cushing's straight pituitary rongeurs with 4 mm bite, punch forceps, hook and knife.

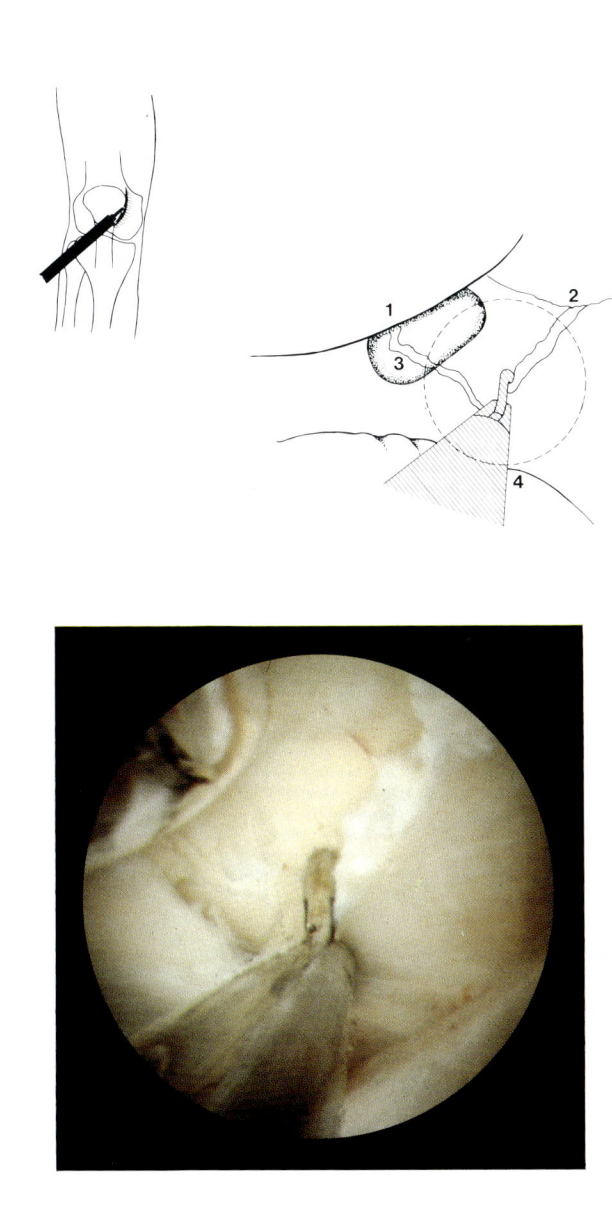

Plate 5.7 Excision of the medial synovial shelf using an operating arthroscope, (1) patella, (2) cut edge of synovium, (3) air bubble, (4) anterior surface of femur.

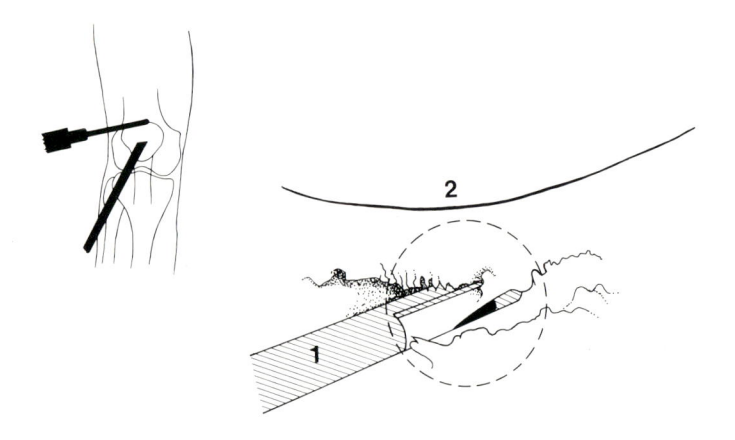

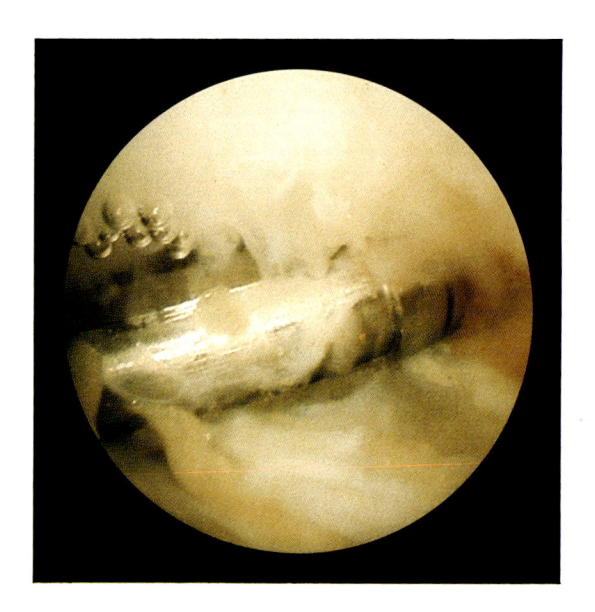

Plate 5.8 Performing a synovectomy using a powered shaver (1), patella (2).

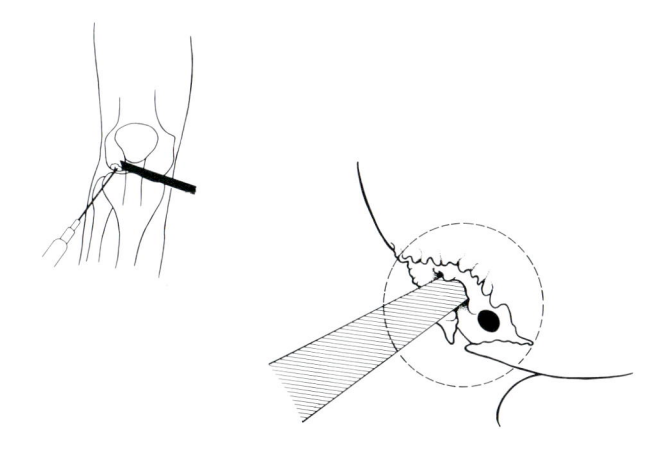

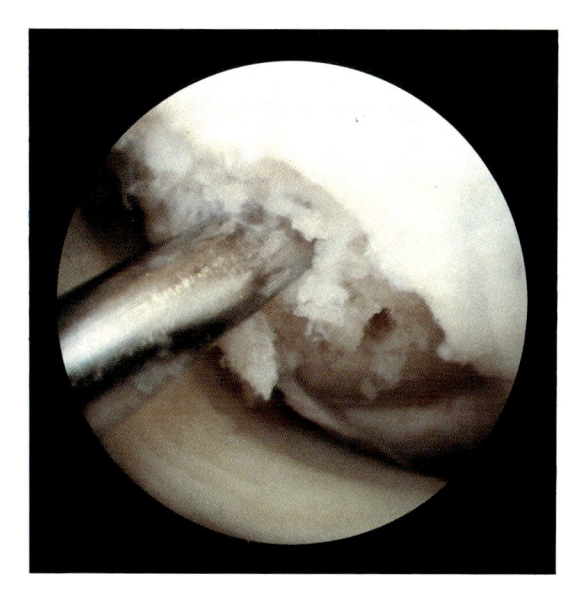

Plate 5.11 Drilling the subchondral bed of a full thickness chondral fracture of the lateral femoral condyle with a thick Kirschner wire.

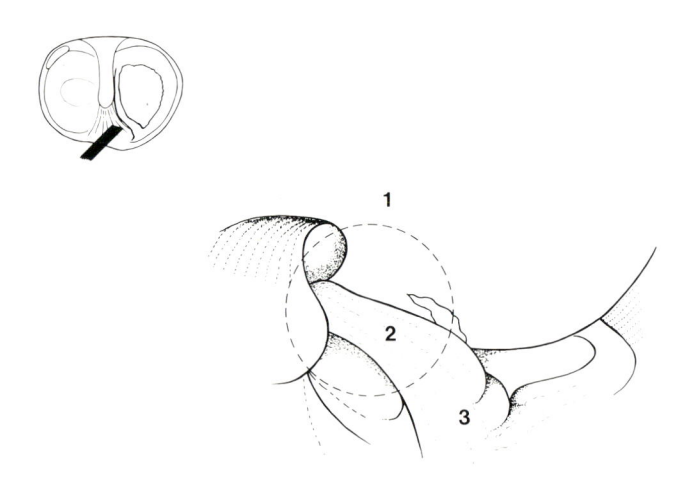

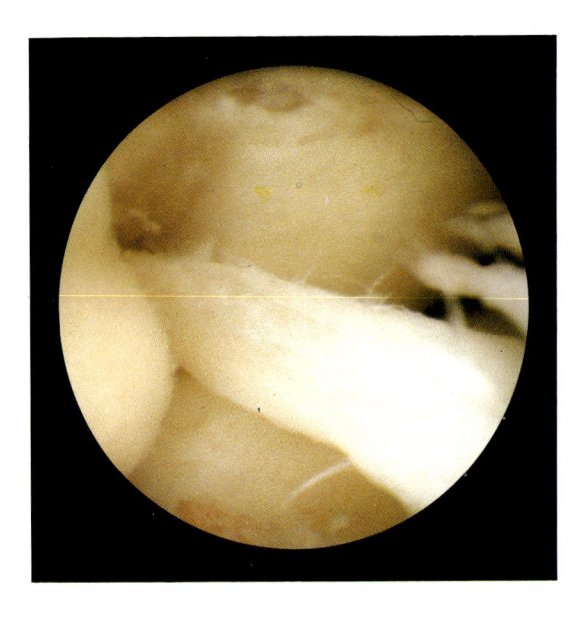

Plate 5.12 A complete (type 1) bucket handle tear of the medial meniscus (2) lying locked in the intercondylar notch beneath the medial femoral condyle (1). The anterior attachment of the fragment (3) is at the anterior horn of the medial meniscus.

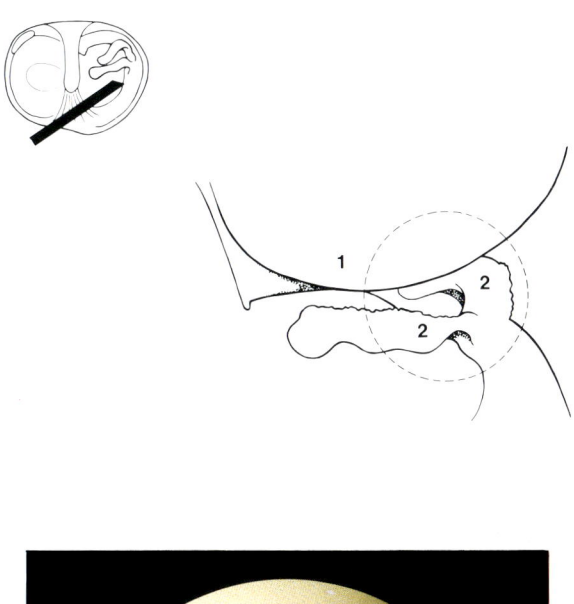

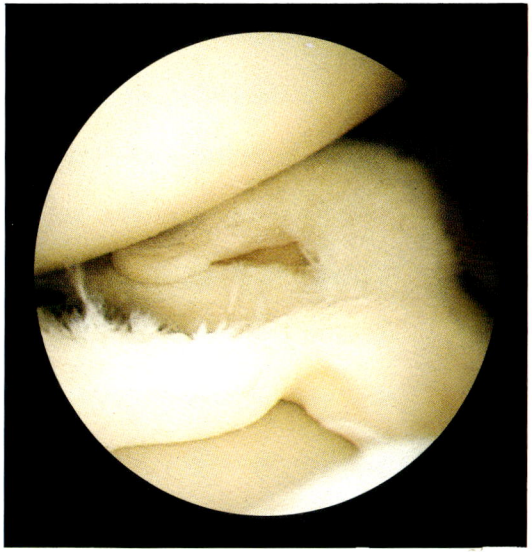

Plate 5.13 Two detached bucket handle fragments of medial meniscus (2) lying in the medial compartment beneath the medial femoral condyle.

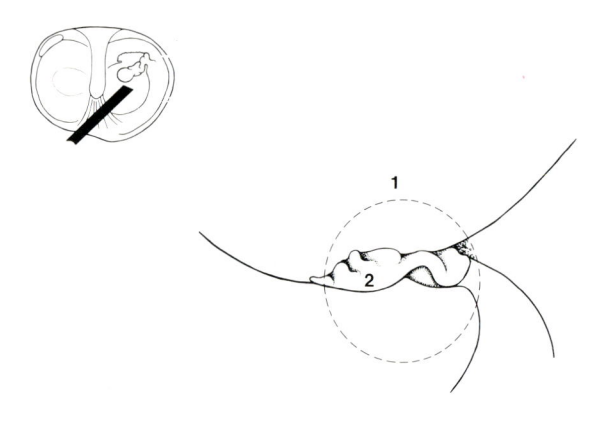

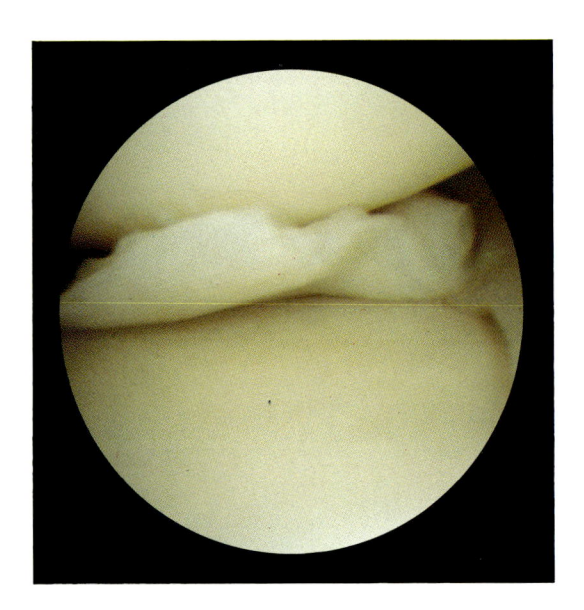

Plate 5.14 A flap of medial meniscus (2) manipulated from beneath the medial femoral condyle (1) by a valgus and external rotation force.

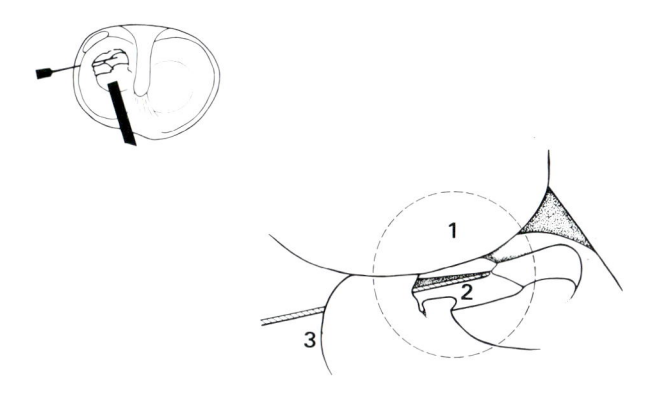

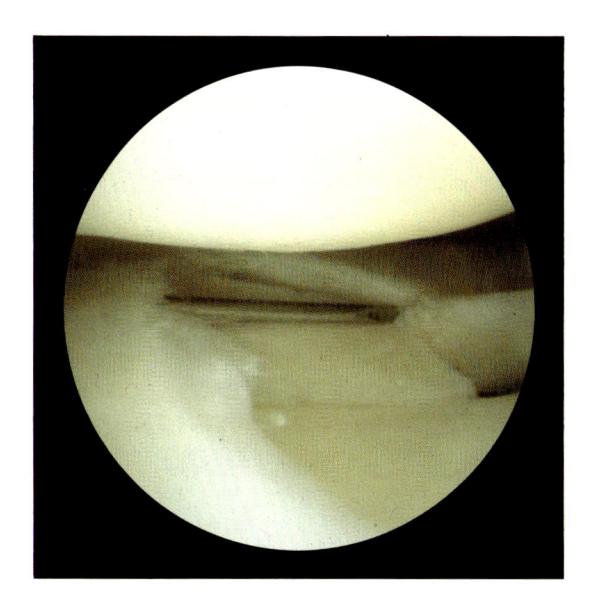

Plate 5.15 A bucket handle fragment of the lateral meniscus ruptured at its centre (2) lying beneath the lateral femoral condyle (1) and probed with a percutaneous needle (3).

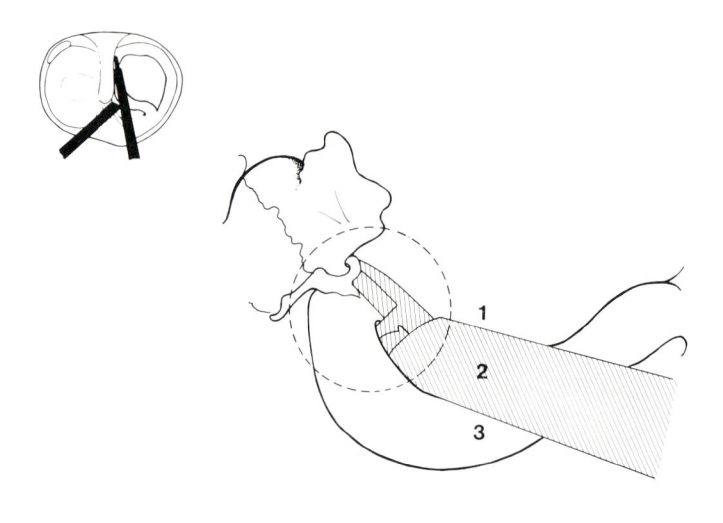

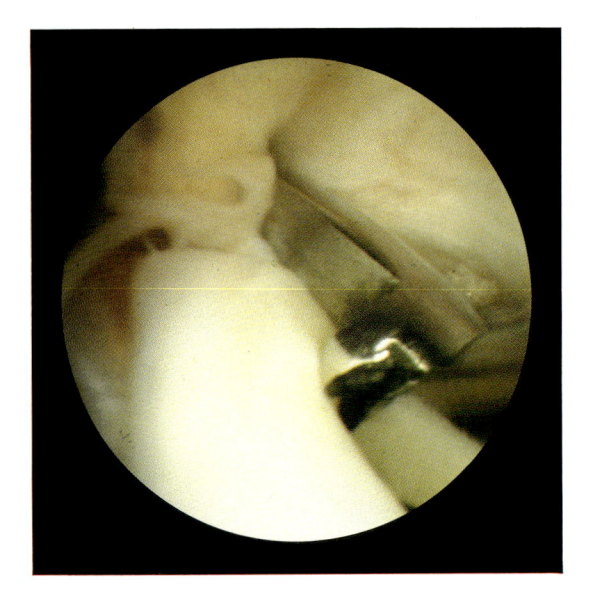

Plate 5.16 A locked incomplete (type 2) bucket handle fragment of medial meniscus being divided at its posterior attachment using arthroscopic scissors (2)–(1) medial femoral condyle.

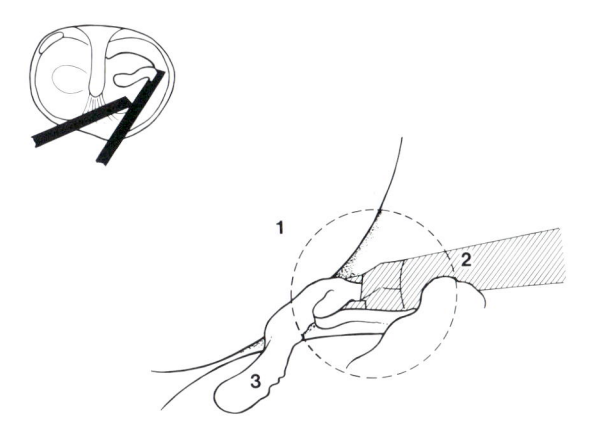

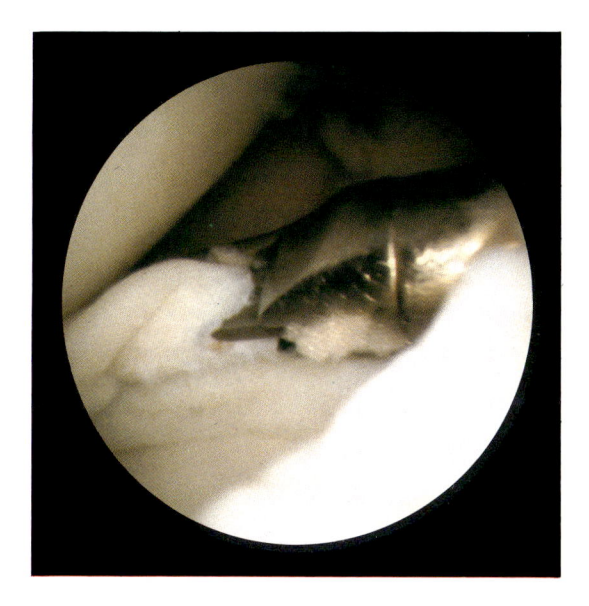

Plate 5.17 A detached bucket handle fragment of medial meniscus (3) is divided with the guillotine (2) as it lies beneath the medial femoral condyle (1).

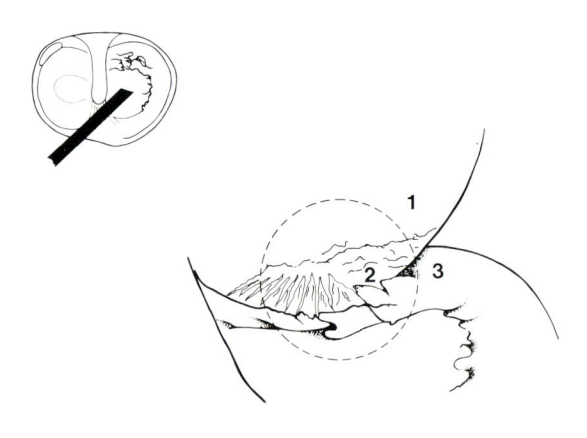

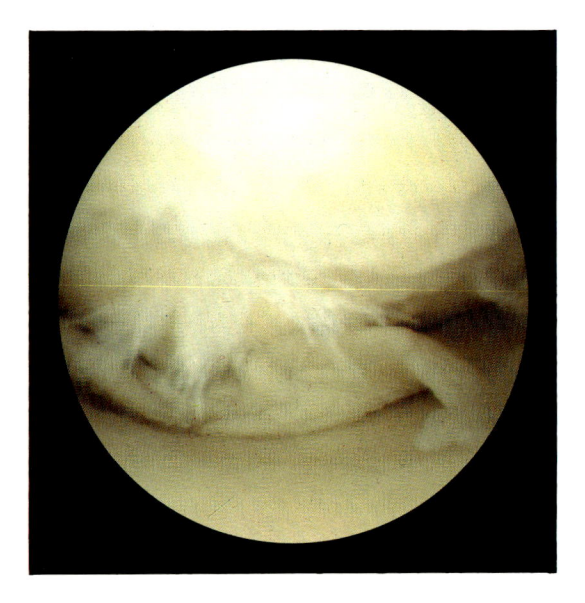

Plate 5.18 A degenerate tear of the posterior horn of the medial meniscus (3) lying beneath an area of degenerate articular cartilage (2) on the under-surface of the medial femoral condyle (1).

Acknowledgment
All Figures from Dandy, D. J. Arthroscopic surgery of the knee. Churchill Livingstone, Edinburgh

5. Arthroscopy and arthroscopic surgery of the knee

D. J. Dandy

History

Arthroscopy was first performed by K. Takagi in Tokyo in 1918 (Takagi, 1933) and was later practised widely in North America and Europe. In 1925, Kreuscher published a paper describing the value of arthroscopy in the diagnosis of meniscus lesions and in 1926 the possibility of performing arthroscopic surgery of the knee was clearly foreseen and described by Geist (Geist, 1926). In the 1930s, Burman and others (Burman, 1931) described the use of the arthroscope in the wrist, shoulder, ankle and elbow, as well as the knee so that, with a history of over 60 years, arthroscopy and arthroscopic surgery can probably claim to be the longest established 'recent advance' in modern orthopaedic surgery.

In the late 1930s, arthroscopy was on the verge of becoming an accepted diagnostic technique but the upheaval of the Second World War brought further progress to a halt. At the conclusion of the war, Masaki Watanabe carried on the work of Takagi in Tokyo and in 1960 became the first surgeon to perform an arthroscopic meniscectomy. At this stage, diagnostic arthroscopy was little known outside Japan until, after working with Watanabe in Tokyo, the technique was brought back to North America by Dr R. W. Jackson of Toronto in 1965. The technique of arthroscopy has since spread to most western countries.

Although arthroscopy for diagnostic purposes slowly gained acceptance, progress was slow largely because the advantages — more accurate diagnosis and more precise surgery — were difficult to measure and did not always seem to justify the tedium and inconvenience of learning a new and difficult technique. It was not until arthroscopic surgery became a reality and patients discovered that they could leave hospital the day after meniscectomy without the need for crutches or plaster immobilisation and return to work within a week, that arthroscopy and arthroscopic surgery gained general acceptance.

In America, the first course on arthroscopic surgery was held in Maine in 1977, and courses on the subject are now so popular in the United States that they are attended by many hundreds of surgeons each year. In Europe, the first course on arthroscopy was held in Nijmegen in 1976 to be followed by others in Scandinavia, and in England in 1978. Today, although there are still a few surgeons who regard arthroscopic surgery as a clinical irrelevance that will not stand the test of time, the principal problem now facing arthroscopic surgery is not that of making the advantages of the technique more widely known, but one of education to ensure that the procedure is performed correctly and safely.

Arthroscopy differs radically from other techniques and involves the surgeon becoming familiar with endoscopes and other instruments that do not normally fall within the province of orthopaedic surgery. To practise the technique safely and confidently requires more patience, precision and meticulous attention to detail than other types of orthopaedic surgery, and is only possible if the surgeon has a firm grasp of the basic techniques of diagnostic arthroscopy.

DIAGNOSTIC ARTHROSCOPY

An arthroscope is an endoscope of similar design to a cystoscope. Because the space between the synovium and the underlying bone is so narrow that a wide angle of vision is an advantage, the standard diagnostic arthroscope has an angle of vision of 70° in saline, instead of the 55° of most other endoscopes (Plate 5.1). The field of vision is increased using a 30° fore-oblique telescope, which can be spun about its long axis to 'sweep' a larger area of the knee. A 0° telescope is also available and is helpful in the learning stages when orientation is difficult within the knee, and a 70° telescope may sometimes be helpful for examining the posterior recesses of the joint.

The telescope of the diagnostic arthroscope also carries a glass fibre light guide, and is mounted in a stout sheath a little larger than the telescope to leave a space for saline to flow along the sheath and leave at its tip. The sheath is as smooth as possible so that accidental damage to intra-articular structures is kept to a minimum. The arthroscope is connected to a light source by a glass fibre or liquid light guide, and has a stop cock for controlling the flow of irrigation fluid.

Sterilisation
The telescope can be sterilised effectively by immersion for 10 minutes in activated glutaraldehyde solution, or by gas sterilisation. Repeated autoclaving will damage most arthroscopes beyond repair, but some designs are now able to withstand repeated sterilisation in a high-pressure steam autoclave.

Anaesthesia
General anaesthesia is preferred by most arthroscopists but local or spinal anaesthesia is also perfectly practicable. General anaesthesia has the advantage that the patient is oblivious to events in the operating theatre, which may be an advantage when the surgeon is learning the procedure. Local anaesthetic has the additional disadvantage that the use of a tourniquet is difficult and the manipulation of the leg may be painful, but spinal anaesthesia is a practicable alternative.

Tourniquet
A pneumatic tourniquet applied to the thigh reduces the amount of bleeding and improves visibility. Exsanguination of the leg is not only unnecessary but a positive disadvantage because it blanches the synovium and makes it difficult to assess the degree of vascularity of the synovium, and even to distinguish synovium from meniscus. Elevation of the leg for a few minutes before inflation of the tourniquet is quite sufficient, and does not interfere with the appearance of the synovium.

Preparation of the leg
Although diagnostic arthroscopy almost always results in some loss of sterility through contact with the eye and eyepiece of the arthroscope, the procedure should always start as a sterile procedure, and the limb should be properly draped with full sterile precautions in a standard operating theatre. The details of draping and other

points of technique are described more fully elsewhere (Dandy, 1981; Jackson & Dandy, 1976; O'Connor, 1979).

Irrigation
The joint cannot be examined unless the synovial cavity is first distended. Saline is the usual medium, but carbon dioxide is preferred in some centres. If saline is used, the joint is distended by placing a needle in the suprapatellar pouch and injecting between 20 and 60 mils of saline. Placement of the needle outside the synovial cavity is surprisingly easy, and makes the operation difficult or impossible. The needle used to distend the knee can be left in the joint and used as an exit channel for the irrigation fluid, but a balance must be struck between the fluid entering the knee through the arthroscope — which depends on the head of saline and the size of the saline channel within the arthroscope sheath — and the rate of outflow, which depends largely on the diameter of the outflow needle. The balance between saline inflow and outflow is one of the details of arthroscopic technique essential for success.

Insertion of the arthroscope
The point of insertion of the arthroscope is critical, and failure to select the correct site is probably the commonest single technical error (Plate 5.2). Although several approaches can be used for routine examination, the antero-lateral approach is most generally used. Insertion of the arthroscope either too high or too low will make visualisation of the knee very difficult indeed.

The central insertion, in the middle of the knee rather than the middle of the patellar tendon, is a good alternative to the anterolateral approach but must also be made carefully and in the correct position (Gillquist & Hagberg, 1976). The notion that the point of insertion should be selected according to the most likely clinical diagnosis is incorrect. If for example, the lateral meniscus is suspected, the arthroscope should still be inserted from the antero-lateral approach because the lateral, as well as the medial, meniscus is seen better from this approach than the anteromedial. In the learning stages, it is advisable to choose one approach and become familiar with it before advancing to others rather than to chop and change between a number of ill-chosen insertions none of which is performed correctly.

Examination of the knee
With the arthroscope in position, the joint can be examined systematically and in an orderly fashion. Although each surgeon will find his own technique, the most popular sequence for examining the knee is to begin in the suprapatellar pouch, including the recess beyond the plica suprapatellaris medialis, the undersurface of the patella, and the medial synovial shelf, taking note of the appearance of the synovium.

The medial compartment can then be entered, the medial meniscus examined, and the surface of the medial femoral condyle inspected. The whole length of the free margin of the meniscus should be clearly seen. The arthroscope is next brought to the intercondylar notch, and the anterior cruciate ligament examined from femoral attachment to the tibial insertion. The arthroscope can then be slipped into the lateral compartment so that the lateral meniscus and condyle can be examined. If the arthroscope is placed in the lateral gutter, the lateral menisco-synovial junction and the popliteus tendon can be seen and the popliteus tunnel entered.

To complete the 'circuit' of the knee described above, the leg must be manipulated about the arthroscope as the arthroscope is manipulated in the knee. Valgus, varus and rotational stresses are applied as appropriate but the exact manipulations necessary to open up the various compartments are complex, and beyond the scope of this chapter.

The postero-medial and postero-lateral compartments of the knee can be entered through the intercondylar notch in almost every patient provided that the arthroscope has been inserted correctly and the correct valgus and external rotational force is applied. With the arthroscope in the medial compartment, the postero-medial recess, the posterior menisco-synovial attachment and the back of the femoral condyle and the superior synovial reflection of the synovium frm the femur can be seen clearly.

When the basic examination has been completed, suspicious areas can be examined in greater detail with the help of probing hooks and percutaneous needles, or by insertion of the arthroscope from other approaches if desired (Plate 5.3).

Different approaches

If the postero-medial compartment cannot be entered, an antero-medial insertion will probably make entrance to this part of the joint more straightforward. If entry is still not possible and there is a real possibility of an abnormality in this area, the compartment can be entered directly from the postero-medial approach (Plate 5.4).

A lateral suprapatellar or lateral mid-patellar approach gives a clear view of the undersurface of the patella and the fatpad from above, as well as the anterior horns of the menisci. Although routine examination of the knee from additional approaches is unnecessarily traumatic, discriminating use of second or even third incisions is often helpful.

Probing hook and percutaneous needle

If a lesion — for example, a tear of the medial meniscus — is suspected on clinical grounds but cannot be seen at arthroscopy, a hook can be passed from the antero-medial approach and used to lift or pull the meniscus to examine its undersurface and confirm the integrity or otherwise of the menisco-synovial junction. Alternatively, an intravenous needle can be passed through the skin over the medial meniscus to lift it so that its undersurface is revealed. Correct placement of the hook or needle is essential for success.

Recording of information

At the conclusion of the examination, a full record of the state of all structures in the knee should be made with particular emphasis on the structures that were considered likely to be responsible for the patient's symptoms. All too often, the notes of arthroscopy include the phrase 'meniscus not seen'. While such honesty is admirable and far preferable to an imaginary account of what the surgeon feels he ought to have seen, to admit that the menisci were not visualised is an admission of technical inadequacy.

Aftercare

At the conclusion of the examination, the tourniquet should be released, the joint irrigated thoroughly, and the wound closed with one stitch. Stitches should be placed deeply to control bleeding in the subcutaneous layers.

A firm wool and crepe dressing is then applied and quadriceps exercises instituted at once. Although patients are usually fit to return home on the day of operation, it is preferable to delay discharge until the following day to ensure that the patient can walk comfortably and easily, and that no haemarthrosis has developed.

ARTHROSCOPIC SURGERY

Before embarking on arthroscopic surgery, the surgeon should be entirely familiar with diagnostic arthroscopy, including the use of the different approaches described above and the probing hook. To attempt arthroscopic surgery without such skills is not only unwise but dangerous and can lead to difficulties for both the patient and the surgeon.

Equipment

The workhorse of arthroscopic surgery is the 5 mm 30° fore-oblique arthroscope but the 70° telescope is occasionally useful, as, for example, when operating in the postero-medial or posterolateral compartment. The 0° telescope is helpful in the learning stages, but should be quickly discarded as the surgeon gains competence and familiarity with the technique.

Operating arthroscopes

The operating arthroscope, in which the sheath of the instrument carries channels for the operating instrument as well as the telescope, light fibre guide and saline channel, makes it possible to cut or grasp objects directly in front of the telescope (Plate 5.5). The use of the operating arthroscope is unfortunately somewhat limited because it is not possible to cut objects from the side unless the structure to be cut is first grasped with another instrument applied through a second incision.

Apart from the limitation imposed by the inability to move the instruments in any direction except parallel to the telescope, the cutting instruments must also be smaller, and therefore weaker, than instruments inserted through a second incision. The telescope in existing models is narrower than the standard diagnostic arthroscope, which restricts the angle of vision and therefore the field of view quite markedly, making orientation more difficult. In short, the present operating arthroscopes are bulky, carry weak instruments that move in one line only, and have a narrow field of vision that makes them difficult to use. Although there is a definite place for the operating arthroscope, it is by no means an essential instrument. To suppose that the purchase of an operating arthroscope is all that is required to perform operative arthroscopy is a depressingly common error.

Powered instruments

Powered instruments, like operating arthroscopes, are occasionally useful but are by no means essential items of equipment. Powered shavers, drills and burrs are available but achieve little that is not accomplished almost as easily with simple hand instruments. The shaver is helpful when levelling an area of chondromalacia patellae and when performing a partial synovectomy, but with these notable exceptions, hand instruments are preferable.

Cutting instruments
A basic set of instruments for arthroscopic surgery should include a blunt probing hook, a straight knife, basket or punch forceps, large and small rongeurs, guillotine, scissors and grasping forceps (Plate 5.6). The instruments should be stoutly constructed to minimise the risk of fracture within the knee and should have smooth surfaces to avoid unnecessary damage to the articular surface.

Most instrument companies now produce a set of such instruments but purchasers should be particularly careful to avoid instruments originally designed for some other purpose, such as laparoscopy, which are seldom suitable for work within the knee.

Technique
The most generally useful technique is the double puncture technique, in which instruments are inserted through a second channel and manipulated under the control of the 30° fore-oblique diagnostic arthroscope. Provided the instruments have been inserted at the point appropriate for the lesion to be treated, the instruments can be brought to bear upon the lesion without difficulty.

There are times, for example when removing a long meniscal flap, when it is helpful to apply traction to the lesion so that it can be cut at its base with a second instrument. This can be achieved either by inserting a grasping instrument through a third channel — the triple puncture technique — or by using the operating arthroscope. The triple puncture technique adds to the difficulties of operating by making it necessary to insert three instruments (cutting instruments, grasping forceps and arthroscope) at precisely determined points and manipulate them in a coordinated fashion. The help of an assistant is required, but unless the assistant can observe the operation with the help of an endoscopic television monitor, he will be unable to appreciate the progress of the operation.

The 'single puncture technique' using the operating arthroscope is subject to the limitations already mentioned, but it is nevertheless a valuable technique. The double, triple and single puncture techniques are not in competition with each other but are complementary and all must be used from time to time.

Triangulation
One of the most difficult skills required for arthroscopic surgery is 'triangulation' or the ability to bring an operating instrument in front of the telescope lens. To 'triangulate' is difficult because the usual visual clues that are available in conventional surgery are absent and the surgeon must develop new visuo-spatial skills if he is to succeed. Apart from the basic technical errors of inserting the arthroscope at the wrong point or failing to manipulate the leg correctly, inability to triangulate probably accounts for most of the difficulties encountered in the learning stages. Some surgeons find themselves quite unable to acquire this skill and are obliged to abandon their attempts to learn arthroscopic surgery, but most surgeons who are able to manipulate fractures or pass guide-wires up the femoral neck while observing their progress on an image intensifier will eventually be able to triangulate.

OPERATIONS ON SYNOVIUM

Synovial biopsy

Of all the arthroscopic operations, synovial biopsy is the simplest and was the first to be performed regularly. Although there are several ways in which the operation can be performed, the best and most commonly used is to take the specimen with pituitary rongeurs or biopsy forceps inserted from the lateral suprapatellar approach and manipulated under the control of an arthroscope from the antero-lateral approach. The synovium should be selected from a representative area of the joint, including if possible red and engorged synovial villi.

Synovial shelf syndrome

Although the synovial shelf syndrome has only recently come into prominence, there is now an increasing body of evidence (Patel, 1978; Sakakibara, 1976; Vaughan-Lane & Dandy, 1982) to suggest that it is a reality. Some reports suggest that up to 75% of patients obtain relief from anterior knee pain following excision of the synovial shelf but in the author's experience, the relief of pain is most reliable in patients with localised pain and tenderness over the medial synovial shelf itself. Provided that the patients are selected carefully the operation is generally successful, but the shelf syndrome is not common and does not provide a universal answer to the eternal problem of adolescent anterior knee pain.

The shelf can be excised using the double puncture technique with punch forceps inserted from the lateral suprapatellar approach, with the operating arthroscope, or by a combination of these techniques, all of which are described at length elsewhere (Plate 5.7).

Synovectomy

Although synovectomy for rheumatoid arthritis and other chronic synovial disorders is less commonly needed than in former years, the need does arise occasionally (Plate 5.8). Arthroscopic partial synovectomy is a straightforward procedure, made easier with a powered shaver. Although the tissue removed consists essentially of exuberant fronds of synovium rather than the full thickness of the synovium, the immediate relief of pain and discomfort that follows is striking. Long-term studies will be needed to determine the duration of this relief and how often the procedure will need to be repeated, but there is no doubt that the rehabilitation is more rapid after an arthroscopic synovectomy. Patients can expect to leave hospital the day after operation and return to work within a week, and are often more prepared to accept such a procedure every six months or so rather than undergo an open synovectomy with all the incapacity and physiotherapy that is involved.

Adhesions and ankylosis

Isolated adhesions are common findings in the knee after arthrotomy or other trauma, and are seldom associated with symptoms, but more extensive adhesions can form in the suprapatellar pouch after a haemarthrosis, fractures of the lower end of the femur, or patellectomy and can limit flexion of the knee quite markedly, sometimes to as little as 30°. If the loss of flexion is due principally to adhesions in the suprapatellar pouch, considerable improvement in the range of movement can be expected to follow release of these adhesions, a comparatively straightforward arthroscopic operation.

Lateral release
Lateral release of the extensor mechanism is indicated if there is excessive lateral tracking or recurrent subluxation of the patella, but performing the operation arthroscopically has no advantages over the standard procedure except that the scar is smaller. The operation also has the disadvantage that a subcutaneous haematoma may form, and infection in such haemarthrosis has been reported. If the operation is done arthroscopically, it is advisable to inject Marcaine 0.5% with added adrenalin along the line of proposed capsular incision, as well as inserting a suction drain and applying a pressure bandage along the line of capsular incision to minimise bleeding and haematoma formation. If these precautions are omitted, it may occasionally be necessary to explore the knee to evacuate blood and control haemorrhage.

Lipomata, ganglia and fatpad lesions
Isolated subsynovial lipomata sometimes develop to form large pedunculated masses within the knee, which can mimic a loose body or even a meniscus lesion. These lesions can easily be removed arthroscopically. Ganglia may also form in the intercondylar notch, from which they can easily be removed, as can areas of intensely inflamed synovium overlying the fatpad, or lesions of the fatpad itself.

OPERATIONS ON THE ARTICULAR CARTILAGE, LIGAMENTS AND BONE

Loose bodies
In principle, the removal of loose bodies is simple but it is considerably more difficult in practice. Whereas synovium and meniscus lesions remain stationary throughout the operation, loose bodies flee to remote fastnesses of the joint at the slightest provocation, and their elusive nature poses problems not met with in other procedures (Plate 5.9).

Apart from the excessive mobility of the loose body, other difficulties can arise from the presence of multiple loose bodies or loose bodies that do not contain calcium, and which are not visible radiologically. Not only can such loose bodies present themselves unexpectedly at arthroscopy but they may be removed only to find that the original loose body, which was visible radiologically, is still present (Plate 5.10).

The problem of mobility can be overcome to some extent by taking the precautions already described elsewhere (Dandy, 1981) but cannot be eliminated. The problem of multiple loose bodies can be minimised by careful examination of all compartments, including the postero-medial and postero-lateral, but despite such elaborate precautions, the possibility of leaving a loose body within the knee remains a source of anxiety.

Drilling
Articular cartilage defects at the site of origin of loose bodies or chondral separation leave exposed cortical bone while osteochondral fractures leave cancellous bone exposed (Plate 5.11). If subchondral cortical bone is exposed, drilling into the

underlying cancellous bone may lead to faster healing of the articular cartilage defect. The indications for drilling cannot be properly established without the results of long-term studies but until these are available reasonable indications for drilling would be the presence of a defect less than 1 cm in diameter surrounded by healthy articular cartilage.

Shaving
Shaving the areas of chondromalacia patellae is an established procedure, even though the results are not universally satisfactory. If shaving of the patella or either femoral condyle is indicated it can be performed just as effectively arthroscopically, without an arthrotomy, as it can by conventional techniques.

Osteophytes
The osteophytes of osteoarthritis can be removed arthroscopically with pituitary rongeurs. Osteophytes in the intercondylar notch are particularly suitable for removal in this way and can lead to a considerable, if temporary, improvement in the patient's symptoms.

Ligament injuries
Rupture of the anterior or posterior cruciate ligament can result in the formation of a large and sometimes oedematous ligament stub that limits flexion or extension of the knee. If the ligament stub is identified when it is too late for a ligament repair to be attempted, the stub can be excised. Excision of the stub, with correction of any associated meniscal lesions, can improve joint movement and make physiotherapy less arduous. If physiotherapy fails to restore quadriceps bulk and function and prevent the collapsing episodes of cruciate insufficiency, reconstruction may be indicated. If anterior cruciate reconstruction becomes necessary, it is technically possible to insert a ligament prosthesis under arthroscopic control. Carbon fibre prostheses were inserted in this manner in 23 patients with restoration of normal stability in 16, (Dandy et al, 1982). Long-term results of the procedure await analysis but early results suggest that ligament instability recurs in some patients and that the carbon fibre acts as a prosthesis only, without the regeneration of a 'new' ligament around the scaffold of the fibres.

OPERATIONS ON MENISCI

In the past, conventional teaching on knee surgery has tended to concentrate on the menisci as the major cause of internal derangement and disorders of the knee. Early work on diagnostic arthroscopy showed that lesions of the menisci were generally diagnosed too often, while other diagnoses were sometimes missed. Experimental work has also shown that the meniscus forms an important part of the weight-bearing mechanism of the knee and that meniscectomy increases the load across the articular surface by up to six times (Seedhom, Dawson & Wright, 1974). As the result of this and other work there has been a swing away from total meniscectomy as the routine treatment for internal derangements of the knee, with an emphasis on partial rather than total meniscectomy whenever possible (Trapper & Hoover, 1969; McGinty,

Geuss & Marvin, 1977). Meniscal reattachment has also been advocated, with encouraging early results.

The operation of arthroscopic meniscectomy depends on accurate arthroscopic diagnosis, and precise use of the operating instruments. To decide only that there is a meniscus lesion without defining it further and then to insert instruments at random points around the knee will not result in success. In arthroscopic surgery, particularly arthroscopic meniscectomy, surgery demands care, precision and meticulous attention to detail.

Arthroscopic meniscectomy proceeds in three stages. The first, the definition of the anatomy of the lesion, is the most important of the three since it determines the surgical strategy and the approach to the lesion. The second, the removal of the fragment, is the easiest provided that the basic groundwork has been done and the anatomy has been defined precisely. The third stage, checking the meniscal rim, is perhaps the most difficult since it is at this stage that a second fragment of meniscus can be left in the knee or partial tears of meniscus made complete by over-enthusiastic trimming of the rim.

Definition of the anatomy

At the conclusion of the diagnostic arthroscopy, a clear picture of the meniscus should have been obtained and enough information gathered to place the lesion in one of several categories, which are described fully elsewhere, (Dandy, 1981). Tears of the medial meniscus usually arise from either circumferential tears that give rise to bucket handle fragments or from horizontal tears that give rise to superficial flaps. Bucket handle tears generally begin as a small tear posteriorly that extends forwards so that the tears can be divided into three types; those that have extended to the anterior limit of the meniscus (complete, or Type 1 tears), (Plate 5.12), those that have not extended all the way to the anterior horn but where the anterior limit is easily seen (incomplete, Type 2 tears) and those in which the fragment lies beneath the medial femoral condyle and cannot easily be detected without a probing hook or needle (concealed or Type 3 tears). Double, triple and even quadruple tears can occur, and the fragment may also rupture to produce a long tag of meniscal tissues. In the medial compartment, these fragments usually rupture at their posterior end to produce a long anteriorly based tag that is easy to remove (Plate 5.13).

Flap tears can arise from either the upper or lower surface of the meniscus and may be based either anteriorly or posteriorly (Plate 5.14). Flap tears usually arise in older patients and are commonest in the posterior third of the meniscus where they can become tucked back beneath the meniscus to produce a tender nodule on the jointline. Other patterns of tear also occur. In the degenerate knee, the meniscus becomes softer in texture, friable, and may show many splits in its free margin, often made worse by the grinding effects of the femoral condyle.

The meniscus can become detached along its periphery and such lesions, which are commonest in the presence of ligamentous laxity or instability, are the most suitable tears for meniscal reattachment provided that the operation is done within two weeks of the injury. In the posterior horn, a variety of horizontal and incomplete splits is found, which present particular difficulty both in diagnosis and removal.

In the lateral meniscus, the pattern of tears is different from that in the medial compartment and is influenced very considerably by the presence of the popliteus tunnel which acts as a localised 'peripheral separation'. Bucket handle tears begin posteriorly and extend forwards either to the popliteus tendon or the anterior horn of the meniscus, but seldom stop at points in between. Furthermore, the bucket handle fragments may involve either the whole or half the width of the meniscus, creating four distinct types of fragment. Bucket handle fragments in the lateral compartment can rupture at any point, to create a range of detached bucket handle fragments not seen in the medial compartment (Plate 5.15).

Apart from circumferential tears complex oblique tears, sometimes called parrot-beak tears, occur and extend obliquely from upper to lower surface of the meniscus, often with a triangular flap of meniscal tissue that varies in size and position according to the relationship of the tear to the popliteus tunnel. Discoid menisci and anteriorly based tags are also found, as well as a wide variety of other meniscal tears not seen in the medial compartment.

Removing the fragments
The recognition of the pattern of tear is of more than academic importance since each lesion demands a slightly different surgical approach. If there is a single 'secret' of arthroscopic meniscectomy it is that the anatomy of the lesion should be defined precisely and both the instruments and the point of insertion selected carefully before any attempt is made to cut the fragment. It is prudent to insert the probing hook first to check that it can be made to reach the desired part of the meniscus; if the hook cannot be made to touch the lesion, then neither can a cutting instrument (Plate 5.16).

Steps to be taken for removal of the meniscal fragments (Plate 5.17) described above are beyond the scope of this chapter. Many approaches are possible and each surgeon will eventually discover his own preferred technique but much tedium and frustration will be avoided if an approach that is known to work is tried before any attempts are made to improve upon it.

Checking the rim
The third stage of arthroscopic meniscectomy is to check the rim carefully to be certain that the loose fragments have been removed. A probing hook and percutaneous needle are useful for this stage of the operation, which is in some ways the most difficult. It is not always easy to decide if a meniscal rim has been trimmed adequately, and attempts to achieve perfect arthroscopic cosmesis can easily result in serious damage to an otherwise intact meniscal rim (Plate 5.18). In general terms, fragments more than $\frac{1}{2}$ cm long should be removed, and anything smaller can be left. It is better to leave a small meniscal irregularity that will become gradually smoother with the passage of time than to divide an intact meniscal rim by over-zealous trimming.

Aftercare
At the conclusion of the procedure, the tourniquet is released, the joint irrigated, the wounds closed and a gauze wool and crepe dressing applied as for diagnostic arthroscopy. Physiotherapy should be instituted when the patient is sufficiently recovered from the anaesthetic. Full straight leg raising and flexion to 90° should be possible within 24 hours of operation, but if it is not, the patient is likely to have a haemarthrosis which should be aspirated.

Results

The results of arthroscopic partial meniscectomy have been reported (Dandy, 1978; Oretorp & Gillquist, 1979; Northmore-Ball & Dandy, 1982). Out-patient physiotherapy is required in approximately one quarter of the patients and return to work is possible after one week for patients in light occupations and approximately two weeks for patients in heavy occupations.

The results after a mean follow-up period of three years are slightly better than those after open partial meniscectomy (Dandy & Northmore-Ball, 1981) and the results of open partial meniscectomy are better than those of open total meniscectomy. In comparing the results of arthroscopic and open partial meniscectomy, some difficulty is encountered in the assessment of flap tears since this category includes complex oblique tears of the lateral meniscus and posterior flap tears of the medial meniscus, which are generally treated by open total rather than partial meniscectomy. In the assessment of the results of bucket handle tears, which were exactly comparable in the two groups, the results of arthroscopic meniscomy were considerably better with a difference reaching statistical significance.

LEARNING ARTHROSCOPIC SURGERY

When learning arthroscopic surgery, it is important to appreciate that the instruments and techniques involved are so different from conventional orthopaedic surgery that even the finest and most experienced technician must begin again and learn basic principles.

Although instructional books and articles are helpful in setting out the basic ideas, complications and techniques, points of detail and operative techniques that make the difference between success and failure can only be learned from experience. The skill of triangulation must also be learned through practice but the learning process can be accelerated with the help of knee models. These devices, some of which are supplied with detachable skin and replaceable menisci, enable the beginner to overcome the problems of monocular vision and the barrel distortion of a wideangled lens without entering the operating theatre, and are also helpful in gaining familiarity with the recognition and excision of various meniscal lesions.

Videotapes, if properly prepared, are helpful in demonstrating the techniques but are intelligible only to those already familiar with the arthroscopic appearance of the knee. Instructional courses, like books, provide a firm basis for further learning but cannot teach the manual skills required as effectively as, for example, can a course on ASIF fixation of fractures which involves the handling of instruments and fixation devices already familiar to the surgeon.

A suitable programme for learning arthroscopic surgery would be to read a book upon the subject, attend a course, perhaps visit a centre where the technique is regularly performed and if possible, gain access to a knee model so that the first fumbling attempts can be made at leisure without the involvement of a patient.

Once embarked on arthroscopy, the surgeon should become thoroughly familiar with the different approaches already mentioned, including the probing hook, and then proceed from simple procedures to the more complex. Synovial biopsy, debridement of anterior cruciate stubs and the removal of detached bucket handle fragments of medial meniscus are suitable for first attempts at arthroscopic surgery.

Loose bodies, though tempting, are often more difficult than they appear at first sight, and should be approached with caution. Complex oblique (parrot-beak) tears of the lateral meniscus are difficult and should be left well alone until the other lesions can be dealt with easily.

At first, it is advisable to allot a fixed period — say 20 minutes — for arthroscopic surgery before deciding to open the knee rather than persevere with the operation regardless of time or lack of progress. In this way, the length of time for each operation will be more or less predictable and more and more will be achieved during the allotted time for arthroscopy until eventually a procedure will be completed successfully.

Problems, complications and general experience

The complications of arthroscopic surgery are few but real. Fracture of instruments within the knee is perhaps the most disturbing; small fragments of metal may break from the tip of a cutting instrument and come to lie in an inaccessible part of the joint. In the author's first thousand arthroscopic operations, instruments fractured within the knee on six occasions and the fragments were retrieved in only four. Every surgeon who embarks on arthroscopic surgery should assume that sooner or later he will fracture an instrument within the knee and be unable to retrieve the fragment.

Infection, which might be assumed to be a major problem in view of the inevitable contamination of the arthroscope, is virtually unknown after arthroscopy and arthroscopic surgery although a few cases have been reported after lateral release and operations performed through dirty or abraded skin. Although some stitch wounds occasionally become red and inflamed, the author has so far performed over 2000 arthroscopic operations without noticeable trouble from stitch abscesses or infection of the joint cavity.

Haemarthrosis is an inconvenience rather than a complication, and has an incidence of approximately 1%. If a haemarthrosis is not aspirated, all the problems of haemarthrosis will be experienced, including pain, stiffness and the prolonged incapacity that the patient hoped to avoid.

Deep vein thrombosis is unusual, and we had an incidence of 0.3% in the first thousand operations. Pulmonary emboli did not occur but one patient had bilateral embolism after a simple diagnostic arthroscopy. The incidence of deep vein thrombosis and pulmonary emboli following arthrotomy is not reported but most surgeons with experience of the knee will have little difficulty in recalling cases from their own experience.

Medico-legal problems

When first introduced in the United States, arthroscopic surgery was regarded with suspicion by those who did not 'believe' in it, and there was considerable anxiety that the introduction of a new technique might bring medico-legal problems in its wake. Since the technique became established, the pendulum has swung the other way with anxiety being expressed about the propriety of proceeding to an arthrotomy for an internal derangement of the knee without a preliminary arthrogram or arthroscopy, and even about the need to advise patients that another surgeon skilled in arthroscopic surgery might be able to perform the same operation in such a way that the patient could return to work within a few days of operation rather than the few weeks often required after the conventional operation. In the United Kingdom it would seem unlikely that medico-legal considerations will reach the same level as in other countries, but surgeons who do not practise arthroscopic surgery should give serious consideration to the wisdom of proceeding directly to an arthrotomy without some form of preliminary investigation.

Workload
The introduction of arthroscopic surgery changes the pattern of work in an orthopaedic unit considerably. While patients admitted for operation on the knee might otherwise have occupied a bed for 1–2 weeks they now occupy a bed for two or at the most three days, with the result that the workload of the unit tends to be pulsatile rather than steady. Demands on the physiotherapy department are also changed with a relative increase in the need for in-patient physiotherapy and a corresponding drop in out-patient requirements.

In the operating theatre, the number of patients treated will fall at first but will increase as the surgeon gains experience. The average time for an arthroscopic procedure is approximately 25 minutes, making it possible to treat six patients in an average operating list of $3\frac{1}{2}$ hours without difficulty but different surgeons operate at different speeds, as in other fields of surgery.

Perhaps the most far-reaching effect of arthroscopic surgery on an orthopaedic practice is the pattern of referral. The advantages of arthroscopic surgery spread quickly among patients and general practitioners with the result that those surgeons practising arthroscopic surgery quickly become overwhelmed with this type of work, as well as those suffering from disorders of the knee not amenable to arthroscopic surgery. Before embracing arthroscopic surgery, the surgeon should consider if he is certain that he enjoys this kind of work, because it will be difficult, if not impossible, to reverse the decision if he eventually discovers that arthroscopic surgery is difficult or uncongenial.

The future role of arthroscopic surgery is a subject of debate, and even controversy. At present, the only indications for arthrotomy in the author's practice are ligament reconstruction, total joint replacement and meniscal reattachment, but it is clearly unreasonable to suggest that this position should be universal. In time, it is to be hoped that any surgeon with an interest in the knee will be adept in the use of an arthroscope, but such a stage of development must await the training of another generation of orthopaedic surgeons who have grown up with the arthroscope as their predecessors grew up with hammers and bone spikes. It may well be that the arthroscope will prove to have the same effect on surgery of the knee as did the cystoscope and trans-urethral resection of the prostate upon urology. While there are many surgeons who practise urology without performing trans-urethral resection of the prostate, it is difficult to imagine a specialist urologist being appointed now unless he is able to perform endoscopic surgery. In the same way, arthroscopic surgery may lead to the establishment of a speciality of knee surgery within the orthopaedic family. Some surgeons suggest that arthroscopic surgery should establish itself as a 'super-specialty', but this would seem undesirable on several counts. There are no gynaecologists who practise only laparoscopic surgery, or urologists who practise only endoscopic surgery, but neither are there urologists who are unable to use the cystoscope. There is no doubt that the arrival of the arthroscope will bring a change in the position of knee surgery within orthopaedic surgery, but only time will tell what that change will be.

REFERENCES

Burman M S 1931 Arthroscopy or direct vieualization of joints. An experimental cadaver study. Journal of Bone & Joint Surgery 13: 669–695
Dandy D J 1978 Early results of closed partial meniscectomy. British Medical Journal 1: 1099–1100
Dandy D J 1981 Arthroscopic surgery of the knee. Churchill Livingstone, Edinburgh and London
Dandy D J, Northmore-Ball M D 1981 A comparative study of arthroscopic and open partial meniscectomy. British Orthopaedic Association April 1981
Dandy D J, Flanagan J P, Steenmeyer V 1982 Clinical Orthopaedics and Related Research 167: 43–49
Geist E S 1926 Arthroscopy: preliminary report. Lancet 46: 306-307
Gillquist J, Hagberg G 1976 A new modification of the technique of arthroscopy of the knee joint. Acta Chirurgica Scandinavia 142(2): 123–130
Jackson R W, Dandy D J 1976 Arthroscopy of the knee. Grune & Stratton, New York
Kreuscher P 1925 Semilunar cartilage disease, a plea for early recognition by means of the arthroscope and early treatment of this condition. Illinois Medical Journal 47: 290–292
McGinty J B, Geuss L F, Marvin R A 1977 Partial or total meniscectomy. A comparative analysis. Journal of Bone & Joint Surgery 59A: 763–766
Northmore-Ball M D, Dandy D J 1982 Long-term results of arthroscopic partial meniscectomy. Clinical Orthopaedics and Related Research 167: 34–42
O'Connor R L 1977 Arthroscopy. J B Lippincott, Philadelphia & Toronto
Oretorp N, Gillquist J 1979 Transcutaneous meniscectomy under arthroscopic control. International Orthopaedics 3: 19–25
Patel D 1978 Arthroscopy of the plicae-synovial folds and their significance. The America Journal of Sports Medicine 6: 217–225
Sakakibara J 1976 Arthroscopic study of Iino's band (plica synovialis mediopatellaris). Journal of the Japanese Orthopaedic Association 50: 513–522
Seedhom, B B, Dawson, D & Wright V 1974 Functions of the menisci — A preliminary study. Journal of Bone & Joint Surgery 56-B: 381
Takagi K 1933 Practical experience using Takagi's arthroscope. Journal of the Japanese Orthopaedic Association 8: 132
Tapper E, Hoover N 1969 Late results after meniscectomy. Journal of Bone & Joint Surgery 60-A: 436
Vaughan-Lane T, Dandy D J 1982 The synovial shelf syndrome. Journal of Bone & Joint Surgery 64-B: 475–476

6. Chemonucleolysis in the treatment of lumbar disc disease

L. L. Wiltse

Chymopapain was first isolated by Jansen and Balls in 1941. It is a proteologic enzyme purified from the latex of the green paw-paw fruit (carica papaya). Louis Thomas (1956) demonstrated that when a solution of crude papain was injected intravenously in rabbits, within 4 hours both ears were observed to curl over at their tips. After 18 hours the ears lost all of their normal rigidity and were collapsed limply on either side of the head rather like those of spaniels. After 3 or 4 days, the ears became straightened and erect again. If at this time a new injection of papain was given, the same bizarre events recurred. Apart from the unusual appearance of the animals, they exhibited no evidence of systemic illness or discomfort and continued to feed and move about in the fashion of normal animals of the species.

These findings were published in 1956. Dr Lyman Smith of Elgin, Illinois, after reading the work of Thomas and in collaboration with Garvin, Gessler and Jennings experimented with chymopapain on animals. They made their initial report in 1963. This report of animal experimentation was followed by a report on human subjects in the Journal of the American Medical Association in 1964 (Smith, 1964). Approval for clinical trials on a wider basis was then sought and from that time until 1975 approximately 15 000 patients were injected in the United States at approximately 75 centres. In 1975 the injections were discontinued in the United States but have continued in many other countries — in particular, Canada, Great Britain, France, Germany, Yugoslavia, Russia and Australia.

Mechanism of action (Stern & Smith, 1967)
Chymopapain dissolves human nucleus pulposus in vitro with liberation of chondroitin sulphate and keratin sulphate. The enzyme is rapidly bound to insoluble components in vitro. The apparent mechanism of action is the hydrolysis of cementing protein of the high molecular weight glycosaminoglycans (Edgar, 1974; Smith et al, 1963).

The enzyme acts on the central contents of the intervertebral disc by hydrolyzing and dissolving the non-collagenous protein that interconnects long-chain mucopolysaccharides (Stern, 1969). There the chondromucoprotein loses some of its water-binding capacity. The specificity is such that it takes some 20 times the dose necessary to react on the chondromucoprotein before there is a visible effect on the fibrous tissues of the adjacent annulus (Stern, 1969).

If the disc space is not already markedly narrowed, narrowing usually occurs and in our studies approximately 80% narrowed at least 0.5 cm during the first 4 months (Edgar, 1974; Garvin & Jennings, 1973, 1965). Garvin and Jennings experimented with dogs to determine among other things the degree of narrowing. They found that in young beagle dogs, narrowing occurred in every case. In dogs receiving 0.1 mg of

104 RECENT ADVANCES IN ORTHOPAEDICS

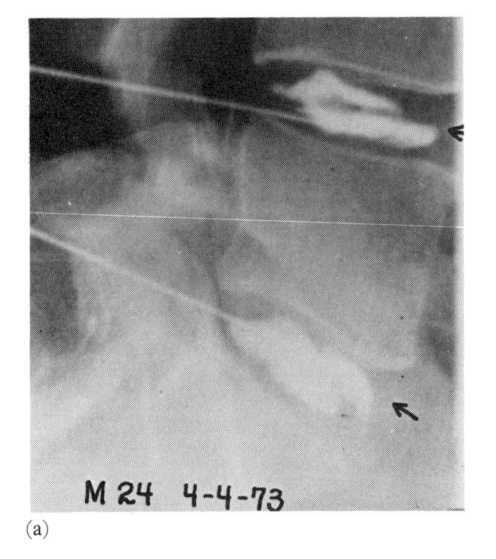

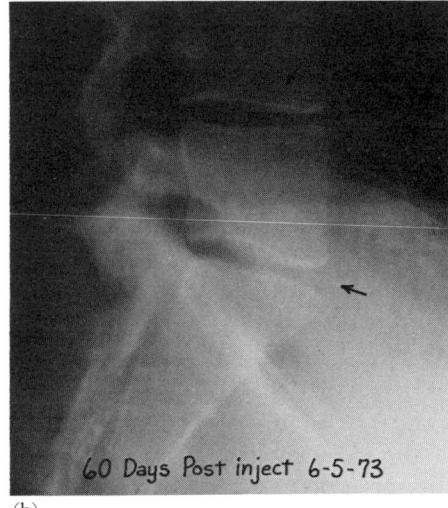

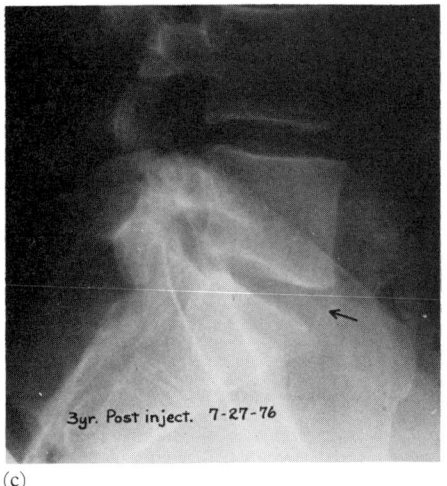

(a) M 24 4-4-73

(b) 60 Days Post inject 6-5-73

(c) 3yr. Post inject. 7-27-76

Fig. 6.1a Discogram of 24-yr old male at time of chemonucleolysis 4–4–73. Both the L4 and L5 discs were injected with 8 mm of chymopapain each.
Fig. 6.1b 62 days post injection. Note rather marked narrowing of both disc spaces.
Fig. 6.1c A little over three years post injection. Rewidening of disc spaces has occurred.

chymopapain in their discs, maximum narrowing had occurred after 9 days and rewidening was complete in about 6 months. Those receiving 1 mg of chymopapain narrowed even more rapidly and did also rewiden but much more slowly. In the human being rewidening is a common phenomenon. At this moment there are no statistics on just how frequently but we believe that in discs which are not too seriously damaged, rewidening is the rule rather than the exception (Fig. 6.1). Toxicologic studies with chymopapain have yielded the following results in rabbits and dogs according to published data:

Doses up to 100 times greater than that required to consistently dissolve the nucleus pulposus in a given animal are tolerated when injected intravenously, intradiscally and epidurally.

Intravenous doses of 5 mg per kilo of body weight in dogs and rabbits have no substantial effect on the cardiovascular system or on blood coagulation factors. Doses of 10 mg per kilo produce hypotension and hypocoagulability. In man, chymopapain injected into the disc leaves the disc and appears in blood plasma very soon. Plasma markedly inhibits the activity of chymopapain (Kapsalis et al, 1974).

Intrathecal injections are toxic and should be avoided. Chymopapain is three times as toxic when injected subarachnoidally just below the foramen magnum as it is when injected down at the L3 level (Wiltse et al, 1975).

Subarachnoid injections cause rupture of the microvascular structures because it dissolves the intercellular bonding substance (Garvin et al, 1965, 1975) of the walls of the capillaries (Wiltse et al, 1975).

We have no way of knowing what the LD50 for chymopapain is when injected subarachnoidally in man but there is little doubt that the human being can tolerate the amount that would ever be injected into one single disc if this were to inadvertently occur.

As an additional safety factor, it has been found that if chymopapain is injected subarachnoidally, immediate decompression of the cord by opening the dura and relieving the cerebrospinal fluid pressure along with massive doses of hydrocortisone given intravenously and intramuscularly will save dogs which had had six times the LD50 (Macnab, 1972). Of course one can tell at the time of discography (before the chymopapain is injected) if the contrast medium is flowing subarachnoidally and so further injection would be halted.

Macnab in 1972 injected chymopapain intrathecally in various sublethal amounts in a series of 25 dogs. These animals were sacrificed at varying intervals up to a year post injection. In no case, when the dog was killed, was there evidence of arachnoiditis in the spinal cord area or above the foramen magnum.

In our own laboratory we injected 60 mg doses in the epidural space of five dogs (Wiltse et al, 1975). The same number of controls were given injections of sterile distilled water. The dogs were sacrificed at 1 hour, 1 week, 3 weeks, 3 months and 6 months. The dura, the neural elements inside the dura, the extradural elements and the spinal nerves before and after exit through the vertebral foramina were carefully studied. In addition in three dogs a needle was inserted into the epidural space but nothing was injected. These dogs were sacrificed at 1 hour, 1 week and 3 weeks. Dr Ann Hamilton, neuropathologist at Irvine, reviewed all the gross and microscopic sections of the central nervous systems of the animals used in this study. In every case all tissues were completely normal. There was no evidence of neural thickening, subarachnoid thickening, haemorrhage or any other abnormality. The areas in which the water had been injected or in fact where nothing was injected but a needle inserted looked exactly the same as the area in which chymopapain dissolved in water had been injected.

This is important because in a severely ruptured disc the contrast material will leak posteriorly at the time of discography in approximately one in four cases. Thus, so also will the chymopapain. It was our custom to go ahead with the chymopapain injection even though the contrast medium leaked out posteriorly into the epidural space. No adverse effects were ever seen.

Computerised axial tomography appears to be a very good diagnostic tool in determining the presence of a ruptured disc and, in the patient with clear-cut symptoms, we tend to use a CAT scan and not a myelogram. If there is doubt, we follow the CAT scan with a myelogram (Fig. 6.2).

106 RECENT ADVANCES IN ORTHOPAEDICS

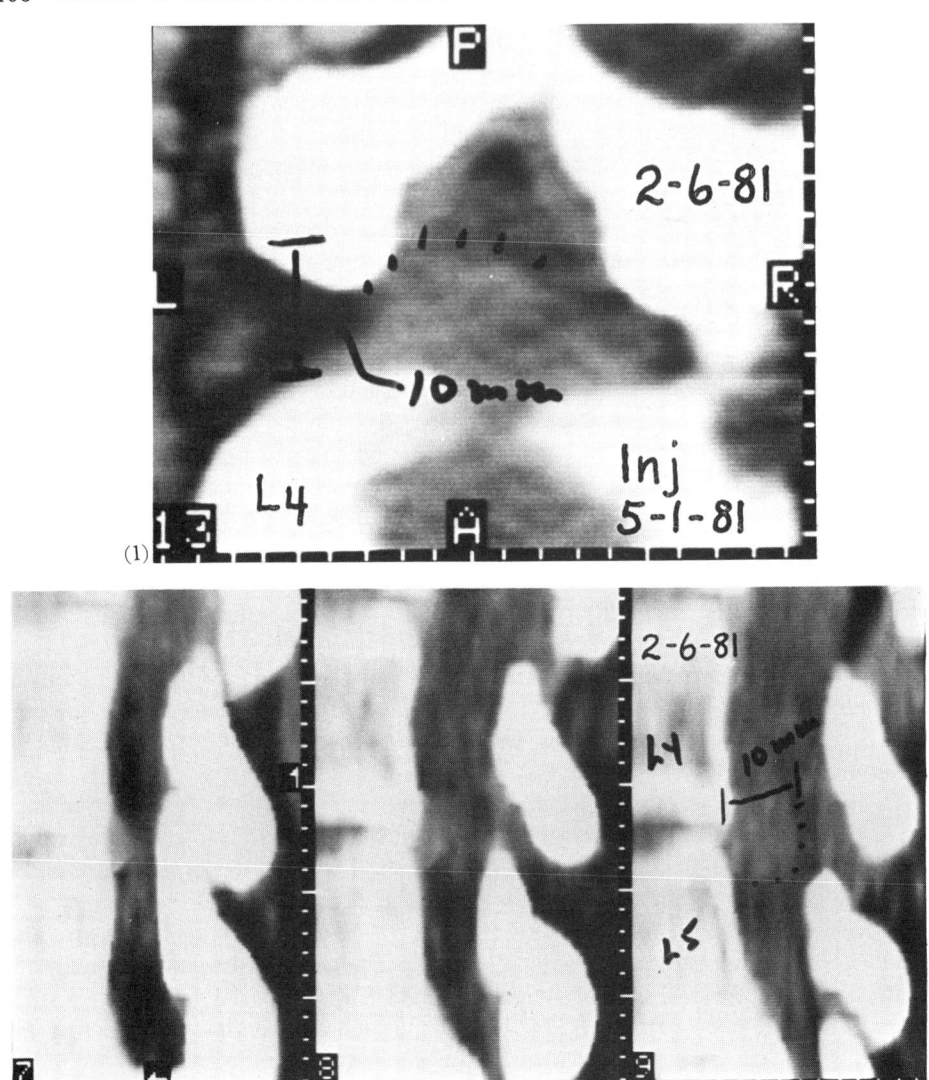

Fig. 6.2a (1) CAT scan at L4/5 junction. Note on axial view disc is 10 mm wide in this 28-year old white female.
 (2) in reconstructed parasagittal view note again the 10 mm disc bulge.

Indications
Indications for chemonucleolysis are very similar to the indications for discectomy. The ideal candidate for a discectomy is usually the ideal candidate for chemonucleolysis. The exception is the patient who is developing a rapidly increasing neurological deficit. These should have a laminectomy.

Absolute contraindications are
a. allergy to meat tenderiser or vegetables and fruit related to the papaya. Also a

TREATMENT OF LUMBAR DISC DISEASE 107

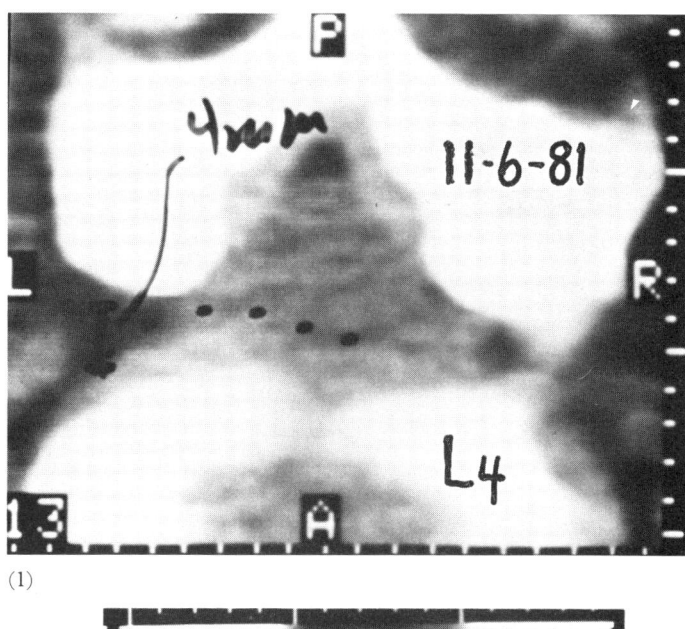

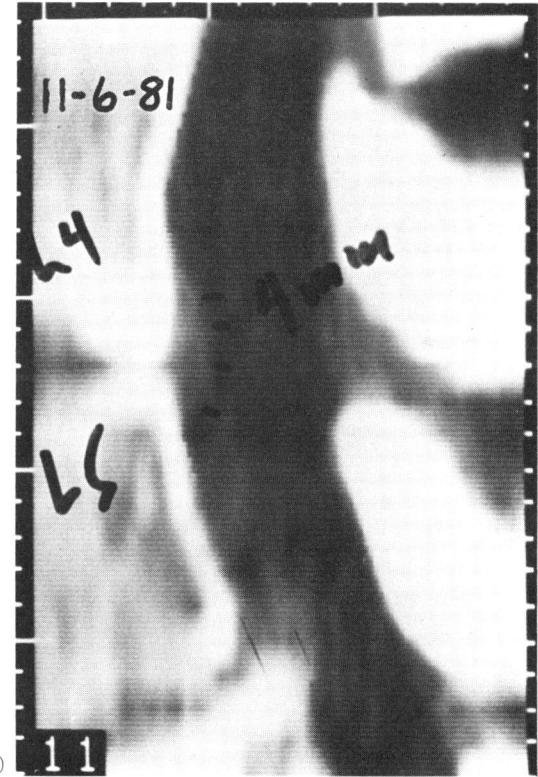

Fig. 6.2b (1) chymopapain injection was done on May 5, 1981. 6 months post injection, the disc has shrunk to 4 mm.
(2) the same reduction in size is seen in the parasagittal view.
In this same patient a disc bulge at L5 measuring 7 mm was not injected and did not change size.

patient with many severe allergies is not considered a good candidate for the procedure.
b. rapidly developing neurological deficit especially if producing bowel or bladder disturbances.
c. possible evidence of spinal cord tumour.

Relative contraindications are:
a. severe spinal stenosis.
b. pregnancy (may not be a contraindication).
c. severe arachnoiditis.

A second injection appears to be contraindicated if the patient has developed a second ruptured disc. Kokan (1982) has reported that from a statistical standpoint, there is an increase in the incidence of allergic reaction on the second injection sufficiently severe to contraindicate the procedure.

A severely extruded disc, as long as it hasn't left the site where it passes through the posterior longitudinal ligament, seems not to be a contraindication. A frankly sequestrated disc probably is (Glossary of spinal terminology, 1980). Our patients with the most severely ruptured discs had the best subjective clinical results. Patients injected during the first year after the onset of symptoms also did better but there may have been other reasons, such as the fact that the patient was held off from injection for many months or years suggesting that the diagnosis was not secure.

Obvious spinal stenosis was considered a relative contraindication although patients with so-called combined stenosis' where a disc bulge occurred in an already compromised space were injected with good results.

Very narrow lateral canals are also a relative contraindication since the injection of chymopapain usually further narrows the disc and the lateral canal. Now that computerised axial tomography is available, it is possible to evaluate the lateral canals much further out from the midline and perhaps tell which patient should not be injected but should have surgery instead.

The technique of injection is extremely important and one cannot urge too strongly the value of having the best possible roentgenographic equipment. Surgeons who have been using discography as part of their diagnostic armamentarium have a great advantage in that they already are skilful in needle placement. If one is to get a good result from chemonucleolysis, it is mandatory that the enzyme be placed into the centre of the disc or at least inside the inner rings of the annulus fibrosis. At the L5 level this is no mean feat even with the best of equipment. Since discography combined with the saline reproduction test is a good diagnostic procedure, I would urge surgeons intending to perform chemonucleolysis to begin by doing discography.

We prefer to use a special procedure room in the X-ray department rather than the operating room since these are usually better equipped.

Either general or local anaesthesia can be used (Fig. 6.3). The patient is placed in the left lateral decubitus position on a stationary fluoroscopy table. He should be taped securely so that he does not roll as even a small amount of change from a true AP or lateral position severely distorts the fluoroscopic image. A portable C-arm is slipped over the stationary unit. This arrangement gives instantaneous bi-planar fluoroscopic control for needle insertion. Ideally the X-ray units should have a so-called memory (video disc recorder) that can be set in such a way that one can have

TREATMENT OF LUMBAR DISC DISEASE 109

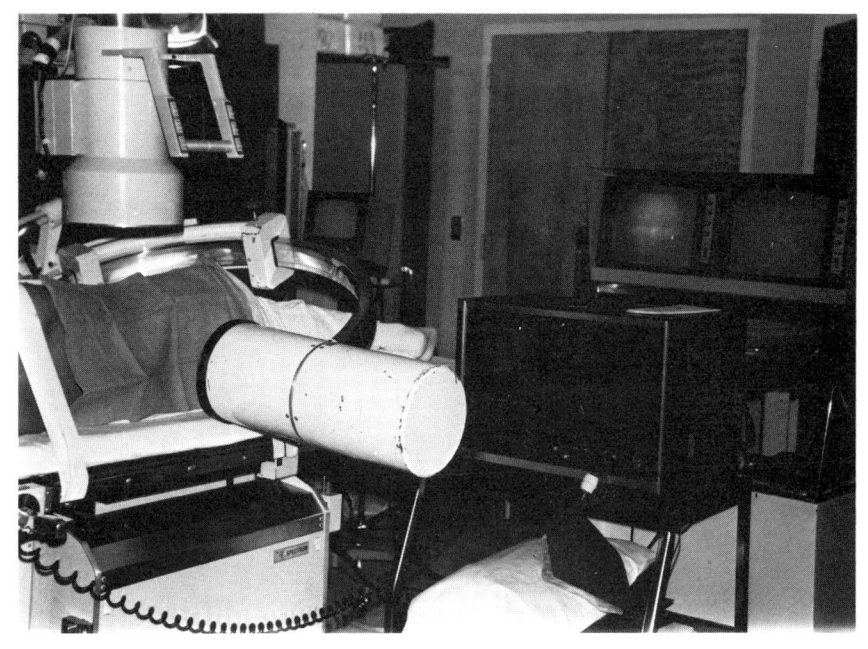

Fig. 6.3 The patient is lying on his side with an inflatable air bag under his left flank. The C-arm of the portable fluoroscope has been slipped over the large stationary X-ray machine. There are two television screens, one for the A–P and one for the lateral view. Each has two screens so that a picture can be held on one while a new image is being generated on the other.

either continuous fluoroscopy or use the memory in which case the image is held on the screen. This cuts down enormously on the amount of radiation which the patient (and the doctor) receive. Skin preparation and draping is the same as for any major surgical procedure. Everyone wears a cap, mask and a full length lead apron under the sterile gown (Fig. 6.4). A plastic drape is put over the overhead X-ray tube. With this

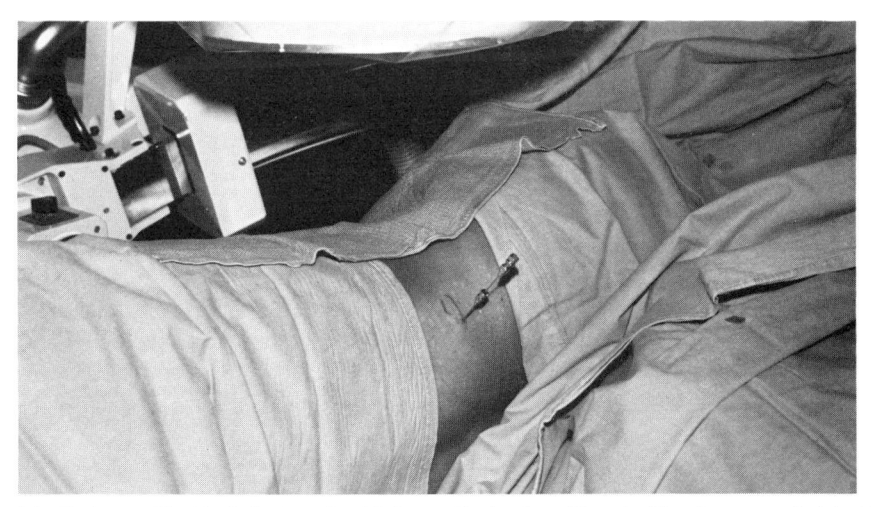

Fig. 6.4 Patient on his side, fully draped, with the needles in place. Note the 22 ga longer needle is inside the 18 ga outer needle. The inner needle should be 4 or 5 cm longer than the outer needle. Note also the sterile plastic drape over the overhead X-ray tube.

110 RECENT ADVANCES IN ORTHOPAEDICS

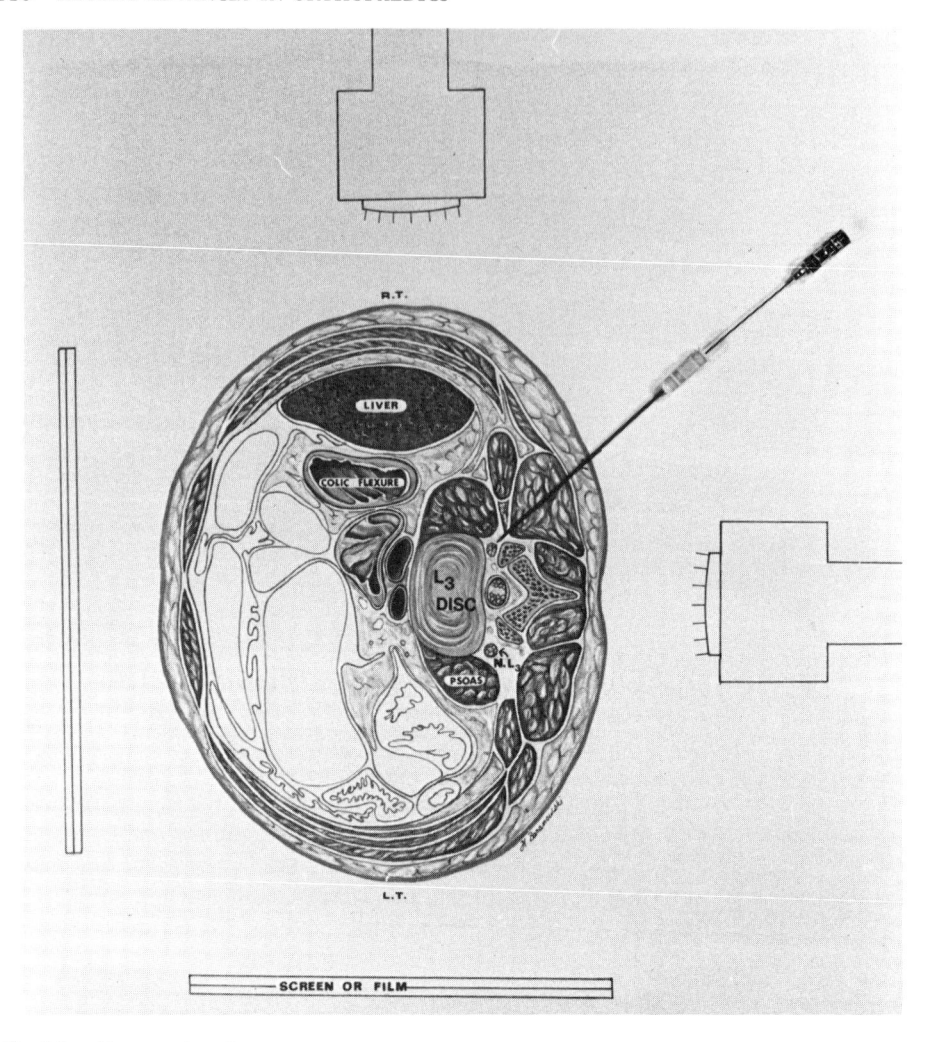

Fig. 6.5a Cross section of the human body at the level of the L3 disc. Note L3 spinal nerve is exactly in the line usually chosen for needle insertion. A small needle passed through the nerve only once or twice seems to do no harm.

arrangement, it is never necessary to move the C-arm unit about. However the top of the table can be moved a few centimetres and thus the surgeon can centre on the disc to be injected. The stationary unit is much more powerful than the portable unit and, in a large person, a good image can be obtained in the lateral projection. Presently available portable units will not give a good lateral image except in small individuals.

We use the double needle technique. An outer 18 ga needle is passed to within a centimetre of the disc and, when the direction seems perfect, the stilette is removed and a 22 ga needle is passed on into the disc. This has the advantage that the needle that goes into the disc can be left in its sterile plastic tube until it is ready for use. Also this inner needle never punctures the skin. The inner needle must be at least 4 cm (and preferably 5 cm) longer than the outer needle. Several companies are making

TREATMENT OF LUMBAR DISC DISEASE   111

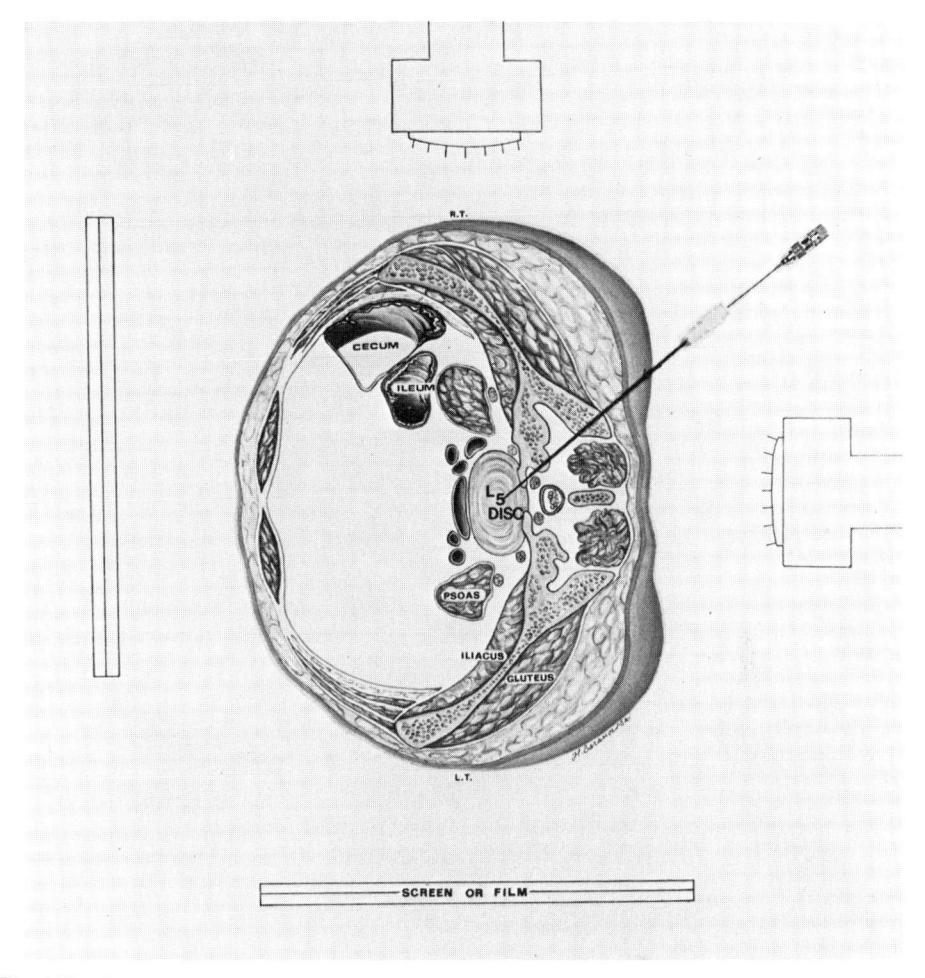

Fig. 6.5b   Cross section at L5. Spinal nerve here is less directly in line of needle but certainly can be hit.

these long thin needles at a very reasonable price. From a point approximately 8 cm lateral to the midline, the needle is angled at 45° toward the centre of the body. Frequent X-ray checks are made as the needle is advanced (Fig. 6.5).

The direction of the needle can be changed slightly by simply rotating it in which case the bevel at the tip will 'sled runner' and change direction. We have never used bent needles although such needles are commercially available. The inner needle with a slight bend will pass down through the outer needle and, when it gets beyond the tip, will spring into the bent position and change direction considerably. This may have real value but one should beware of bending the needles oneself as they may break off. The professionally bent needles are probably safe.

When the surgeon is satisfied that the needle is in proper position, a contrast medium, iothalamate (Conray 60) is injected for discography. A 50 cm plastic tube is used to inject this so that the operator can watch the material flow in, yet keep his hand out of the X-ray beam.

As to which contrast medium is the best, there may be argument. We use iothalamate (Conray) because this seems to be the least irritating if it should accidentally be injected into the subarachnoid space. (We have never had this occur, but such an accident is possible.) The question arises, do these contrast media in any way partially inactivate the chymopapain? Apparently they do not. Mark Brown, Arthur Naylor (1982) and Ivan Stern (1967) have investigated this and none feel that the action of chymopapain is in any way compromised by the contrast.

Getting the needle into any disc space above L5 is quite easy while L5 is the difficult level. We put an inflatable air bag in the patient's flank. Thus, if necessary, we can laterally flex his spine by pumping up the air bag. We prefer the spine to be straight. People with narrow hips often don't need such a bag but a person with very wide hips does. If one has difficulty getting into a disc space, the following things can be done:

1. Laterally flex the patient by pumping up the air bag, thus opening up the space.
2. Use a bent discogram needle.
3. As a last resort, one can turn the patient on his abdomen and pass the needle directly through the midline. (During the first few years of discography, this is the way it was always done.)

As regards inadvertent stabbing of other structures other than a spinal nerve there seems to be little danger of damage. There is a small chance of passing the needle through an abdominal visus, and then changing the direction of the needle insertion, thus carrying infection on into the disc. By using the double needle technique, this danger is eliminated.

We virtually never insert the same outer needle twice. If we have reason to pull it out, we simply discard it and use a new needle. We have never had a case of disc space infection and have done over 1700 cases, counting both the chymopapain injection and the plain discography done over the past 25 years.

It is very possible to hit a nerve with the needle as it is being advanced. Using local anaesthesia, the patient knows if a nerve is touched but not so under general. Sometimes it can be difficult to avoid the nerve. If one has difficulty, I would strongly advise against repeated stabbing with a large 18 ga needle as this can seriously damage the nerve which lies snugly against the side of the disc and vertebral body. Once the outer sleeve is in perfect position, the inner needle can be passed on into the disc. Even though the small needle passes through the spinal nerve a time or two, no harm will come to the nerve. For this reason I have come to believe that general anaesthesia is as desirable as local.

It is very important to have an experienced anaesthesiologist at the head of the table even when one is using local anaesthesia. (At this time we believe that hydrocortisone 2000 mg should be given intramuscularly $2\frac{1}{2}$ hours before the chymopapain is injected (this can be given i.v. at the time the patient is on the table) and benadryl 50 mg i.v. at the time the procedure is started. I strongly believe this cuts down the severity of anaphylaxis. A large intracath should be fastened securely in the vein and an infusion of Ringer lactate should be started.) At the slightest sign of allergic reaction, treatment should be instituted. The earliest sign is usually a rash on the neck. For this reason, the drapes are removed immediately after the injection of the enzyme so that the skin can be observed. If a rash appears, along with an increased pulse rate and a drop in blood pressure, one should institute treatment. Briefly, the steps are as follows:

1. Turn the patient on his back.
2. Check cardiac function by an electrocardiogram and by palpating the carotid arteries. If there is no heart beat, then start closed chest cardiac massage.
3. Give 0.3 to 0.5 ml of epinephrine (1:1000) i.v. and allow a mixture of epinephrine and saline to flow into the vein so the patient gets 0.3 to 0.5 ml of epinephrine per minute. (Halothane should not be used as an anaesthetic for chemonucleolysis because epinephrine with halothane is contraindicated.)
4. See that there is a proper airway. Intubate if necessary. Give oxygen by positive pressure. Perform tracheostomy if necessary (we have never had to resort to this).
5. Give 5% dextrose in lactated Ringers solution as rapidly as possible.
6. Give hydrocortisone sodium succinate (Solu-Cortef), 2–3000 mg by rapid intravenous injection.
7. If bronchospasm is a problem, give 250–500 mg of aminophylline by slow intravenous injection.
8. Give an antihistamine such a diphenhydramine hydrochloride (Benadryl) intravenously.
9. A vasopressor may be used with caution if hypotension persists.
10. Electrical defibrillation may be used if necessary.

Post operative care

The patients are allowed up as soon as they wish. They usually want to walk to the bathroom the same day. They are allowed to go home as soon as they feel able. We train all our patients in isometric abdominal and squatting exercises. No exercises that are painful are done.

Between August 1968 and July 1975, 1446 patients had their lumbar spines injected with chymopapain by our group. All were done in one hospital, Long Beach Memorial Hospital Medical Center. All but one were done in one room of the Radiology Department, using almost ideal equipment. There were 35 physicians involved, 30 orthopaedic surgeons and five neurosurgeons (Wiltse, 1969).

As nearly as possible our series was done in accordance with a rigid protocol. All patients were seen at intervals until they were one year post injection and detailed clinical records were kept. This group was reviewed in detail. The records in the surgeon's files in conjunction with questionnaires gave sufficient information to arrive at a valid rating. Some patients were lost to follow-up and could not be evaluated. About 80% were available for rating. The following criteria were used in rating the patient's subjective clinical result:

1. excellent — normal activity, no pain and no analgesics.
2. good — able to work but with some limitation of activity and occasionally some pain. May sometimes need a mild pain medication.
3. fair — unable to work except at very light work and has frequent pain needing a strong analgesic. Not bad enough to want open surgery.
4. poor — much limitation by pain, very minor improvement.
5. failure — severe pain and limitation of activity. No improvement or even worse.

The overall results of the whole group, giving no consideration to age, sex, compensation connection, number of levels injected, etc., are shown in Table 6.1 and Table 6.2.

Table 6.1 No previous low back surgery

excellent	108 (34.1)
good	111 (35%)
fair	38 (12.7%)
poor/failure	60 (18.9%)

Table 6.2 If a patient had had one or more previous low back operations, the results were poorer as seen here in Table 6.2

excellent	26.2%
good	19.6%
fair	16.8%
poor/failure	37.4%

One of our requirements before doing chemonucleolysis was that the patient's pain should be bad enough and of long enough duration that he would have had open surgery if chemonucleolysis had not been available. In the original total group, approximately one in ten came to surgery. Chemonucleolysis did not seem to prejudice the chances of a good result from subsequent surgery if such was necessary.

Complications
We had almost exactly one case of anaphylaxis per hundred injections. After the first 500 cases, we learned to control these satisfactorily with routine care as noted previously under *Technique*. Transient rash occurred in one case in 200. We also had a few cases of temporary foot drop and one case of permanent moderately severe dorsiflexor weakness. There were no disc space infections. A few cases already had thrombophlebitis due to a long period of bed rest and traction pre-injection. No deaths occurred.

Reversibility of neurologic deficit
Patients who had a definite neurologic deficit immediately before injection were re-evaluated neurologically one year post injection (Wiltse et al, 1975). The deficits evaluated were deep tendon reflexes, motor weakness and sensory deficit. Of those with absent tendon reflexes, 60% reverted, having returned to normal when rated a year post injection. Of those with gross muscle weakness, 85% had reverted to normal by the end of the year. Of the cases with sensory deficit, 75% had reverted.

Time required to achieve the best results
It was of interest that, while the relief of sciatica was frequently immediately following chemonucleolysis, the presence of back pain and spasm persisted for days or even weeks. 51.8% of the total stated that they had achieved their optimal results within the first 4 months. 74% had achieved their optimal results within the first 6 months but 12% required the passage of at least 1 year before attainment of the optimal symptomatic end result.

Because of the problems in evaluating subjective clinical results in a group of patients who are fairly diverse (e.g. a few had three levels injected, some had a possibility of monetary gain by staying ill, others had few organic findings), it was decided to study the results in patients who would be ideal candidates for surgical discectomy, had not chymopapain been available. Dr Abdelmonen A. Afifi (biostatistician) assisted in this study. The follow-up was done by questionnaire an average of 3.5 years post injection. All questionnaires were evaluated by an unbiased professional (non physician) who had had no previous contact with the patient.

One might ask if such a study is statistically acceptable. It was the opinion of Dr Afifi that, since patient selection was made prior to sending out the questionnaire that the study met the demands of a reliable statistical evaluation (Wiltse, 1978).

Fundamentally we were interested only in what the patient thought of his result and not what the doctor thought. Organic disability in these patients was of little consequence. With a questionnaire sent out by a third party, the patient is under no emotional pressure to report a better result than he actually has.

Criteria for selection of the ideal candidate

1. all were private patients with no industrial or other liability connection.
2. all were between the ages of 21 and 65.
3. none had had previous back surgery of any type.
4. all injections were confined to the lowest two lumbar vertebrae. No patient had a 3-level injection.
5. every case had a strongly positive myelogram with a diagnosis of herniated lumbar disc. All myelograms were reviewed by Dr Oas, Radiology Department, Long Beach Memorial Hospital and he confirmed that it was indeed strongly positive.
6. every patient had psychological studies and was given a pyschological rating preoperatively. However, a case was not eliminated from the study on the basis of his psychological study results. A separate study was made of this.
7. every case had at least two 'hard' organic findings besides the strongly positive myelogram. 'Hard' organic findings were considered to be as follows:
   a. sensory deficit which followed a definite dermatomal pattern.
   b. motor changes such as calf weakness, dorsiflexor weakness or extensor hallucis longus weakness.
   c. change in the achilles reflex. In this study differences in the patellar reflex were not considered.
   d. elevation of the spinal fluid protein to no less than 50 mg/dl.
   e. definite electromyographic changes in the lower legs as determined by Dr Druckman, neurologist.
8. all had a classical ruptured disc syndrome with sciatica.
9. all had had what was considered an adequate trial with conservative treatment without relief prior to injection, the shortest interval from the onset of symptoms being 6 weeks.
10. no disc that was even remotely normal by discography was injected with chymopapain.
11. all had a series of X-rays of the low back taken during the year after injection.
12. a final physical examination was done at the end of one year.

Finding enough perfect candidates among 1472 would on the face of it seem easy but that was not true. The final number of questionnaires sent out was 174 of which 135 were returned, a return rate of 77.5%. Those who did not answer or could not be

Table 6.3 Months from day of injection to final rating in a group considered to be ideal candidates for laminectomy

Median	36
Mode	36
Mean	42
Range	12–84 months

Table 6.4 Rating an average of 3.5 years post injection in ideal candidates

	No.	%
Excellent/good	115	85.2
Fair	9	6.6
Poor/failed	11	8.1

Table 6.5 Correlation of duration of symptoms before injection with an excellent or good subjective clinical result
(Rating averaging 3.5 years post injection)

	6 weeks–6 months	7 months–12 months	over 12 months
Number of patients	71	45	19
% with E or G results	90	91	52

Note the rather marked drop in the quality of results when the patient had had his symptoms for more than one year.

Table 6.6 Further low back surgery

	N–10
	7.4%
Average time from day of injection to day of laminectomy	11.1 mo
Range	1 to 35 mo

Table 6.7 Correlation of number of organic findings with subjective end result (rating averaging 3.5 years post injection)

Number of organic deficits	Total patients with this number of defects	N with E or G rating	% with E or G rating
3	47	33	70.2
4	53	42	79.2
5	25	22	88.0
6	10	8	80.0

Table 6.8 This group of ideal candidates was further refined and only those who were also excellent or good candidates from a psychological standpoint were included. The results were as follows

		N–80	
Excellent/good	N–72		92.5%
Fair	N–3		3.75%
Poor/failed	N–2		3.75%

Dr Patrick Rocchio gave the patients their psychological rating pre-injection.

reached were studied by going to the chart and using the surgeon's rating at the patient's last visit. The results in this group are reported separately.

The purpose of selecting such a group was to obtain a homogeneous study population so severely affected that members would be unlikely to become symptom-free without a long wait and (Hakelius, 1970), because of the severity of their pain, would probably demand surgery. Tables 6.3 through 6.8 show the results of this study.

We recognize of course that many patients who are not ideal candidates have serious symptoms and need the relief that surgery or chemonucleolysis affords. So treatment need not be withheld just because the person is not 'ideal' for the procedure.

SUMMARY

Chymopapain chemonucleolysis was found to be an effective means of providing relief of symptoms due to lumbar disc herniation. Of those patients who had definite neurological change in the form of reflex, sensory or motor disturbance, 74% had reverted to normal by the time of evaluation one year post injection. The most significant complication (anaphylaxis) was found in 1% of our first 500 patients but, after we started using preoperative steroids along with other safeguards, we were able to control this complication. It is still something to constantly be on guard against.

An extruded nucleus pulposus is not a contraindication in chemonucleolysis. A sequestrated one is (Glossary of spinal terminology, 1980).

Patients who have had previous low back surgery have a lower percentage of satisfactory results than those who have had no previous surgery. Chemonucleolysis does not prejudice the chances of a good clinical result in a subsequent open surgical procedure.

Pre-operative psychometric testing is a very effective predictor of results in relation to pain relief.

Studies in our laboratory again confirm beyond a doubt that, in the dog, injection of very large amounts of chymopapain in the epidural space of the lumbar spine has no effect on the subarachnoid contents, the dura, or the spinal nerves as they lie outside the dura and exit through the intervertebral foramina.

The rare case where there is a direct communication between the disc space and the subarachnoid space can be detected as the contrast medium is injected.

If by chance chymopapain were inadvertently injected intrathecally, the top dose of 8 mg which would be injected at any one level would be well within the tolerable range in the human being.

It is my belief that the procedure is safe and effective.

List of credits
This investigation was supported in part by research projects 135B–71 and 147C–72 from the Long Beach Memorial Hospital Medical Center Foundation, Long Beach, Cal.
Our thanks to:
Michael Edgar, M.D. of Stanmore, England who did the research on disc-space narrowing and its relation to subjective relief, while working at the Rancho Los Amigos Hospital, Downey, Ca.

Ann Hamilton, M.D. neuropathologist at the University of California, Irvine, for reviewing all of the gross and microscopic sections of the central nervous systems of the animals used in this study.

Dr Abdelmonen A. Afifi, Chairman of the Department of Biostatistics, University of California at Los Angeles for his assistance in the statistical studies.

Dr Richard A. Oas, Department of Radiology, Long Beach Memorial Hospital Medical Center for reviewing the myelograms.

Dr Ralph I. Druckman, neurologist, Long Beach Memorial Hospital Medical Center for reviewing the electromyograms.

Dr Patrick Rocchio, clinical psychologist, Long Beach Memorial Hospital Medical Center for supervising the clinical psychological examination of the patients in this study.

REFERENCES

Brown M 1982 Personal communication
Edgar M 1974 Personal communication
Ford L T 1969 Experimental study of chymopapain in cats. Clinical Orthopaedics 67: 68–71
Garvin P J, Jennings R B 1973 Long term effects of Chymopapain on Intervertebral Disks of Dogs. Clinical Orthopaedics 92: 281–95
Garvin, P J, Jennings, R B, Smith, L et al 1965 Chymopapain: A pharmacologic and toxicologic evolution in experimental animals. Clinical Orthopaedics 42: 204–223
Glossary of spinal terminology, American Academics of Orthopaedic Surgeons, 1980
Hakelius A 1970 Prognosis in sciatica. Acta Orthopaedica Scandinavica (Suppl) 128
Jansen E F, Balls A K 1941 Chymopapain: New crystalline proteinase from papaya latex. Journal of Biology Chemistry 137: 459
Kapsalis, A A, Stern I J Bornstein I: The fate of chymopapain injected for therapy of intervertebral disc disease. Journal of Laboratory Clinical Medicine 532–540
Kokan P 1982 Personal communication
Macnab I 1972 Personal communication
Naylor A 1982 Personal communication
Sorbie C 1981 Chemonucleolysis in the treatment of lumbar disc protrusion. CMA Journal, 124
Smith L 1963 Enzyme dissolution of the nucleus pulposus. Nature 198
Smith L 1964 Enzyme dissolution of nucleus pulposus in humans. Journal of the American Medical Association 187: 137
Smith L, Brown J E 1967 Treatment of lumbar intervertebral disc lesions by direct injection of chymopapain. Journal of Bone and Joint Surgery (Britain) 49B: 502
Smith L, Garvin P J, Gesler R M et al 1963 Enzyme dissolution of the nucleus pulposus. Nature 198: 1311–1312
Stern I J, Smith L 1967 Dissolution by chymopapain in vitro in tissue from normal or prolapsed intervertebral disc. Clinical Orthopaedics 50: 269–277
Stern I J 1969 Biochemistry of chymopapain. Clinical Orthopaedics 67: 42
Thomas L 1956 Reversible collapse of rabbit ears after intravenous papain, and prevention of recovery by cortisone. Journal of Experimental Medicine 104: 245
Wiltse L L, Widell Jr E H, Yuan H A 1975 Chymopapain chemonucleolysis in lumbar disk disease. Journal of the American Medical Association 231: 474–479
Wiltse L L 1978 Chemonucleolysis in the ideal candidate for laminectomy. Report to Spectator Club, June
Wiltse L L 196: Report to the research committee, Long Beach Memorial Hospital Medical Center

7. Chronic osteomyelitis in adults

P. J. Kelly

INTRODUCTION

This essay will discuss chronic osteomyelitis in adults. The major categories are: hematogenous osteomyelitis, osteomyelitis associated with fractures, and postoperative osteomyelitis. In an arbitrary fashion, closure of the growth plate is a convenient dividing line between adult and child. This chapter will deal with osteomyelitis of the femur and tibia. Past studies indicate that femoral and tibial osteomyelitis represent 77% of the osteomyelitis seen by the orthopaedic surgeon (West et al, 1970) at this clinic. Uncommon infections, such as the granulomatous, have been discussed by Pritchard (1975). Infections of the upper extremity, especially the hand, have been reviewed recently by Linscheid & Dobyns (1975). Osteomyelitis of the foot ordinarily represents a complication of diabetes mellitus or circulatory disease (Kelly, 1972).

CLASSIFICATION AND INCIDENCE OF OSTEOMYELITIS

Chronic hematogenous osteomyelitis for the years 1951 through 1961 accounted for 44% of osteomyelitis of the femur and tibia. A review of this category of osteomyelitis for the years 1967 through 1980 reveals an incidence of 28% when averaged for these 14 years.

Almost invariably, these patients date the onset of infection to childhood. A flare-up of the infection may occur after a long period of quiescence. Interestingly, in a majority of these patients (60%), deep cultures at surgery show a staphylococcus that is susceptible to penicillin G.

Acute hematogenous osteomyelitis is uncommon in adults. However, acute osteomyelitis in drug addicts, especially with involvement of the spine, has been reported (Wiesseman et al, 1973). In 1979 we saw seven patients with osteomyelitis of hematogenous origin. Four of these dated their original infection to an episode of osteomyelitis from 40 to 55 years prior to consultation at this clinic. However, two patients (age 17 and 24) were diagnosed with osteomyelitis of hematogenous origin with a duration of 4 and 6 months, respectively. In the 7th patient (age 69), osteomyelitis developed in association with long-standing ulcerative colitis. There is nothing in the histories of any of these patients to directly implicate drug abuse as a cause of the osteomyelitis.

Osteomyelitis associated with a united fracture has remained at an incidence of about 40%. This incidence was observed for the years 1953–1961, and from 1967–1980 the average was 37.5% when plotted on a yearly basis. No trend seems apparent.

As regards nonunion associated with osteomyelitis, the incidence for the years 1953–1961 was 16%, while for the years 1967–1980 the average was 28%. Postoperative or post-traumatic chronic osteomyelitis not associated with fractures represents a small fraction of osteomyelitis and averaged only 7% for the years 1967–1980; this is very similar to the incidence in the series reported for the years 1953–1962, which was 8.6%.

The total number of patients of all categories seen during this 14-year period is 298, with the yearly average being approximately 21 patients with chronic osteomyelitis of the femur and tibia.

MICROBIOLOGY

Since the last review (Kelly, 1977) of chronic osteomyelitis from this clinic, the pattern has changed very little. The predominant organism cultured is *Staphylococcus aureus* in about 40%; in 18% the infection is polymicrobic — that is, *S. aureus* and gram-negative rods. About 30% of the positive cultures grew gram-negative rods. The remaining category includes anaerobic organisms such as *Corynebacterium diphtheriae* or *Propionibacterium acnes* (Morrey et al, 1977). Regarding isolates of gram-negative rods, the most common species were *Pseudomonas* sp., *Proteus mirabilis*, *Enterobacter* sp., and *Escherichia coli*, in that order of frequency. This pattern again varies little from the last report from this clinic in 1977.

SURGICAL MANAGEMENT

In viewing osteomyelitis of a long bone, in particular that involving the femur or tibia, certain objectives are evident. The first is removal of any dead bone. Sequestra that are retained in a cavity will keep osteomyelitis smoldering for years. Often as a consequence of removal of dead, devitalized, and infected bone, a sizeable cavity or 'dead space' will exist. Therefore, the second objective is consideration of a method to obliterate any dead space. When one deals with an infection of soft tissue, after debridement or drainage of an abscess the soft tissue collapses to fill in the defect. On the other hand, bone, a very rigid structure, does not collapse and scar as does soft tissue. Therefore, a method of obliterating dead space can be a very major aspect of the surgical considerations. A third objective is to obtain soft tissue coverage of exposed bone. Often this is part of the objective of obliterating dead space. Table 7.1 lists the surgical procedures that have been employed to manage chronic osteomyelitis in 213 patients during the period 1971–1980. Fundamentally, the surgical procedure is designed to obtain closure and obliteration of dead space. This includes patients who have had bone grafts in order to fill in a defect. In these patients, finely divided bone grafts of cancellous bone are employed to fill a saucerized cavity. The technique is often termed a Papineau procedure (Papineau, 1973).

Suction irrigation and delayed closure

A review of the data in Table 7.1 indicates that approximately 46% of the patients were treated by closure over suction irrigation tubes. After an initial enthusiastic reception for this technique, it became apparent that the method, although useful, has some serious drawbacks. First, it is not a technique for the delivery of antibiotics to a

CHRONIC OSTEOMYELITIS IN ADULTS   121

Table 7.1 Patients (213) and surgical procedures (220)* 1971–1980

Year	Closure with suction irrigation	Delayed closure	Free flap	Muscle pedicle	Bone graft	Secondary intent	Skin graft	Patients (No. of procedures)
1971	16					2	2	20 (20)
1972	10	1				3	7	23 (23)
1973	11				2	2		13 (13)
1974	14						3	17 (17)
1975	14	4		2	1	3	1	25 (25)
1976	6	4			1	7		18 (18)
1977	10	3		6	1			23 (23)
1978	6	5		10	1		3	23 (23)
1979	2	3	1	11†	5†	1	1	24 (26)
1980	12†	2	6†	9	2	1	3	27 (32)

* Represents patients with hematogenous, fracture with union, or posttraumatic or postsurgical chronic osteomyelitis.
† Multiple procedures.
For the years 1974–1979, those treated with suction irrigation had a successful arrest of infection of 92%. For the years 1974–1979, for all other forms of treatment (delayed closure, free flap, muscle pedicle, bone graft, secondary intent and skin graft), when these were considered as a single group the arrest rate was 86%.

bone. Parenteral administration of antibacterials is the route of choice. With certain nephrotoxic antimicrobials, irrigation of freshly saucerized long bone can lead to levels in the bloodstream that are toxic. The suction irrigation technique can allow entry of organisms into the saucerized cavity and can lead to superinfection. For this reason a note of warning — the suction irrigation method is useful mainly as an addendum to a delayed closure four to five days after initial saucerization of the wound. The principal effect is to minimize accumulation of wound hematoma and to draw soft tissues into the saucerized cavity. The irrigation and suction should be limited to a period of three to four days. One might argue that simply a delayed closure with simple drainage and no irrigation could accomplish the same thing. A review of Table 7.1 suggests that this is a choice elected by the surgeon in a sizeable percentage of patients.

A delayed closure with suction irrigation or simply a drain seems most suitable for diaphyseal osteomyelitis, if soft tissues are suitable, especially in non-union or hematogenous osteomyelitis. If the closure 'tents' over the saucerized cavity much like a drum, then it is likely that failure will occur, especially if the soft tissues and skin are tight at the time of closure.

Free flap (composite graft and microsurgery)
The experience with this technique is growing at this clinic, and Drs M. Wood and W. Cooney of our division of hand surgery provide the expertise to accomplish this demanding technique. Figure 7.1 illustrates a difficult problem in a young man with bone loss and persistent drainage following a crushing injury to the proximal tibia. Osteosynthesis was obtained by bone grafts placed posteriorly between the tibia and the fibula. However, a large cavity in the proximal and anteromedial leg region persistently drained. A composite graft from the latissimus dorsi region was vascularized by microsurgical methods and yielded a brilliant result for the patient. At this time, as Table 7.1 reveals, follow-up on this category is insufficient for evaluation of this method.

Muscle pedicle grafts
Twenty-eight muscle pedicle procedures were performed from 1971 through 1979. Twenty-one involved the tibia and seven the femur. For assessment of effectiveness, at least a two-year follow-up is required; for that reason, it is too early to evaluate patients who were treated in 1980. In only three instances was the method considered a failure, and in the remaining 25 there was no clinical evidence of infection after two years or more. The technique employed at this clinic has been reviewed by Woods et al (1977) and Irons et al (1980).

Technically, the method is ideal for management of defects involving the diaphysis of the tibia. The muscle is freed up, with particular attention to preservation of the blood supply to the muscle. Figure 7.2 illustrates the procedure in a diagrammatic fashion. If skin closure is not easily performed, it is preferable to skin graft the surface of the muscle graft with a meshed graft of split skin. The gastrocnemius muscle seems best suited for proximal tibial defects and the soleus for distal tibial defects.

Bone grafts
Employment of bone grafts has to be viewed in two contexts: first, as a method of

CHRONIC OSTEOMYELITIS IN ADULTS   123

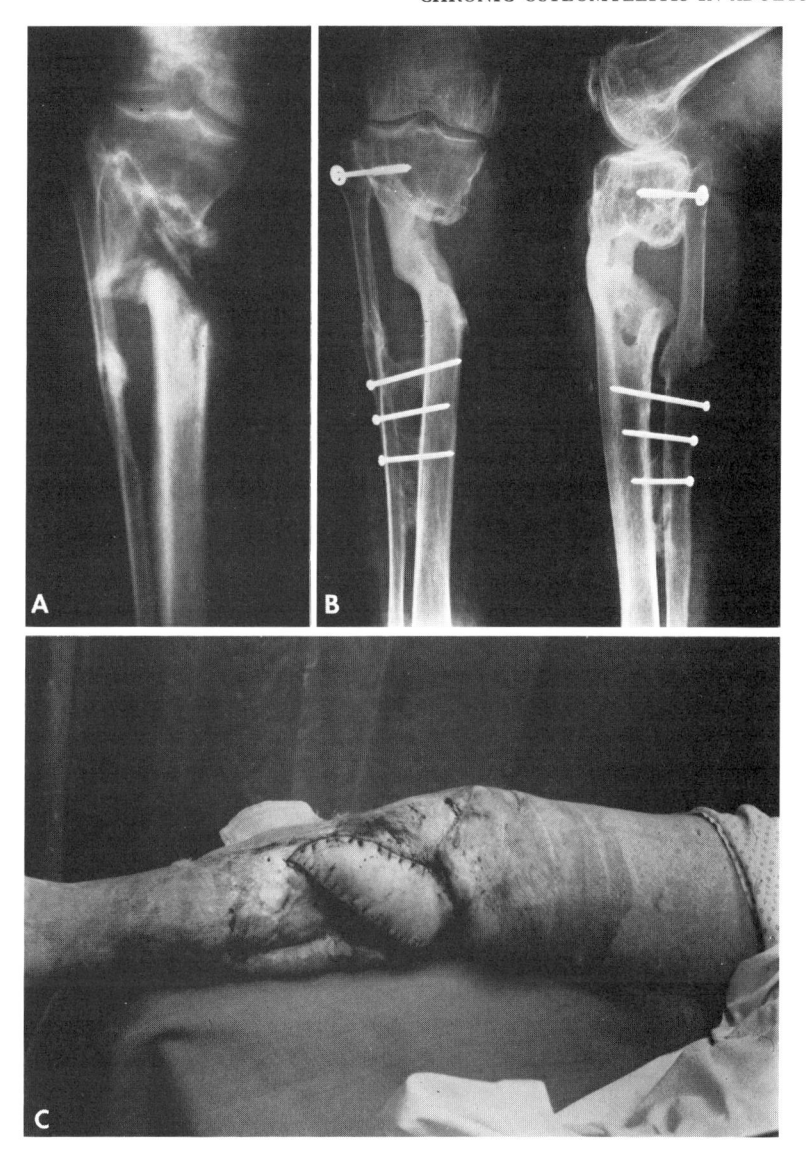

Fig. 7.1 (A) & (B)   Bone graft to infected nonunion. Procedure performed by a posterior approach. (C) Free flap covered soft tissue defect anteriorly.

obliterating a defect or dead space after saucerization; second, to establish union if nonunion exists. It is for the management of a chronically draining osteomyelitis that the greatest interest has been shown recently in this technique. As mentioned, the eponym Papineau is used frequently at this institution to describe this procedure. The technique was employed extensively in World War II on military casualties (Rhinelander, 1975).

The infected area is saucerized and then packed open until the entire cavity has become covered with healthy granulations. Then the cavity is filled with fine cancellous bone. Cortical bone should be avoided. In the category of patients so

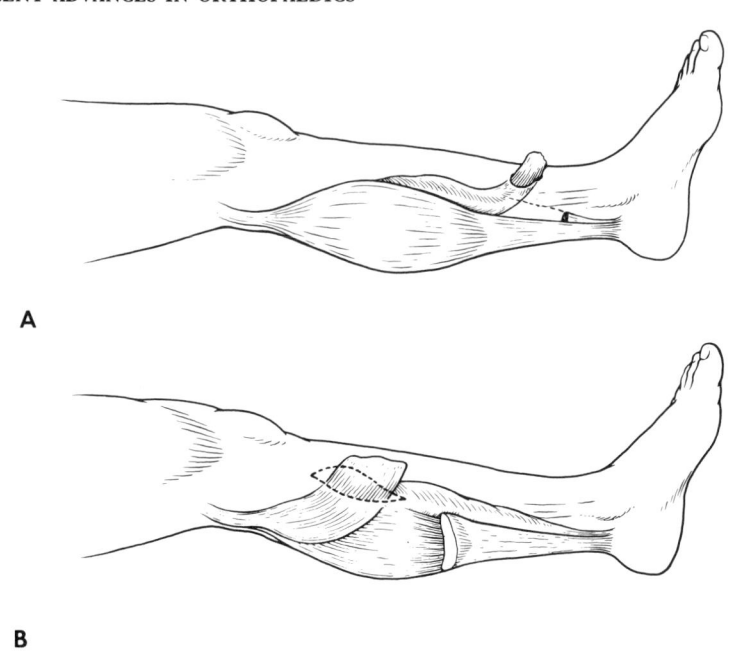

Fig. 7.2 (A) Soleal muscle flap for coverage of a distal tibial saucerized cavity. (B) Gastrocnemius flap for coverage of a more proximal cavity. (From Woods J E, Irons G B Jr, Masson J K 1977 Use of muscular, musculocutaneous, and omental flaps to reconstruct difficult defects. Plastic and Reconstructive Surgery 59: 191–199. By permission of the American Society of Plastic and Reconstructive Surgeons.)

treated there is often lack of sufficient soft tissue for closure. Therefore, the technique has its greatest utility in obliterating deep cavities in the ends of long bones. The surgeon must be patient and wait until clean granulation tissue lines the cavity. The bone grafts are prepared from cancellous bone and should be in uniform small pieces. Unless this requirement is followed, the bone grafts will not revascularize. The method appears promising for the most difficult osteomyelitis of the tibia and femur, those infections involving the ends of a long bone.

Secondary intent

Saucerizing an infected area and allowing it to heal by secondary intent is a most ancient technique. As Table 7.1 illustrates, the method has been resorted to less often recently; only two patients were managed in this fashion during 1977–1980. It will continue to be employed as a method of last resort. However, at this time other methods should be considered if at all possible; if technically possible, composite grafts and microsurgery may be the choice or, alternatively, the use of bone grafting without closure.

The employment of a split-thickness graft to cover a saucerized cavity, if shallow, is a reasonable technique. The disadvantage is that the skin is laid on granulation bone and leaves an unstable scar. Subsequent minor trauma often injures this poor covering and leads to recurrence of ulcers. For this reason, if it is feasible, one of the other methods of obtaining coverage is preferable.

MANAGEMENT OF NONUNION

An evaluation of success or failure of the category of osteomyelitis with nonunion is summarized in Table 7.2. It includes patients treated from 1971 through 1979. The patients evaluated are summarized as to treatment and results. There were 45 patients, 10 with nonunion of the femur and 35 with nonunion of the tibia.

Table 7.2 Infected nonunions (1971–1979)

Procedure	No. of procedures	No. known successful	No. known failures
Femur (10 procedures)			
Intramedullary fixation	5	5*	0
External fixation	2	1	1
Immediate bone graft	1	0	1
Saucerization only	1	1	0
Compression plate	1	1	0
Tibia (35 procedures)			
Saucerization (brace or cast)	10	6	4
Saucerization (external fixation)	7	6	1
Saucerization (delayed bone graft)	9†	8	0‡
Saucerization (immediate bone graft)	9	6	3

* Two with supplemental iliac bone graft
† Delay of 12 weeks or more
‡ Lost to follow-up

These data support the view that initial saucerization of the infected bone and then delayed bone grafting gives superior results to saucerization and early bone grafting. Immediate bone grafting — that is, within a few days or weeks of saucerization — failed in one instance when used in a femoral nonunion and in three of nine instances when used in tibial nonunions. Review of the records suggests that of the four failures, three of the procedures were poorly conceived in the light of present knowledge; that is, not enough care had been taken in preparing the area for bone grafting and using finely divided cancellous bone combined with a suitable external fixator. Treatment of a nonunion can be successful if, after complete saucerization, stability is achieved by a brace or cast, external fixation, or even intramedullary nailing without bone grafting. Failure in this category of patients is in the main due to failure to control the infection.

ANTIBACTERIAL AGENTS IN THE MANAGEMENT OF OSTEOMYELITIS

Treatment of bone infections with antibiotics is one of the major advances in this century. Before the introduction of antibiotics, one-third of the patients died of acute hematogenous osteomyelitis, and a high proportion of patients with chronic osteomyelitis came to amputation. In this clinic, successful treatment of chronic osteomyelitis (arrest for two years of evident infection) was about 50% for the patients seen from 1951 to 1963. Since we began a regimen of four weeks of parenteral antibiotic therapy, the rate of success in recent years has been nearly 90% for chronic osteomyelitis in the categories of hematogenous infection, postoperative (exclusive of fracture) osteomyelitis, and osteomyelitis in united fractures (Table 7.2), and it is 78% for osteomyelitis associated with nonunion. It would be difficult to prove that this was attributable to a standardized regimen of antibacterial treatment. On reflection, however, it seems likely that careful selection of antibacterial agents based on sensitivity determination of the organisms cultured from the depths of the osteomyelitis focus is an important aspect of treatment. The regimen used, when possible, is four weeks of parenteral therapy and eight weeks of oral therapy if in vitro susceptibility tests and the choice of antibacterials does not contraindicate such a regimen.

The polymicrobic nature of chronic osteomyelitis may require more than one antibacterial agent. If the flora changes, selection of the antibacterial may need to be changed also. It is the patients with residual infections, especially those due to species of *Pseudomonas*, *Proteus*, *Enterobacter*, and *Escherichia*, who are the most difficult to treat.

Antibiotics exert their effect in tissue in the interstitial fluid space. The degree of lipophilia and the molecular weight influence movement of antibacterials across the capillary and into the interstitial fluid space. Furthermore, antibacterials can probably be best monitored in bone by plasma assay (Bloom et al, 1980). Transport in osteomyelitic bone is similar to that observed in normal bone (Hall et al, 1980).

Therefore, circumstantial evidence favours the use of antibacterial agents for the treatment of osteomyelitis, and there is no barrier to transport of antibacterials into bone.

INFECTION IN BONE AND METAL FIXATION

How should the surgeon view internal fixation and infection? Should internal fixation be removed in the face of osteomyelitis? If the fixation is offering stability to a fracture, the fixation can be left in until union occurs. If the fixation is loose and not efficient, it should be removed and another form of fixation employed if casts or braces are unsuitable (Fig. 7.3). External fixation has been used at this clinic for years (Fig. 7.4) and may be the only treatment needed to obtain union following saucerization of an infected nonunion. Ordinarily, after the fracture has healed, the fixation will have to be removed.

An evaluation of fracture site fixation in a dog model (Rand et al, 1981) with external fixation is underway at this clinic. Our initial experiments have been with a Sukhtian-Hughes fixator compared with a dynamic compression plate (Lewallen et al, 1982). Although the external fixator is not as rigid a fixation device as a plate, it does offer enough fixation to allow healing.

SUMMARY

Treatment of chronic osteomyelitis demands a combined approach; that is, it is a surgical problem and a condition requiring experience with a powerful array of drugs — antimicrobials. Treatment has advanced in the last 20 years, and it would appear that arrest of the infection and return to useful activity can be expected in the vast majority of patients.

CHRONIC OSTEOMYELITIS IN ADULTS 127

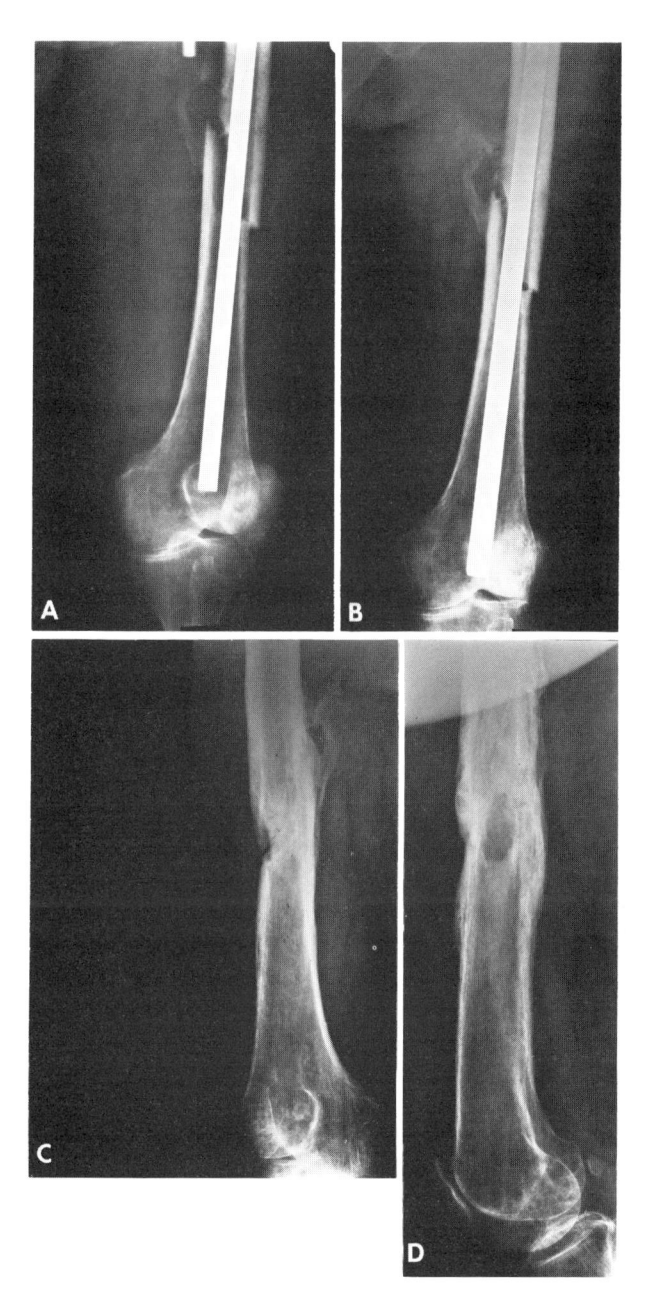

Fig. 7.3 (A) Infected femoral nonunion with a loose intramedullary nail. (B) Replacement with a tighter-fitting nail. (C) Anterior and (D) lateral views after removal of intramedullary nail.

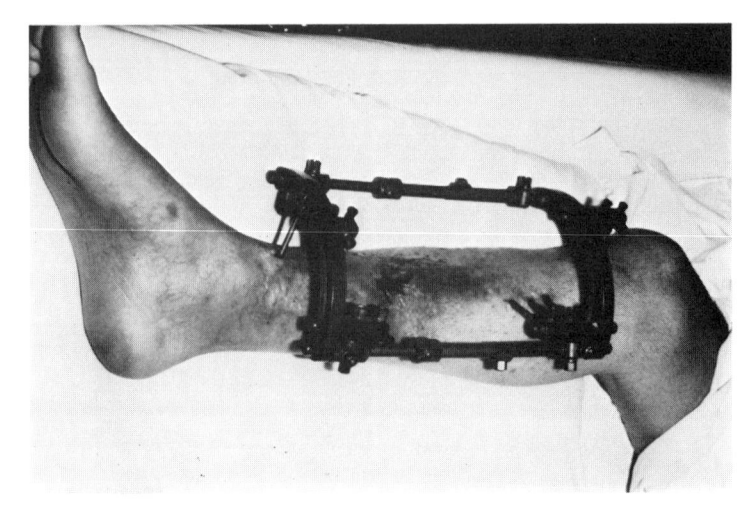

Fig. 7.4 Presently, an external fixator (Fischer type) is probably a better method of achieving stability of an infected ununited diaphyseal fracture.

Since the last review from this clinic in 1977, the changes that are worth noting are:
1. the reintroduction of muscle flaps to obtain closure of saucerized wounds;
2. the introduction of more efficient external fixation devices to treat unstable infected nonunions;
3. the promising early results from cancellous bone grafting of carefully prepared saucerized cavities in osteomyelitic bone;
4. the development of methods for the study of transcapillary transport and distribution of antibiotics in bone.

REFERENCES

Bloom J D, Fitzgerald R H Jr, Washington J AII, Kelly P J 1980 The transcapillary passage and interstitial fluid concentration of penicillin in canine bone. Journal of Bone and Joint Surgery. American Volume 62: 1168–1175

Hall B B, Fitzgerald R H Jr, Kelly P J, Washington J A II 1980 Pharmacokinetics of penicillin in canine osteomyelitic bone (abstract). Orthopaedic Transactions 4: 175

Irons G B, Arnold P G, Masson J K, Woods J E 1980 Experience with 100 muscle flaps. Annals of Plastic Surgery 4: 2–6

Kelly P J 1972 Orthopedic principles of amputation, rehabilitation, and skin grafting in occlusive arterial disease. In: Fairbairn J F II, Juergens J L, Spittell J A Jr (eds) Allen-Barker-Hines peripheral vascular diseases, 4th edn. W B Saunders Company, Philadelphia, p 707

Kelly P J 1977 Infections of bones and joints in adult patients. Instructional Course Lectures, American Academy of Orthopaedic Surgeons 26: 3–13

Lewallen D G, Chao E Y S, Kelly P J 1982 External skeletal fixation vs. dynamic compression plating of canine tibial fractures: a comparison of the biomechanics, histology, and physiology of fracture healing. Present at the Twenty-Eighth Annual Meeting of the Orthopaedic Research Society, New Orleans, Louisiana, January 19 to 21

Linscheid R L, Dobyns J H 1975 Common and uncommon infections of the hand. Orthopedic Clinics of North America 6, no. 4: 1063–1104

Morrey B F, Fitzgerald R H Jr, Kelly P J, Dobyns J H, Washington J A II 1977 Diphtheroid osteomyelitis. Journal of Bone and Joint Surgery. American Volume 59: 527–530

Papineau L-J 1973 L'excision-greffe avec fermeture retardée délibérée dans l'ostéomyélite chronique. Nouvelle Presse Medicale 2: 2753–2755

Pritchard D J 1975 Granulomatous infections of bones and joints. Orthopedic Clinics of North America 6, no. 4: 1029–1047

Rand J A, An K N, Chao E Y S, Kelly P J 1981 A comparison of the effect of open intramedullary nailing and compression-plate fixation on fracture-site blood flow and fracture union. Journal of Bone and Joint Surgery. American Volume 63: 427–442

Rhinelander F W 1975 Minimal internal fixation of tibial fractures. Clinical Orthopaedics and Related Research 107: 188–220

West W F, Kelly P J, Martin W J 1970 Chronic osteomyelitis. I. Factors affecting the results of treatment in 186 patients. Journal of the American Medical Association 213: 1837–1842

Wiesseman G J, Wood V E, Kroll L L 1973 Pseudomonas vertebral osteomyelitis in heroin addicts: report of five cases. Journal of Bone and Joint Surgery. American Volume 55: 1416–1424

Woods J E, Irons G B Jr, Masson J K 1977 Use of muscular, musculocutaneous, and omental flaps to reconstruct difficult defects. Plastic and Reconstructive Surgery 59: 191–199

8: The electrical stimulation of bone healing in cases of nonunion and delayed union

J. Watson

INTRODUCTION

In 1853 the US Medical Times and Gazette described how a Mr Holl, House Surgeon at York County Hospital, had treated an ununited fracture of more than a year's duration (Stillings, 1974). Apparently he 'introduced a needle from each side of the limb into the interspace between the bones, and then passed a continuous galvanic current through. The operation was repeated every day for about a fortnight, and a cure ultimately resulted'.

A few years ago, a natural reaction to such a report might have been to dismiss it as yet another example of nineteenth century quackery, but recently, impressive and well-documented evidence has shown that just such a system is capable of producing union in some 70 to 80% of cases treated. Unfortunately, the scientific basis of this and associated forms of electrical treatment is still obscure in spite of the wide-ranging investigations of the past two decades.

Surgically, a number of clinical tests of various systems has been carried out, and in order to appreciate the factors and protocols involved, it is necessary to have some familiarity with basic electrical phenomena and how they are produced.

BASIC ELECTRICAL PHENOMENA

An electrical circuit is said to be linear if it obeys Ohm's Law; that is, if the electric current flowing is directly proportional to the voltage applied. (In hydraulic terms, this can be thought of as analagous to the flow of water in a pipe being proportional to the pump pressure applied.) If the voltage is V volts, and the current is I amps, then for a linear system V/I is a constant called the resistance of the circuit R ohms (Fig. 8.1).

If the cross-sectional area A of the circuit at some point is taken, then a current density J could be calculated:

$$J = \frac{I}{A} \text{ amps per unit area (assuming a perfectly homogenous current flow in the material).} \quad (1)$$

If living tissue obeyed Ohm's Law, then simple calculations such as that above could be adapted to define the current density at any point between two implanted electrodes, having regard for the geometry of the system. However, as soon as a voltage is applied between two such electrodes, various electrochemical processes take place, including polarization, which severely limit the current. Also, though it is technically possible to force a higher current to flow, it is still extremely difficult to determine current density at a given point, partly because of the heterogeneous nature

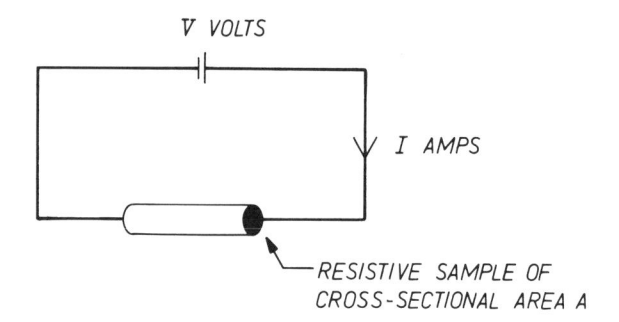

Fig. 8.1 Ideal specimen obeying Ohm's law (Total resistance of sample R = V/I)

of living tissues, each component of which presents a different (average) resistance. Consequently, it is not possible, except in hypothetical 'ideal' cases, to determine the distribution of the current flow in a living system. This accounts for the fact that most reports have quoted only values of current magnitude as opposed to values of current density, even though the latter would be expected to have the greater electro-biological significance.

Although it has been found that the *passage* of current across a nonunion can be efficacious in stimulating healing, the most successful methods involve actually placing the (negative) electrode between the bone ends. Here, consistent osteogenesis is observed very close to the electrode surface itself.

In addition to the use of smooth one-way or *direct current*, fluctuating direct current has also been employed, as has true *alternating current* in which a series of current direction reversals occur (Hassler et al, 1977, 1979; Spadaro, 1977).

There are three methods of providing current to electrodes. Firstly, a battery pack may be implanted along with the electrodes; or the electrodes may be inserted percutaneously with the power pack mounted externally; or finally, an implanted coil may have a current *induced* in it via a pulsing magnetic field generated externally. The latter technique — magnetic induction — may also be used to induce a current within the tissues themselves without involving electrodes or any other implanted devices whatsoever. A brief description of magnetic induction now follows.

A magnetic field is always produced by a current-carrying wire, and takes the form shown in Figure 8.2a if that current-carrying wire is formed into a coil. If two such coils are juxtaposed parallel to each other and carry the same current, then they can produce a common magnetic field as depicted in Figure 8.2b. If the coil diameters are greater than their distance apart, they form a *Helmholz Pair*, and the magnetic field near their common axis is very uniform.

An alternative way to define the location of a magnetic field is to wind a coil of wire around a core of magnetic material (such as soft iron), in which case the two ends of this core are known as the *poles* and the whole arrangement is an *electromagnet*. In the case of a C-shaped core as shown in Figure 8.2c, the magnetic field will be largely non-uniform except for a small region half-way along the axis between the poles. The magnetic material itself can be thought of as concentrating most of the magnetic field within its boundaries (apart from leakage, which is usually quite large) and this field bulges out into the space between the poles as is also shown in Figure 8.2c.

If an aqueous-based material of moderate electrical conductivity, such as living

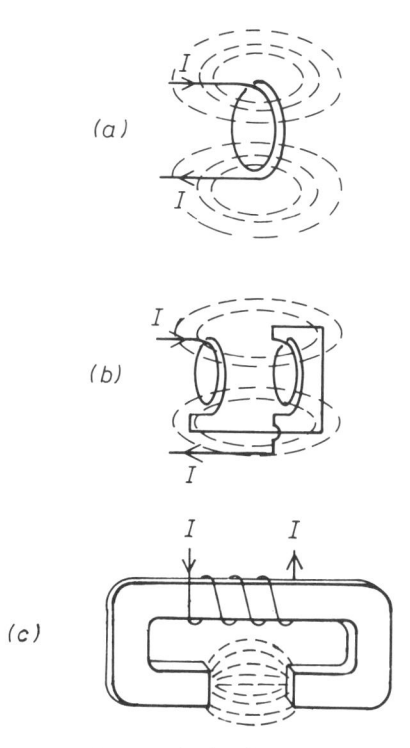

Fig. 8.2 Magnetic fields produced by (a) a single coil (b) a Helmholz pair and (c) an electromagnet

tissue, is placed in a magnetic field — either between the coils of a Helmholz Pair or between the poles of an electromagnet — then provided the field is constant there will be no observable effect: the field will simply permeate the material. However, should the field change, then during the time it is actually in process of changing, an electric current will be induced within the material. Figure 8.3, which represents a limb containing a fracture, shows that this induced current actually rotates around the axis of the magnetic field, and in fact, the direction of rotation is dependent upon whether the field is rising or falling. Thus, if the magnetic field is continuously pulsing, then the induced current pulses rotate in each direction successively.

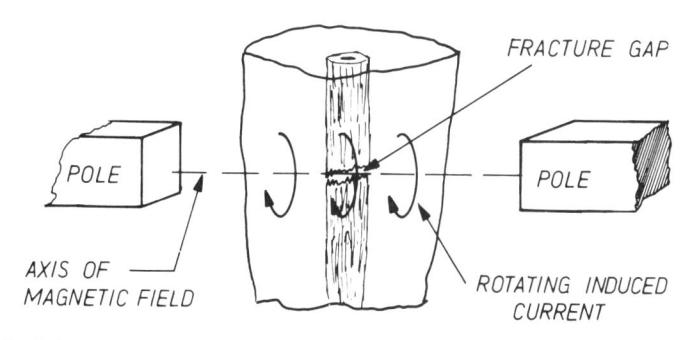

Fig. 8.3 Idealised sketch showing induced currents rotating about magnetic-field axis in limb with fractured long bone

Strictly speaking, a voltage is produced which is directly proportional to the rate of change of the magnetic field; and if the material is purely resistive, a current flows which is proportional to that voltage:

$$i \propto v \propto \frac{d\Phi}{dt} \qquad (2)$$

In a resistive material, there will actually be a *voltage gradient*, measured in volts per unit length. This is called an *electric* field E, and it can be measured by inserting a calibrated search coil into the magnetic field, and measuring the voltage appearing between its ends. The current density is then given by:

$$J = E/\varrho \qquad (3)$$

where ϱ is the resistivity of the material.

In order to pulse the magnetic field, the current through the field-producing coils must also be pulsed — in fact, the shape of the magnetic field wave is identical to that of the current producing it. Usually, a voltage waveform is applied across the coil in order to accomplish this, and Figure 8.4 shows what happens when a square voltage wave is applied to the two systems under consideration.

In Figure 8.4a, it will be seen that the current I in the coil follows the voltage V across it almost exactly, and it can be assumed that the magnetic field waveform has the same shape as this current waveform. The induced current i will appear only whilst the magnetic field is changing, so that a series of sharp current pulses appear as shown, and these decay rapidly.

In Figure 8.4b it will be seen that the coil current I rises much more slowly than does the voltage, and this results from a phenonenon known as *inductance*, which is very much greater in a system with an iron core than in one without. The coil current rises and falls exponentially as shown, and hence, so does the magnetic field. This in turn results in an induced current which takes the form depicted: at any point, its magnitude is proportional to the rate-of-change of the field. The final result is that whereas the current induced by the core-less coils is high but lasts a short time, that in the iron-cored system is lower in magnitude, but lasts longer.

In practice, the inductance of the core-less coils can be increased by using a large number of turns, and that for the electromagnet can be reduced by judicious choice of the magnetic material and its dimensions. So, should it be so desired, the performance of each can be made quite similar to the other, within limits.

The magnitude of the induced current i is proportional *only* to the rate-of-change of the magnetic field, and not to the field strength itself. Thus, a magnetic field which rises from zero to a few gauss* very rapidly will induce a larger instantaneous current than will a field which rises to (say) several hundred gauss, but slowly. When the field falls, the direction of the induced current reverses, as indicated by those portions of the i-waveform below the horizontal axis. In Figure 8.4, these 'negative' pulses are symmetric with their 'positive' counterparts, but this is solely because the waveform of the magnetic field is assumed to fall at the same rate as it rises. If this field were to fall more slowly than it rose, the 'negative' parts of the induced current would be lower in magnitude, but longer in time. In fact, the area under the i-waveform below

---

* The gauss is a convenient, albeit old-fashioned unit of magnetic field strength. The modern (SI) unit is the Tesla, which is 10 000 gauss.

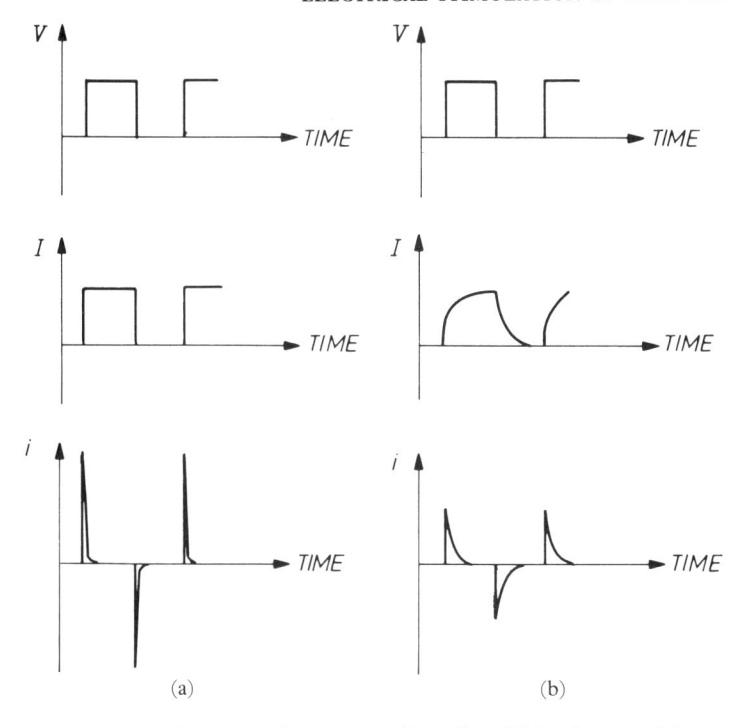

Fig. 8.4 Application of a square voltage wave to (a) a coil, and (b) an iron-cored electromagnet

the horizontal axis must always be identical to that above it on average. Asymmetric waveforms have been used in some stimulatory equipment, and will be further described later.

The induced current so far described has been assumed to flow in the material which lies in the magnetic field. However, if a coil of (highly conductive) wire is implanted within that material, then a *secondary voltage* will be induced within that coil, and this can be used to drive a spatially more concentrated current between two electrodes connected to the coil ends. By this means it is possible to produce an electrode system which is powered via the magnetic field rather than by either an implanted or an external battery pack. This current is inherently alternating, though it is possible to make it unidirectional by the inclusion of a rectifier in the secondary coil circuit.

Based on the technology so far outlined, several different forms of stimulatory apparatus have been developed, all of which depend upon a very tenuous body of bioelectrical theory and experiment, and this will first be considered.

THE BASIS OF BIOELECTRICAL BONE STIMULATION

When bone is stressed, it produces an electrical charge separation (that is, a voltage), and in terms of a whole long bone under bending, this voltage appears as shown in Figure 8.5. The source of the voltage is widely held to be due to the phenomenon of piezoelectricity, and a large amount of evidence has been accumulated for this, ranging from early reports (Fukada and Yasuda, 1957; Bassett & Becker, 1962) to

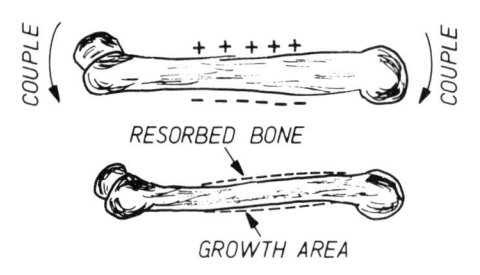

Fig. 8.5 Stressed bone showing charge separation (upper) and growth pattern (lower) according to Wolff's Law

very subtle interpretations based on investigations at the osteonic level (El Messiery, 1981). However, there is also evidence that another phenomenon, that of streaming potentials, is also at least contributory, and this mechanism has been reported to be particularly relevant to wet bone (Ericsson, 1976; Pienkowsky & Pollack, 1981; William & Gross, 1981).

The mechanism by which stress-generated voltages appear is of secondary importance clinically speaking; the major point is that these voltages have been postulated as mediating the stress remodelling of bone described by Wolff's Law (Bassett & Becker, 1962; Bassett, 1971), as is indicated in Figure 8.5.

To test this suggestion, battery packs were used to drive small currents between electrodes implanted through the cortices of dog femora, and bone growth was observed — predominantly near the negative electrode — within the intermedullary cavity (Bassett, Pawluk & Becker, 1964).

This work led to a large number of very diverse experiments being carried out in succeeding years, using various models and sundry forms of electrical stimulation. A survey (Hassler et al, 1977) concluded that there was little to choose between direct or alternating current methods, or between the various waveforms employed in the latter cases (Hassler et al, 1977; Spadaro, 1977). However, it did become evident that certain current levels (usually some 5 to 20 microamps) were more efficacious than others in mediating osteogenesis; and that higher current levels (approaching 100 microamps) could lead to tissue necrosis, particularly at the positive electrode.

Most of the reports dealt with current levels, rather than current densities, because the latter are very difficult to determine, as has been pointed out. However, there was a remarkable consistency discernable, to the effect that irrespective of the geometry of each system (including the electrode surface areas), the above-mentioned current levels of 5 to 20 μA continued to be the most efficacious. It has only recently been suggested that the solution to this unlikely agreement may be that the initial surface area presented by each electrode is rapidly covered by a film of organic material except for a small remaining active region which gives rise to a current density of the order of 1 milliamp per square millimetre (Black & Brighton, 1979). This is considerably greater than would be expected at the electrode surface as calculated simplistically from equation (1).

In addition to the empirical establishment of optimum current levels, investigations relating to electrode positioning have shown that the best results appear to be obtained when the negative electrode is placed actually within the fracture gap itself (Friedenberg et al, 1971), as has been mentioned. This results in osteogenesis very close to the electrode surface, and again suggests that not only current flow, but electrochemical reactions may be involved. For example, it has been suggested that oxygen depletion near the negative electrode, and an increased pH level due to the production of hydroxyl radicals may be involved (Brighton et al, 1977; Black & Brighton, 1977). Also, it has been shown that if a silver electrode is used at a positive potential, silver ions are released, which are bactericidal. Hence, the possibility arises of first using the electrode in this way to reduce infection, then reversing the polarity to stimulate osteogenesis (Becker, Spadaro & Marino, 1977; Becker & Spadaro, 1978).

Although the various models have shown that osteogenesis may indeed be stimulated by electrical phenomena, the relationship between these models and the initial concept involving Wolff's Law, has become increasingly tenuous. Indeed, it is difficult to see what stress-related remodelling has to do with fractures, which are certainly not subject to stressing in their early stages. However, it is at least conceivable that some naturally-occurring electrical phenomenon may be involved here too, and in this context, measurements of skin potentials appearing over the anterior tibial surface for both normal and fractured tibiae have been made (Friedenberg & Brighton, 1966), in which negative-going dips were observed over the fracture. More comprehensive measurements are presently under way (Watson, 1979), for it may be that such voltage patterns could be related also to the normal resorption/deposition balance, apart from which an eventual clinical apparatus may have value in the determination of the progress of fracture healing.

At a more basic level, *in vitro* experiments are beginning to contribute somewhat to an understanding of preosteogenic mechanisms. For example, it has been reported that pulsed electric fields (which imply pulsed high voltages applied between two plate electrodes insulated from the experimenal material) can lead to increased production of collagen in mouse fibroblasts (Bassett & Herrman, 1968) and to morphological changes in rat calvaria (Norton & Moore, 1972) and embryonic chick tibiae (Watson, de Haas & Hauser, 1975); and that also in the chick tibia model, pulsed magnetic fields can result in both the inhibition of chondrogenesis and the stimulation of calcification (Archer & Ratcliffe, 1981; Fitton-Jackson et al, 1981).

The work described so far is quintessentially empirical, and though some very basic electrochemically-oriented studies have begun (Pilla, 1981), the fundamental bioelectricial mechanisms relating to the stimulation of osteogenesis remain obscure. Nevertheless, various forms of apparatus for the treatment of non-union have been developed, and a survey of these now follows.

ELECTRICAL BONE STIMULATION

The various forms of apparatus which have been used to stimulate healing in cases of nonunion can be categorized under headings which relate to the number and type of operative procedures which must be carried out. Thus, the term 'doubly-invasive' means that two procedures must be carried out, as where a battery pack must be both implanted and removed; 'semi-invasive' means that electrodes may be inserted percutaneously (usually under local anaesthetic); and 'non-invasive' implies that no surgical procedure whatsoever is necessary.

Note that in all cases, the application of electrical stimulation is relevant to nonunion or delayed union: the acceleration of normally-healing fractures is (at the time of writing) regarded as not proven (Becker, Spadaro & Marino, 1977; Connolly, Hahn & Jardon, 1977; De Haas, Lazarovici & Morrison, 1979), though some reports to the effect that acceleration is possible have appeared (Jorgensen, 1977; Shim, 1981).

Doubly-invasive procedures

The technique of complete implantation of apparatus which will produce direct current at the site of a nonunion is at present represented by two commercially-available devices, the Telectronics Osteostim™ and the DePuy Orthofuse™.

The Osteostim™ has its origins in work performed in Australia on the use of direct current in spinal fusions (Dwyer & Wickham, 1974), and later on long bone nonunions (Paterson, Lewis & Cass, 1980). It is available in both single and quadruple cathode versions for long-bone and spinal use respectively (Lunceford, 1981a; Kane, 1981) and the former is shown in Figure 8.6. It consists of a cylindrical titanium case (hereafter called the power pack) some 11 mm in diameter by 53 mm long, from one end of which projects the cathode lead.

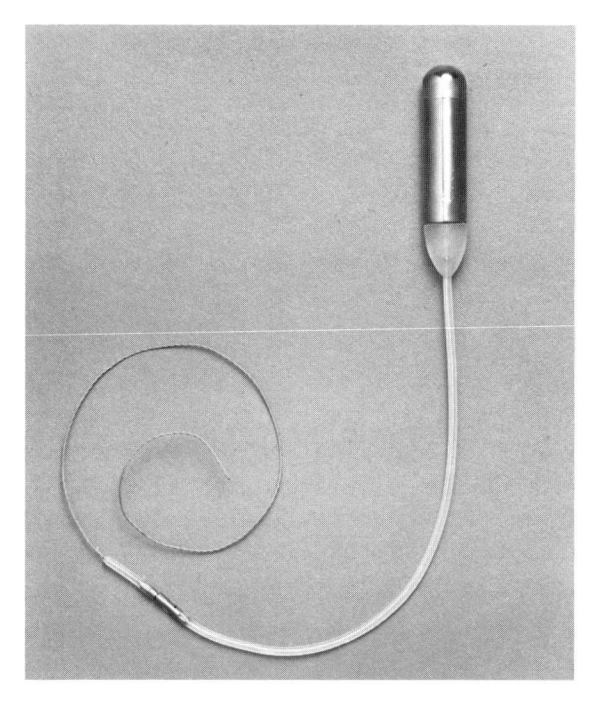

Fig. 8.6 The Telectronics Osteostim™ (reproduced by permission)

This power pack contains a pair of silver oxide/zinc cells and an electronic circuit, which act as a constant current generator providing $20\,\mu A$ to the cathode. The cathode lead consists of 15 cm of silicone-insulated, twisted stainless steel wire terminated by a titanium connector socket. The cathode itself is 25 cm of 3-stranded uninsulated titanium wire terminated with a connector pin which plugs into this socket. The hemispherical opposite end of the power pack is platinum-plated to form the positive anode of the system.

In use, the Osteostim™ requires that a block of bone some 2 cm to 3 cm long and about 1 cm in width is excised longitudinally across the fracture site, leaving a slot (Lunceford, 1981a), after which the adjacent intermedullary cavity is cleared. Then a second incision is made some 10 cm distant, so that the power pack can be placed in soft tissue close to the skin surface. A haemostat is passed from the second incision to the first, and the cathode is threaded through to the nonunion site. The tube is then removed, and the uninsulated cathode wire is formed into a spring-like helix by winding it over a disposable mandrel. This helix is inserted into the slot, and fragments of cancellous bone may be placed in the coils to assist healing.

Routine closure is then performed, after which post-operative care and limb immobilization are as normal.

For certain versions of the Osteostim™, the correct functioning of the implant may be checked by use of a hand-held monitoring receiver. Provided that it can be held within 8 cm of the implanted power pack, the monitor will pick up a small signal which is continuously emitted by that power pack, and indicate the current being delivered to the electrodes. It will also show whether the batteries are nearing exhaustion (which is normally after some 20 to 24 weeks).

After five to six months, the second incision is reopened for power pack removal. This may be done under local anaesthesia, and a pull on the cathode lead will disconnect the socket from the cathode pin, the cathode spiral being thus left *in situ* (no adverse effects resulting from titanium implants are reported (Leventhal, 1951)).

The main precaution during implantation is to avoid the use of electrical haemostasis when the Osteostim™ is in position, and the use of short-wave diathermy thereafter: both may damage the Osteostim™ circuitry.

The manufacturer reports a success rate of 87% based on 180 cases, and breaks the classification down into several groupings having regard to the time between injury and implantation, and whether other procedures were involved. Perhaps the most significant column involves cases treated more than a year after injury, with no procedures other than implantation of the Osteostim™, which indicates 85 successes out of 104, or 82%. Further, the manufacturer apparently does not regard infection as a contraindication, and quotes a similar success rate in such cases.

The DePuy Orthofuse™ is similar to the Osteostim™ and the application thereof has also been described by Lunceford (1981b). Figure 8.7 shows a typical orientation for the device in use.

Semi-invasive methods

The necessity for a second surgical procedure to extract a power pack can be avoided if the unit is mounted externally and the anode is attached to the skin surface. Then, only the cathodes need be implanted, and this procedure can be simplified if these cathodes are designed for percutaneous insertion under X-ray control, and possibly using only local anaesthesia. This entire 'semi-invasive' technique has been described at length (Brighton et al, 1981) and the series of clinical trials quoted — both in the originating medical school and elsewhere — have demonstrated success rates exceeding 83% and 72% respectively.

Commercially, the 'semi-invasive' method is represented by the Zimmer® DCBGS™ Osteogenesis System, which consists of a QUADPAK® power supply which delivers $20\,\mu A$ to each of four cathodes, the total $80\,\mu A$ being returned via a

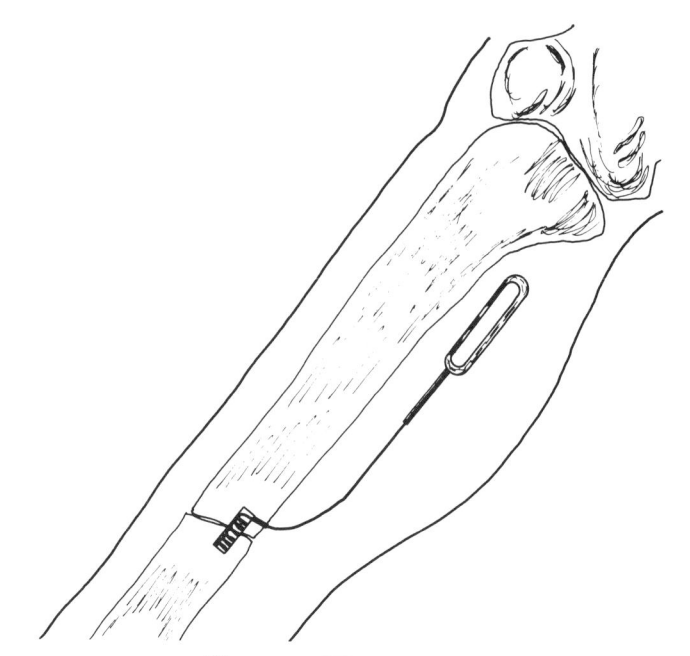

Fig. 8.7 The Osteostim™/Orthofuse™ in position for tibial nonunion treatment

skin-surface mounted anode. This current can be directly monitored using a QUADPAK® Test Meter which is also provided. The anode itself consists of a gel-soaked pad which adheres to the patient's skin; whilst each cathode is essentially a stainless steel Kirschner wire some 23 cm long, 1.2 mm diameter, and TEFLON insulated except for the sharpened, diamond-shaped tip.

The recommended method of usage involves the marking of a line on the skin surface (after normal preparation and draping) to define the position of the nonunion. After this, the proposed cathode entry sites are injected with an appropriate local anaesthetic and then reinjected down to the periosteum and the nonunion itself.

A specially modified drill is used to hold the blunt end of a cathode, and a DELRIN sleeve is threaded over part of this cathode to prevent bending. The sharp end of the cathode is then inserted percutaneously and drilled through part of the cortex until it lies within the nonunion as evidenced by image-intensified X-ray control.

Depending on the bone involved, from one cathode (for the medial malleolus, for example) to four (for large long bones), are so implanted. Figure 8.8a shows a sketch of the DCBGS system and Figure 8.8b shows four cathodes *in situ* in a tibial nonunion.

An appropriate ointment with squares of sterile dressing are applied at each point of entry, the limb is encased in sterile WEBRIL and a special tool is used to bend the protruding cathodes through 90° to lie parallel with the long axis of the limb. They are then cut off to about 2.5 cm and cushioned with WEBRIL pads. The leads from the power pack are clipped to the cathodes and the pack itself cushioned and fixed over an area of soft tissue, as shown in Figure 8.8c.

A non-weight-bearing cast is applied with the anode lead and monitoring leads protruding. Both the adhesive anode pad and its site are changed by the patient every alternate day to prevent skin irritation, for which reason an appropriate press-stud contact is attached to the end of the anode lead.

Precautions to be taken during the procedure are largely concerned with the proper positioning of the cathodes, and establishing that no undue stress is placed upon them, or upon any of the leads. Ideally, the cathode tips should all lie in the nonunion and be about 0.5 cm apart. Also, they must not touch any metallic implant which may be present. A further precaution involves the checking of current level at the monitoring point to establish not only that the power pack is operative, but that none of the cathode circuits has become open-circuited (i.e. broken).

Contraindications for the use of the device include pathological fractures due to any form of tumour, congenital and synovial pseudarthroses and active infection including osteomyelitis. Also, the patient should not be sensitive to nickel or chromium. If superficial or deep infection at a cathode occurs, that cathode should be removed; and should osteomyelitis or thrombophlebitis develop, treatment should be terminated.

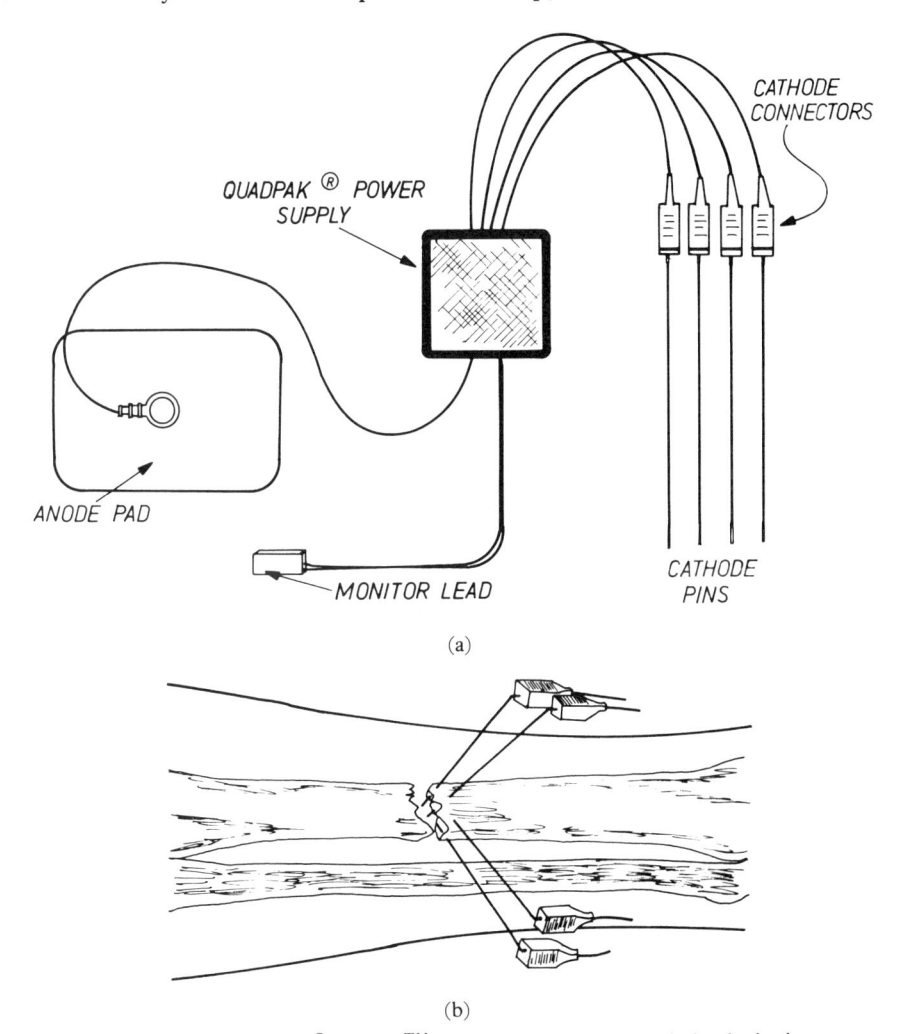

Fig. 8.8 (a) The Zimmer® DCBGS™ osteogenesis system (b) typical cathode placement

142 RECENT ADVANCES IN ORTHOPAEDICS

(c)

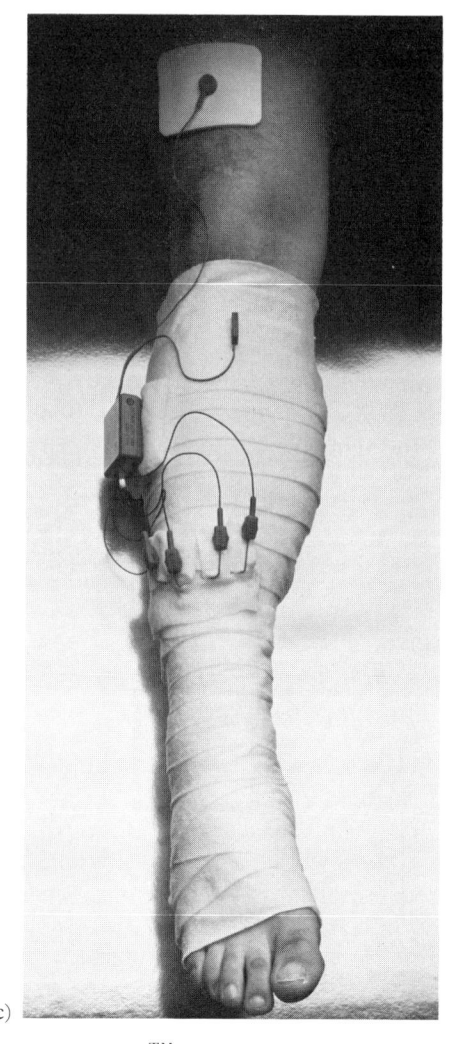

Fig. 8.8 (c) The DCBGS™ system in situ (reproduced by permission)

Non-invasive methods

As has been explained, a Helmholz pair of coils can be used to produce a changing magnetic field, and a limb positioned between such coils will have electric current induced in it which will rotate around the axis of that field (Figs. 8.2b and 8.3). This method has been extensively used for the stimulation of long-bone nonunions (Bassett, Pilla & Pawluk, 1977; Bassett, Mitchell, Norton & Pilla, 1978; Mulier & Spaas, 1980), and the commercial form of the relevant apparatus is the Electro-Biology Inc. Bi-Osteogen™ system. Figure 8.9 shows the device in use and in this case the two coils are strapped to the anterior and posterior surfaces of a lower leg cast, and positioned so that the tibial nonunion under treatment lies inside the uniform portion of the magnetic field. The lead from the coils is plugged into an electronic control unit which provides the voltage pulses which drive these coils.

The shape, magnitude and frequency of the voltage pulses are said to be critical by

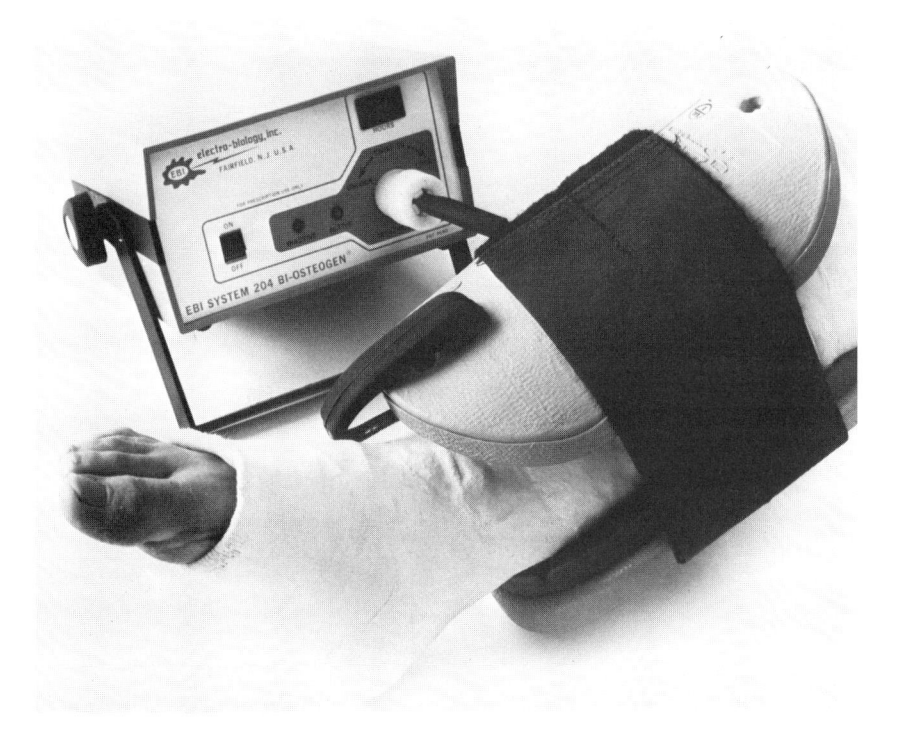

Fig. 8.9 The E.B.I. bi-osteogen™ apparatus in situ (reproduced by permission)

the manufacturer, and are defined in the relevant patents (Ryaby & Pilla, 1981). Further, the distance between the coils, as given by the outside diameter of the relevant plaster cast, defines the magnitude of the applied voltage wave. Therefore, at the time of writing, a coil/control unit system is pre-adjusted for each case on the basis of information provided by the surgeon-in-charge, and the system is leased for the treatment of the case in question. It is then returned and may be re-adjusted and re-leased for further cases.

It has been claimed (Bassett, Mitchell, Norton & Pilla, 1978) that certain sequences of pulses may be more appropriate for the treatment of congenital pseudarthroses than others recommended for acquired nonunions, and this is reflected in the patents relating to the commercial instrument.

For the treatment of pseudarthroses, a series of voltage pulses to the coils (called 'Mode 1') are used, and these result in an induced current of the shape shown in Figure 8.10a. It should be noted that this induced current can be detected by a small 'search coil' placed inside the magnetic field and connected to a cathode-ray oscilloscope. The voltage induced in this search coil will have the same waveform as the current induced in a resistive medium — the limb under treatment in this case.

Some explanation is needed at this point to reconcile Figures 8.4a and 8.10a. Because of the low inductance of the Helmholtz pair of coils, the current I in them can change very rapidly, and in fact it follows the applied voltage wave V as in Figure 8.4a. But because the *induced* current i exists only during the time the magnetic field is changing, there is no point in maintaining the horizontal tops of the V and I

144 RECENT ADVANCES IN ORTHOPAEDICS

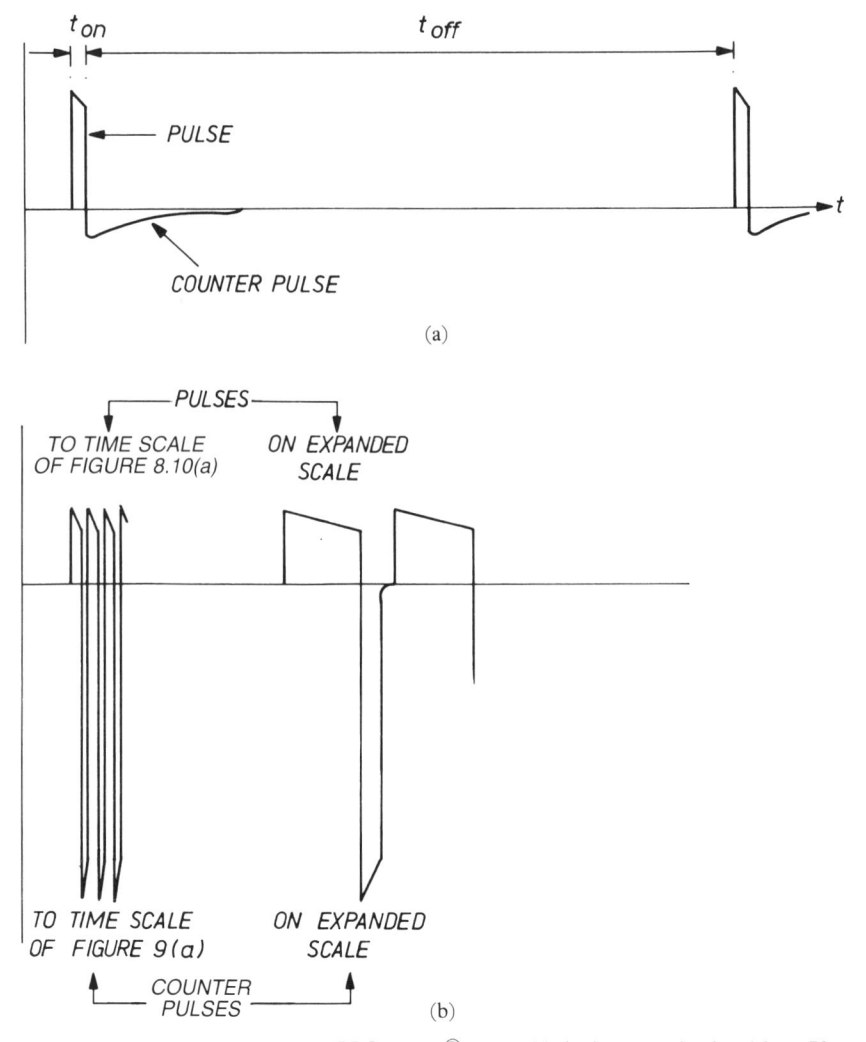

Fig. 8.10 Induced pulses produced by EBI Osteogen® system (a) single repeated pulses (about 72 per second) (b) pulse bursts (about 15 per second)

waveforms for very long. In the present case, this time t_{ON} is very short – some 0.3 mS — and this is shown in Figure 8.10a, which has a very much expanded time axis scale compared with Figure 8.4a. The beginning of the decay of i is clearly shown over the period t_{ON}, and when the applied voltage is cut off, the induced current also falls rapidly, and in fact reverses, as shown by the excursion below the time axis. (It will be recalled that this means that the induced current first rotates one way, then the other, around the axis of the magnetic field.) The magnitude of the counter-rotating current is quite small because a 'fly-back' diode has been incorporated into the driving circuit, making the i-waveform markedly asymmetrical. However, the area of the counter-pulses plotted below the time axis must be equal to the area of the pulses plotted above, which means that each low-magnitude counter-pulse must last much longer than each high magnitude pulse. In the waveform recommended for the treatment of pseudarthroses, these ('Mode-1') pulses are repeated about 72 times per second, so that the time between pulses is about 13.2 mS, and according to the relevant patent, 3.3 mS of this is alloted to the counter-pulse. The 'Mode 2' waveform, which is said to be preferable for the treatment of acquired nonunions, actually consists of a series of rapid pulse bursts, with a repetition rate of some 15 bursts per second. In order to accommodate a large number of pulses in each burst (which lasts about 5 mS), the fly-back diode is omitted, so that a high-magnitude but brief counter-pulse appears, as shown in Figure 8.10b. In fact, the counter-pulse exceeds the pulse in magnitude, and appears as shown in the expanded sketch on the right.

In use, the outside diameter of the plaster cast adjacent to the nonunion is measured, and this along with other relevant data, is submitted for the procurement of an appropriate coil pair along with a pre-adjusted drive unit, as has been mentioned. Under X-ray control, a locator block is positioned on the surface of the cast and centred over the nonunion. It is then firmly fixed by further p.o.p. bandaging. One of the coils is placed over this locator block, the other is placed diametrically opposite to it, and webbing is wound around the two, and fixed with Velcro™ pads. The result is exemplified by Figure 8.9.

The patient is instructed in the home use of the apparatus, which involves some 12 to 16 hours per day of stimulation, with no weight-bearing. Each month, radiographic examinations are carried out with the plaster *in situ*, and if healing is taking place, it should be evident after three or four months.

It is noteworthy that in treatments such as this, very good immobilization is necessary, and if this is difficult using plaster (as in some cases of femoral nonunion, for example) internal fixation is permissible *provided* that the plate, intramedullary nail or external fixation device are non magnetic.

Typically, endosteal bone healing is observed, with little or no external callus. When evidence of healing is present, a progressive regime of loading and weight-bearing is begun. Here, further patient training is necessary.

The presence of infection, including osteomyelitis (and draining sinuses) is not a contraindication for this treatment, because no foreign material is introduced into the tissue. In fact, it has been noticed that non-invasive magnetic treatment using either coils or electromagnets (see below) appears to contribute to the clearing of such infections. Conversely, the technique should not be used where a true synovial pseudarthrosis is present, or where the gap approaches 1 cm, for success is unlikely under such circumstances.

At the time of writing, over 3000 patients have been treated by this method, and the manufacturer quotes an overall success rate of 75.7%. Further, 89.6% had undergone prior (failed) surgical intervention, some 31% had existing (non-magnetic) internal fixation in place, and 33% had a prior history of infection or were actively draining at the commencement of treatment.

Several comparatively small clinical trials have been described using an iron-cored electromagnet (Watson & Downes, 1979; de Haas, Morrison & Watson, 1980), and employing the waveforms shown in Figure 8.4b. In the more recent work, a squared-off, C-shaped electromagnet weighing 1.8 kg was used for tibial nonunion, along with a smaller version for use with the upper extremities or with children (Watson, 1981), and a larger version for adult femoral nonunions.

A mains-operated electronic drive unit produced a square wave of voltage which was applied to a coil wound around the electromagnet, and the resulting coil current produced the requisite pulsing magnetic field. A frequency of about one induced pulse per second was chosen, on the grounds that this is a common 'biological' frequency, being of the same order as the frequencies of walking, breathing and cardiovascular pulsing. Further, it was known that the piezoelectric transfer function of bone also involved time constants of the order of a second.

The amplitude of the induced current pulse was about an order of magnitude below that produced by the Helmholz coil system described above, but lasted much longer, the electromagnet being highly inductive.

In use, the electromagnet was lowered into guides mounted on each side of the plaster cast, and could be removed at intervals by the patient, who was allowed short periods of weight-bearing. However, very good immobilization was again called for, and the recommended treatment time was 12 hours per day for 12 weeks.

Over several years, the original, rather heavy electromagnet has been refined, and a recent (small-scale) clinical trial* (Watson & Downes, 1981) has shown that a success rate of more than 70% can be achieved with much lighter electromagnets, and using an empirically-determined minimum waveform amplitude. On the basis of this work, a new, completely portable unit has been developed using a very lightweight (0.5 kg) electromagnet, and at the time of writing, clinical trials of this have just commenced. Figure 8.11 shows a version of this unit, and the electromagnet is of the same shape as

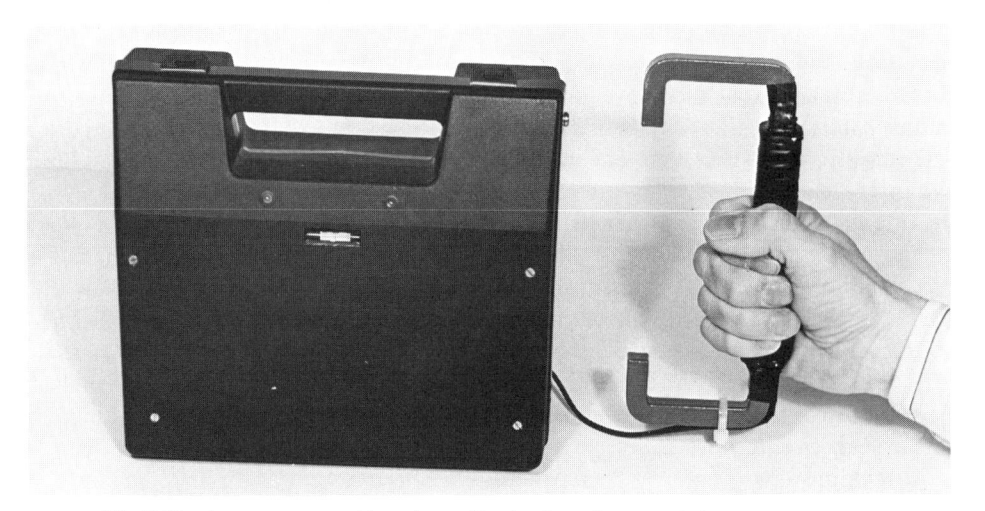

Fig. 8.11 A prototype portable orthopaedic stimulator (iron-cored electromagnet type)

its heavier predecessors, but has a much smaller cross-sectional area. The drive unit is operated from an internal 12 volt battery which will run the device for some 30 hours, and can be recharged (during use) overnight.

The prime advantage of the iron-core electromagnet system is that it requires no setting-up procedures, because the poles being always he same distance apart, the electronic drive unit need not be adjustable. The prime disadvantages — those of

* Supported by Howmedica International Inc.

weight and the necessity of a mains-operated drive unit — have been overcome in the portable version, but its efficacy has yet to be demonstrated.

Because the method is entirely non-invasive, the presence of infection, including osteomyelitis, is not a contraindication, and as has been mentioned, there is subjective evidence of beneficial results.* However, success is unlikely where large gaps are present, or in most cases of congenital or synovial pseudarthrosis. However, the presence of *non-magnetic* internal fixation is not a contraindication.

An example of use of the iron-cored electromagnet is depicted in Figure 8.12, which refer to a sixteen-year-old boy who sustained a displaced, closed, oblique fracture at the junction of the middle and distal thirds of the right tibia and fibula in a road accident. Initial treatment was by conservative means, with manipulation and the application of a long leg plaster cast. Nine months later, there was obvious mobility of the tibial fracture, and radiographs showed features of hypertrophic nonunion (Figure 8.12a).

Treatment with the iron-cored stimulator was initiated on a 12-hour-per-day basis, and filling in of the fracture line was evident after some three months (Fig. 8.12b). Mobilisation was commenced, and after a further two months, sound consolidation was achieved (Fig. 8.12c).

The concept of electromagnetic induction can also be extended to an invasive technique by including an implant which consists essentially of a secondary coil of wire. The voltage induced in this coil may be applied to two of the screws which hold a compression plate in place, and which are insulated from the plate itself, so that the resulting current flows through the bone and adjacent tissues. If these two special screws are positioned at each side of the nonunion, then at least part of this current would be expected to cross that nonunion to effect stimulation. The overall success rate of this method is said to exceed 90% (Lechner, Ascherl, Kraus & Blumel, 1981).

In this method, the current must of course be alternating, and in practice, frequencies between 2 and 30 Hz have been used, and the current densities involved have been quoted at 2 to $5 \mu A/mm^2$.

CONCLUSIONS

The foregoing material has been concerned largely with stimulators which are now commercially available, and it should be noted that a considerable amount of other work has also been done in the laboratory, and clinically, by individual groups. However, insofar as the surgeon is concerned, his main interest must be related to the immediate practicability of patient treatment, and in this context, a number of questions need to be asked, as follows.

Is the electrical treatment of nonunion effective?
To answer this question, it is first necessary to define nonunion, and this continues to be a point of contention. Nonunion has been defined as a condition which exists when the surgeon considers that the fracture will not heal without surgical intervention; but to determine a success rate based on this sort of subjective definition is to open the results of the relevant study to criticism, and this has indeed happened. To introduce

* Personal communication from E M Downes, Consultant Orthopaedic Surgeon.

148 RECENT ADVANCES IN ORTHOPAEDICS

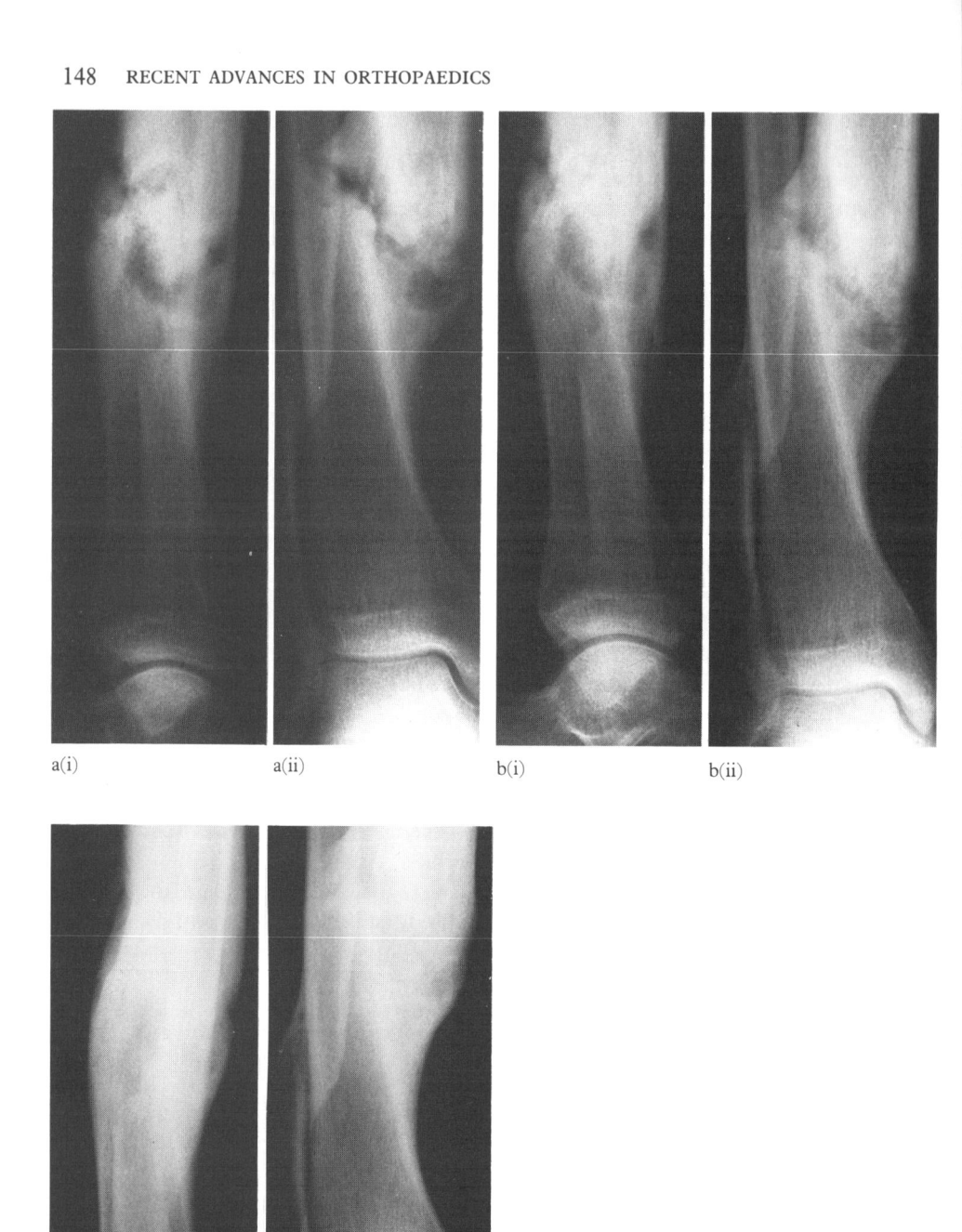

a(i)　　　　　　a(ii)　　　　　　b(i)　　　　　　b(ii)

c(i)　　　　　　c(ii)

Fig. 8.12 A tibial nonunion at commencement of treatment with iron-cored orthopaedic stimulator (a), after three months (b), and at five months (c)

a degree of objectivity, the A–O Group suggest that an interval of nine months must elapse from the time of injury before a nonunion is diagnosed (and that four to nine months designates a delayed union).

Those techniques which involve operative procedures, sometimes including the insertion of bone fragments into a slot, are also subject to criticism on the grounds that sufficient surgery has been performed to effect union without electrical stimulus. However, a considerable number of case histories are now available in which failed surgical intervention has been followed by successful electrical treatment — *and* vice versa!

Some manufacturers and the associated research teams have gone to considerable lengths to show how the success rate depends upon such factors as the nature and location of the initial injury (or the form taken by any congenital pseudarthrosis), whether prior treatment was involved, the absence or presence of infection, and the time from the initial injury to the commencement of electrical treatment. In the fullness of time, such studies will no doubt be independently collated and subjected to proper statistical analysis.

The definition of 'success' has been also somewhat obscure, but sound bony union, clinically and radiologically, along with an absence of pain can hardly be considered disputable criteria.

Most of the trials so far conducted quote figures ranging from 70% to 90% success rates (using each group's definitions), the disparities being related to the factors mentioned above, the equipment used, and the experience of the centres involved. If such figures are accepted at their face value, then electrical treatment would seem to offer much the same chance of success as the various forms of surgical intervention.

Frequently, the question of the double-blind trial arises, and this has also proved a contentious issue. Though such a trial would normally be considered a scientific prerequisite to the acceptance of a technique, it is ethically difficult to justify the random non-treatment of any person presenting with a clinically-treatable condition. Moreover, it could be said that each patient for whom a nonunion or delayed union has been diagnosed, is his own control, so that some form of treatment is indicated. Whether this should be surgical or electrical (or either one following a failure of the other) is clearly a matter for clinical decisions based upon experience.

Certainly, the evidence so far available which supports the efficacy of electrical stimulation in cases of nonunion, is no less convincing than that appertaining to any other form of treatment, to which it will be found that similar caveats to the ones above, also apply.

What factors determine the choice of method?
In the first instance, a choice must be made between an invasive, semi-invasive or non-invasive technique, and the factors involved include the nature of the nonunion and the bone involved, the condition of the surrounding tissue and skin, and the degree of co-operation expected of the patient. For example, in the case of a tibial or femoral nonunion and for a patient for whom some degree of mobility was essential and/or who could not be expected to co-operate effectively where accessible equipment was involved, a fully implantable device might be preferred. (The manufacturers list of contraindications must of course be taken into account.)

Where the patient can be relied upon to perform treatment procedures at home, there may be grounds for choosing the semi-invasive technique. For example, where poor vascularity or soft tissue trauma exists, the percutaneous insertion of cathodes may be possible whereas open surgery may not. In the case of the DCBGS, the patient must be competent to change his anode pad on alternate days; and though he may move about during the basic treatment period, the fracture must be immobilized, and weight-bearing must not commence until the cathodes have been extracted following evidence of union.

Although it is claimed that recurrence of osteomyelitis during the treatment period has presented no problems, its presence is nevertheless regarded as a contraindication, and this may lead to the choice of a non-invasive method, even apart from the fact that the avoidance of any form of surgery, no matter how minor, is desirable *per se*, and especially so where there has been significant soft tissue damage and skin loss. In the case of the Bi-Osteogen™, the patient must be relied upon to effect regular treatment over the described period, keeping in mind that he must use a mains supply to power the drive unit.

The primary requirement of this method is that of extremely good immobilization, and except for a few cases of very stable nonunion, or where (non-magnetic) internal fixation is present, weight-bearing is prohibited until there is evidence of bony union. A listing of casts appropriate to various conditions is supplied by the manufacturer.

At the time of writing the alternative technique using an electromagnet is still in the development stage, but it is hoped that it will allow a solution of the portability problem, and it has the inherent advantage of not requiring adjustment on a case-to-case basis.

Where electromagnetic induction methods are concerned, questions relating to optimum values of induced current density, frequency and waveshape continue to arise, and it has to be admitted that there is very little evidence to show that one set of parameters is better than another, or if indeed an optimum set exists at all. However, as is frequently the case in medicine, empirical observations are beginning to show that certain combinations are somewhat more effective than others; but it is unlikely that this vexed question will be resolved for some considerable time.

Are the various techniques safe?

At the time of writing, and as far as is known, there are no reports of adverse effects resulting from the clinical use of electrical methods of bone stimulation. However, it must be recognised that these techniques are all in their infancy, and that long-term follow-ups are still in progress. Also, it should be noted that where adverse reactions *are* known from animal experimentation — such as observed tissue necrosis at current levels approaching $100\,\mu A$ — the relevant clinical devices contain built-in protection to prevent current flow at such levels. Furthermore, the lists of contraindications offered by manufacturers include purely precautionary items where prior work is lacking.

Insofar as the application of magnetic fields are concerned, the flux densities used are much smaller than those for which limits have been published (Battocletti, 1976), but nevertheless, it has not been recommended that the relevant devices be used for treatments other than to the extremities.

Summarizing, it is clear that normal caution should preclude the use of electrical methods of treating nonunion, except where prior work has been performed and reported.

CONCLUDING COMMENTS

As will have been deduced from the discourse above, it is becoming clear that the three basic techniques are not necessarily competitive, but can be considered complementary, the choice being dependent upon the case under consideration. Certainly, the interpretation of 'success rate' being so arbitary, this factor cannot at present be used as a first criterion, though when sufficient independent trials have been carried out, it may become so. The major point is that, at the time of writing, the electrical treatment of nonunion has progressed from being not only a last resort of salvage for failed attempts to achieve union by traditional methods, but has become a viable alternative to those methods.

ACKNOWLEDGEMENTS

Grateful thanks are due to E Malcolm Downes F.R.C.S., Consultant Orthopaedic Surgeon, for assistance with the manuscript and for the case history and X-rays included; and Messrs. Telectronics, DePuy, Zimmer and Electro-Biology for information provided and permission to use the selection of plates and diagrams.

REFERENCES

Archer C W, Ratcliffe N A 1981 The effects of pulsed magnetic fields on bone and cartilage in vitro. Transactions of the First annual meeting, Bioelectrical Repair and growth society, Philadelphia, 1: 1

Bassett C A L 1971 Biophysical principles affecting bone structure. In: Bourne G H (ed) Biochemistry and physiology of bone, 2nd edn vol 3, Academic Press, New York. ch 1, p 1–76

Bassett C A L, Becker R O 1962 Generation of electrical potentials in bone in response to mechanical stress. Science 137: 1063–1064

Bassett C A L, Pawluk R J, Becker R O 1964 Effect of electric currents on bone in vivo. Nature 204: 652–654

Bassett C A L, Herrman I 1968 The effect of electrostatic fields on macromolecular synthesis by fibroblasts in vitro. Journal of Cell Biology 39: 9a

Bassett C A L, Pilla A A, Pawluk R J 1977 A non-operative salvage of surgically-resistant pseudarthroses and non-unions by pulsing electromagnetic fields. Clinical Orthopaedics & Related Research 124: 128–143

Bassett C A L, Mitchell S N, Norton L, Pilla A A 1978 Repair of non-unions by pulsing electromagnetic fields. Acta Orthopaedica Belgica 44: 706–724

Battocletti J H 1976 Electromagnetism, man and the environment. Elek Book, London

Becker R O, Spadaro J H, Marino A A 1977 Clinical experiences with low intensity direct current stimulation of bone growth. Clinical Orthopaedics and Related Research 124: 75–83

Becker R O, Spadaro A A 1978 Treatment of orthopaedic infections with electrically-generated silver ions. Journal of Bone and Joint Surgery 60-A: 871–881

Black J, Brighton C T 1977 Treatment of nonunion with constant direct current. Clinical Orthopaedics and Related Research 124: 106–123

Black J, Brighton C T 1979 Mechanisms of stimulation of osteogenesis by direct current. In: Brighton C T, Black J, Pollack S R (eds) Electrical properties of bone and cartilage, Grune and Stratton, New York

Brighton C T, Friedenburg Z B, Mitchell E I, Booth R E 1977 Treatment of nonunion with constant direct current. Clinical Orthopaedics and Related Research 124: 106–123

Brighton C T et al 1981 A multicentre study of the treatment of non-union with constant direct current. Journal of Bone and Joint Surgery 62-A: 2–13

Connolly J F, Hahn H, Jardon O M 1977 The electrical enhancement of periosteal proliferation in normal and delayed fracture healing. Clinical Orthopaedics and Related Research 124: 97–105

De Haas W G, Lazarovici M A, Morrison D M 1979 The effect of low-frequency magnetic fields on the osteotomized rabbit radius. Clinical Orthopaedics and Related Research 145: 245–251

De Haas W G, Morrison D M, Watson J 1980 The non-invasive treatment of ununited fractures of the tibia using electrical stimulation. Journal of Bone and Joint Surgery 62-B: 465–470

Dwyer A F, Wickham G G 1974 Direct current stimulation in spinal fusion. Medical Journal of Australia 1: 73–75

El-Messery M A E 1981 Physical basis for piezoelectricity of bone matrix. Proceedings of the Institution of Electrical Engineers 128-A: 336–346

Ericsson C 1976 Electrical properties of bone. In Bourne G H (ed) The biochemistry and physiology of bone, 2nd edn vol 4, Academic Press, New York, ch 8, p 271–297

Fitton-Jackson S, Jones D B, Murray J C, Farndale R W 1981 The response of connective and skeletal tissues to pulsed magnetic fields. Transactions of the First annual meeting, Bioelectrical repair and growth society, Philadelphia, 1: 85

Friedenburg Z B, Brighton C T 1966 Bioelectric potentials in bone. Journal of Bone and Joint Surgery 48-A: 915–923

Friedenburg Z B, Roberts P G, Didizian N H, Brighton C T 1971 Stimulation of healing by direct current in the rabbit fibula. Journal of Bone and Joint Surgery 53-A: 1400–1408

Fukada E, Yasuda I 1957 On the piezoelectric effect of bone. Journal of the Physical Society of Japan, 12: 1158–1162

Hassler C R, Rybicki E F, Diegle R B, Clark L C 1977 Studies of enhanced bone healing via electrical stimuli. Clinical Orthopaedics and Related Research 124: 9–19

Hassler C R, Cummings K D, Clark L D, Rybicki E F, Diegle R B 1979 Augmentation of bone healing via electrical stimuli. In: Brighton C T, Black J, Pollack S R (eds) Electrical properties of bone and cartilage, Grune and Stratton, New York

Jorgensen J E 1977 Electrical stimulation of human fracture healing by means of a slowly-pulsing asymmetrical direct current. Clinical Orthopaedics and Related Research 124: 124–127

Kane W J 1981 A technique for the insertion of the totally-implantable bone growth stimulator for lumbosacral fusion via a mid-line approach. Telectronics Pty Ltd, Colorado

Lechner F, Ascherl R, Kraus W, Blumel G 1981 The electrodynamic field therapy of pseudarthroses — principles of the process and a ten-year follow-up. Proceedings of the First annual meeting, Bioelectrical repair and growth society, Philadelphia, 1: 17

Leventhal G S 1951 Titanium — a metal for surgery. Journal of Bone and Joint Surgery 33A: 473–474

Lunceford E M 1981a A technique for the insertion of the totally implantable bone growth stimulator. Telectronics Pty Ltd, Colorado

Lunceford E M 1981b Orthofuse — a surgical procedure. De Puy, Indiana

Mulier J C, Spaas F 1980 Out-patient treatment of surgically-resistant non-unions by induced pulsing current — clinical results. Archives of Orthopaedic and Traumatic Surgery 97: 293–297

Norton L A, Moore R R 1972 Bone growth in organ culture modified by electric fields. Journal of Dental Research 51: 1492–1495

Patterson C C, Lewis G N, Cass C A 1980 Treatment of delayed union and nonunion with an implanted direct current stimulator. Clinical Orthopaedics and Related Research 148: 117–127

Pienkowski D, Pollack S R 1981 The effect of fluids on stress generated potentials in bone. Proceedings of the First Annual Meeting, Bioelectrical repair and growth society, Philadelphia. 1: 7

Pilla A A 1981 Electrochemical kinetic correlates for low-level pulsating current modulation of cell and tissue function. Proceedings of the First annual meeting, Bioelectrical repair and growth society, Philadelphia. 1: 62

Ryaby J P, Pilla A A 1981. US Patents 4, 266, 532 and 4, 266, 533

Shim S S 1981 Effect of electromagnetic pulse applications on fracture healing with emphasis on vascularisation. Proceedings of the First annual meeting, Bioelectrical repair and growth society, Philadelphia. 1: 19

Spadaro J A 1977 Electrically stimulated bone growth in animals and man. Clinical Orthopaedics and Related Research 122: 325–332

Stillings D 1974 Healing fractures electrically. Journal of the Association for the Advancement of Medical Instrumentation 8: 259–259

Watson J 1979 The electrical stimulation of bone healing. Proceedings of the Institute of Electrical and Electronic Engineers 67: 1339–1352

Watson J 1981 Electricity and bone healing. Proceedings of the Institution of Electrical Engineers 128-A: 329–335

Watson J, De Haas W G, Hauser S S 1975 Effect of electric fields on the growth rate of embryonic chick tibiae in vitro. Nature 254: 331–332

Watson J, Downes E M 1979 Clinical aspects of the stimulation of bone healing using electrical phenomena. Medical and Biological Engineering and Computing 17: 161–169

Watson J, Downes E M 1981 Stimulation of long bone nonunion healing using iron-cored electromagnets. Proceedings of the First annual meeting, Bioelectrical repair and growth society, Philadelphia 1: 39

Williams W S, Gross D 1981 Is streaming the source of strain related potentials? Proceedings of the First annual meeting, Bioelectrical repair and growth society, Philadelphia 1: 87

9. Recent advances in total hip resurfacing

H. C. Amstutz

INTRODUCTION

The increasing incidence of complications occurring after conventional stem-type total hip replacements, such as prosthetic loosening, stem fractures and the inherent difficulties of adequate revision, reawakened an interest 10 years ago in devising an alternative approach to existing stem designs. The fact that such complications occur more frequently in younger, more active, or heavier patients accentuates the need for improved durability.

Modern acrylic fixation surface replacements were introduced in 1971 by Paltrineri and Trentani in Italy. Later, Furuya, Eicher, Tanaka, Freeman, Wagner, and Amstutz developed surface replacements and initiated clinical trials prior to the mid-1970s. In addition, since 1976, the list of other innovators who have implanted various designs has grown. This chapter outlines the design and development of the Total Hip Articular Replacement by Eccentric Shells (THARIES) surface replacement system and discusses indications, techniques, and results. The world-wide experience is reviewed and related to the variables of design and technique.

DESIGN AND DEVELOPMENT

The design and development of the THARIES surface replacement was based on five main objectives (Clarke et al 1977):

1. Use of eccentric shells to optimize socket durability and fixation.
2. Optimal reaming of the femoral head using specialized cylindrical and chamfer reamers to provide a reproducible technique.
3. An adequate range of components providing interchangeability and custom-fitting capabilities for improving fixation with minimal loss of bone stock.
4. Positioning of the femoral and acetabular components as anatomically as possible.
5. Use of a trans-trochanteric approach to obtain optimal visualization of the acetabulum and femoral head for careful reaming and component orientation, and to facilitate trochanteric advancement when the neck requires shortening.

In considering plastic-on-metal components, thin, ultra-high molecular-weight polyethylene is now known to perform best in the female bearing socket rather than in the male component (femoral cup) of a surface replacement (Freeman, 1978). However, the minimum wall thickness for polyethylene sockets previously used in conventional replacements varied from 5 to 11 mm or more, depending on the ball diameter and patient size. With less thickness the polyethylene may deform significantly and loosen, especially if it is not adequately supported by bone. Therefore, taking minimum metal and plastic wall thickness as 1 and 5 mm respectively, the minimum space required is at least 12 mm on a diameter for the surface replacement. It was obvious that space was at a premium in optimizing the patient's range, with adequate mechanical strength and fixation capability.

Based on these data, eccentric shell designs were proposed for the surface replacement to minimize bone resection and put the bulk of the material where it was required most, i.e., on the superior load-bearing areas. prototype eccentric metal cup has a minimum wall thickness of 1.25 mm, approximately 50% greater than that of the earlier Smith–Petersen cup. The superior shell is 2.5 mm thick, providing strength and deep fixation channels of 1.5 mm in depth, tapering to 0.75 mm of the thin section. The thick wall also allows a relatively greater range of motion at the superior bearing surfaces, where they are required.

In designing for the 40- to 60-mm range of head diameters (Clarke & Amstutz, 1975), five sizes were initially selected. In this way the size increments were kept small (3 to 4 mm), thus permitting the surgeon maximum scope in fitting the device. The larger the cup fitted, the less femoral bone will need to be resected. Moreover, the resulting range of motion will be enhanced, regardless of original femoral head size. The metal selected was cast cobalt–chrome–molybdenum, Zimaloy. Clinical experience dictated a need for one larger and one smaller component to accommodate the complete range of pathological entities encountered.

The ultra-high molecular-weight polyethylene shell is also eccentric. To aid the surgeon in this custom-fitting, each of the seven sizes of femoral cups has three polyethylene sockets of varying wall thicknesses: small, medium and large. Each size relates to those above or below for maximum fitting selection, e.g., an SR4 large liner has the same outside diameter as an SR5 small socket shell. The smallest shell size throughout the range is designed so that it fits the patients acetabulum with minimal reaming, thereby assuring a fit except in dysplastic acetabulae. If more bone stock is available, the correspondingly thicker shells can be used. Alternatively, if the acetabulum can take an SR4 small shell but the femoral head has to be reamed to an SR3 metal cup, the SR3 large shell can be substituted, thus keeping the cement volume to the required minimum.

In our early clinical experience we seldom used the large-socket component to preserve acetabular stock, so that only the small and medium sockets were manufactured in the regular line. However, the large components are useful in some revision cases, if loss of femoral bone stock requires the use of a smaller femoral component or larger socket shell.

The initial THARIES sockets were designed to a depth of 1 mm over a hemisphere. These were used in 73 hips. With favourable clinical experience and no dislocations, the depth was reduced to 1 mm under a hemisphere for 43 hips. Since stability was still satisfactory, the depth was further reduced to 3 mm under a hemisphere. In two patients with grossly abnormal muscle and bone stock, stability remains excellent, with only two dislocations. One patient underwent a takedown of an arthrodesis, with massive heterotopic bone completely replacing the abductor muscles, and the other had a short neck owing to extensive post-trauma osteonecrosis. After reduction, both have remained stable for over one year postoperatively.

INDICATIONS

Our initial indications for THARIES replacement included lifestyles or hip problems that might prejudice the fatigue life of conventional stem-type femoral prostheses or component fixation.

1. Osteoarthritis secondary to slipped capital femoral epiphysis, congenital hip dysplasia (CDH), dwarfism, coxa vara, Legg-Calve Perthes disease or post-trauma conditions with significant symptoms and functional loss. The CDH group were especially young and active and had the highest complication rate initially. However, markedly improved results were achieved using shallower sockets and bone grafting to cover and contain the socket fully within the pelvis together with better patient selection.

Patients with dysplasia prior to the onset of severe osteoarthritis are best treated with pelvic shelving procedures. Older patients with high-riding dislocations often require special conventional replacements.

2. Nontraumatic or traumatic osteonecrosis: In patients with nontraumatic osteonecrosis the disease is often bilateral; these are generally young or middle-aged adults. While the group that suffered traumatic necrosis has had no loosenings, those with nontraumatic necrosis (particularly if taking steroids) have had a higher rate of loosening. This is not surprising in view of the poor bone stock on the femoral side, the youth of these patients and their high activity levels. Measures such as reducing the femoral component size, resecting most of the necrotic bone and shortening of the head combined with new fixation techniques have improved durability. Older patients with severe necrosis may be best treated with conventional replacement while younger patients, before extensive collapse, may be amenable to core decompression or the rotational osteotomy of Sugioka.

3. Multiple joint arthropathy: Juvenile and rheumatoid patients, and those with other arthritides who have increased risk of postoperative sepsis owing to steroids or other immunosuppressive drugs and general debility. The management of infection and salvage, if necessary, are far simpler and require less traumatic procedures than conventional stem THRs. The results obtained in this group have been among our best. However, techniques should include hypotensive anaesthesia to promote a dry field, compression containment for acrylic fixation and, in addition, a slight shortening of the lever arm when there is severe osteoporosis to reduce the risk of neck fracture. Avoidance of neck fractures implies avoidance of neck notches and proper trochanteric removal.

4. Primary osteoarthritis: As we improved our technique and confidence in the procedure we extended our indications to include patients 60 and older, occasionally even 70, at their option, after careful explanation of the risks, advantages and disadvantages of both THARIES and conventional replacement. This older group, whose activity level is lower, has experienced the fewest complications. The procedure offers a distinct advantage over the conventional replacement because of its initial and permanent stability, absence of sepsis and ease of revision. However, care should be taken when recommending the procedure for the older patient who has significant osteoporosis unless the surgeon has confidence in his technique. If such a patient suffers a fall, he would have virtually the same hazard of neck fracture as he would without a replacement, and a fracture in an area that had been resurfaced

would require a total hip replacement. It is probably true that this same population could sustain fractures below conventional total hip replacement prosthetic stems or precipitate loosening of the femoral component, and thus there may well be a positive trade-off in favour of the surface replacement.

In the event of a neck fracture, we have designed a series of conversion conventional stem-type replacements available on custom order. These would be indicated in situations where the socket shell was tight within bone. Inasmuch as it is desirable to select an optimal stem and neck length, we have available combinations in Micrograin high-strength cobalt-chrome stems to match SR-0 to SR-6 anthropometrically. However, any combination of neck length can be obtained.

CONTRAINDICATIONS

There are only two absolute contraindications: Active sepsis with high-virulent gram-negative organisms and open epiphyseal plates. The many relative contraindications include active sepsis with low-virulent gram-positive organisms, marked loss of bone stock, and severe leg-length discrepancy.

SURGICAL TECHNIQUE

The lateral transtrochanteric approach is utilized to provide wide access (Amstutz, 1981). The trochanteric osteotomy is performed with a Gigli saw placed extracapsularly, using the Gigli saw passer guide to ensure that the amount of trochanter removed is smallish. It should be based below the vastus tubercle so that the vastus lateralis tendon can be subsequently repaired and enhance trochanteric reattachment. Hemostasis is aided by Gelfoam paste compressed into the trochanteric bone base (sterile Gelfoam mixed with saline). The greater trochanter is reflected and held proximally by three short 4-in Steinmann pins placed 2–3 cm apart into the pelvis, and at least 1 cm proximal to the acetabular rim. The pin placed posterior to the other two should be placed more proximally into the ilium so that it will not interfere when the pin-centring guide is applied to the femoral neck.

The maximum width of the femoral neck is carefully determined with a caliper (Fig. 9.1). This should be less than the internal dimension of the smallest reamer to be used for femoral component insertion. The surgeon decides whether to begin reaming on the femoral or on the acetabular side. Generally, acetabular preparation is commenced by reaming, with the reamer just under the femoral head size and expanded so as to permit at least 2–3 mm of acrylic all around. The operative worksheet is used to determine the optimal size reamer for a given component (Table 9.1). We now prefer to use debris-retaining reamers, reaming to a depth where approximately 50% of the bed is cancellous. Final reaming should await careful inspection and preliminary reaming of the femoral head to ensure optimal reconstruction. The socket gauge is used to assess the depth by carefully observing the spatial relationship of the rim and socket gauge, so that when the socket shell is pressed in, this will not 'bottom out' during acrylic insertion. If the acetabulum is dysplastic, consideration should be given to adding an iliac crest graft to provide socket shell containment.

We now recommend making *four* holes into the superior ilium and one each into the

RECENT ADVANCES IN TOTAL HIP RESURFACING 159

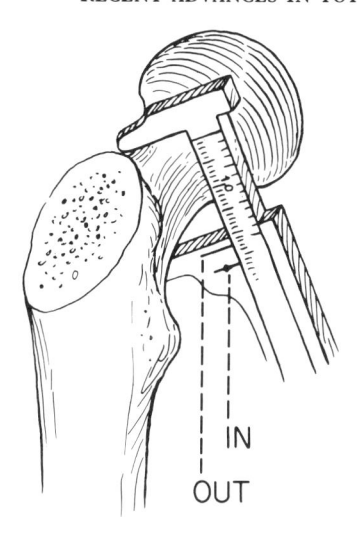

Fig. 9.1 Measurement of greatest neck diameter with caliper

ischium and pubis (total six) (Fig. 9.2). The holes should be about 6 mm in diameter, approximately the same size as the tip of the syringe gun nozzle, so that the acrylic can be contained by sealing the nozzle to the bone when injected. Curettes are preferred for making fixation holes because the holes must never penetrate into the pelvis. All debris and fractured trabecules are removed with a slightly angled curette. Thrombin-soaked Gelfoam sponges are inserted into these fixation holes to assist in controlling haemorrhage.

Table 9.1 Working dimensions of the THARIES system for surface replacement

THARIES component	Neck width (mm)	Reamed head diameter (mm)	Femoral shell ID/OD (mm)	Acetabular shell OD (mm)	Reamed acetabulum ID (mm)
*SR-0	<26	26	29/33	41-s 43-m 45-l	44 46
SR-1	<29	29	32/36	44-s 46-m 48-l	47 49
SR-2	<32	32	35/39	47-s 49-m 51-l	50 52
SR-3	<36	36	39/43	51-s 53-m 55-l	54 56
SR-4	<40	40	43/47	55-s 57-m 59-l	58 60
SR-5	<44	44	47/51	59-s 61-m 63-l	62 64
*SR-6	<47	47	50/54	62-s 64-m	65 68

* Available on a custom order basis

160 RECENT ADVANCES IN ORTHOPAEDICS

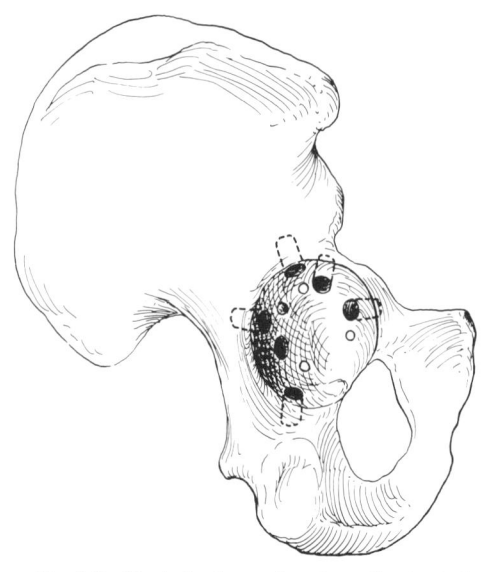

Fig. 9.2 Maximized cancellous bone fixation holes

In order to help the surgeon preserve femoral neck integrity, the pin centring guide was designed to assist in inserting a 4-in Steinmann pin down the central axis of the neck relative to its widest dimension (Fig. 9.3). It is important to realize that the central neck axis is located superiorly and anteriorly with respect to the head; i.e., the head will tend to overhang the neck both inferiorly and posteriorly. Osteophytes may exaggerate the offset. Since the major axis of the neck lies close to the coronal plane, the integrity of the inferior and superior cortices will be at risk while the head is being reamed. In particular, it is essential to avoid notching the much thinner superior

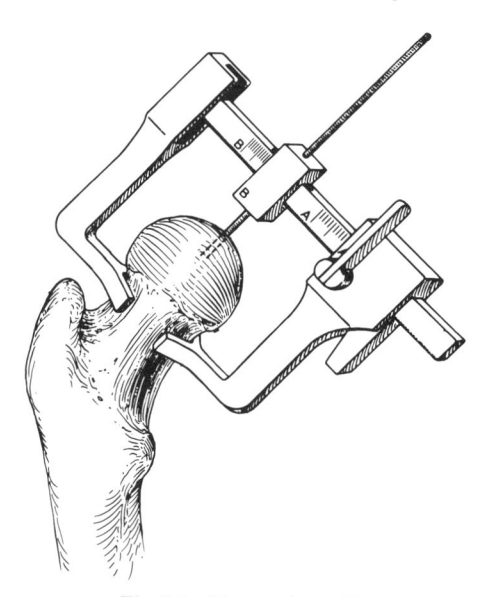

Fig. 9.3 Pin centring guide

RECENT ADVANCES IN TOTAL HIP RESURFACING 161

cortex, where the maximum tensile stresses can be anticipated. The pin-centring guide jaws are generally attached to the neck across the major axis, which generally runs from superior and slightly anterior to inferior and slightly posterior toward the lesser trochanter. Osteophytes which may keep the pin-centring guide from fitting snugly should be rongeured to ensure tightness. The centring device itself should be positioned by setting the same number of notches on the B scale as indicated on the A scale.

The guide pin should be driven in about 5–15 mm. The cylindrical reamer gauge can be rotated about the central axis pin to indicate the limits of the particular reamer to be used. If the pin is off centre several millimetres, it is easy to reposition; if it is only off a millimetre, then replacement is impractical because the original pin track will be followed.

Proper pin placement will avoid the selection of a reamer that is smaller than the neck or one displaced from the neck axis, possibly causing notching of the neck during the remaining process (Fig. 9.4).

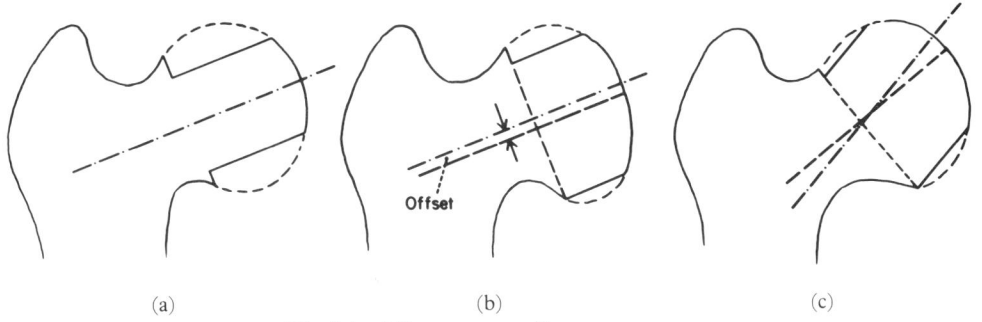

Fig. 9.4 A Reamer too small
B Reamer too low or deformed head
C Poor reamer orientation

An oversized reamer (generally two sizes larger) is selected initially to remove a minimal amount of bone, and successive reamings are made with appropriate smaller reamers to the final reamed head diameter. It is desirable to assess the reaming process accurately, both visually and by palpation, to ensure that there were no positioning errors and that the reamer will not invade the neck as it is advanced. The diameter of the final reamer should exceed the largest dimension of the neck. It is helpful to post the THARIES working dimensions on the wall of the operating room for reference. Each reamer has an intrinsic stop to keep the teeth from cutting into the intertrochanteric area (Fig. 9.5). These anthropometrically designed stops are effective as long as

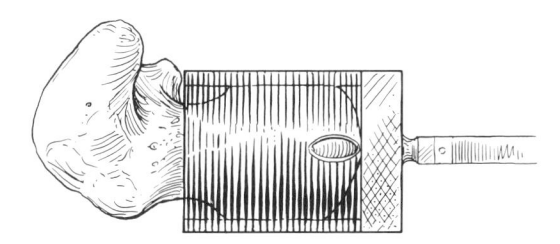

Fig. 9.5 Cylindrical reamer gauge

the largest cylindrical reamer is two sizes or less than the final reamer based on neck dimension, and the neck is not abnormally short. If pin placement is not precisely down the central axis or if final reaming is coming close to neck notching, then final reaming should be done carefully freehand (Fig. 9.6). The final reamer should be

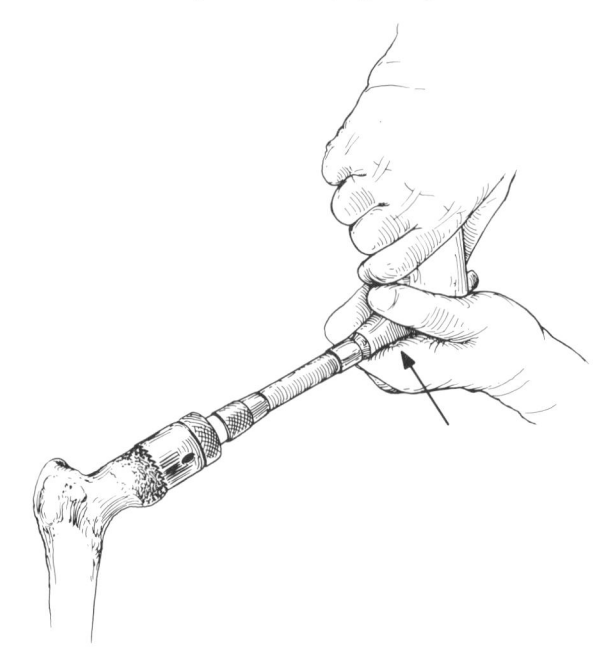

Fig. 9.6 Completion of final reaming with hand pressure to protect and avoid a notch into the superior neck

started for about 5 mm with the pin in place and then removed. Final reaming is performed by using hand pressure on the reamer, being careful not to notch the neck interiorly and anteriorly.

The saw guide is then applied and positioned so that the inferior margin will cover the reamed portion of the head. The dome of the head is removed with a sabre saw; sectioning the dome at this level ensures that the femoral component will cover the reamed surface and minimizes the risk of a head–neck junction stress riser. This is especially important if there is severe osteoporosis. The next step is bevelling the margins of the proximally cut femoral head with the chamfer reamer. The final shape of the reamed femoral head is checked with a template (Fig. 9.7) corresponding to the internal dimensions of the femoral component. If there are remaining cysts, the membrane linings should be meticulously removed. We have found that a high-speed burr effectively removes tenacious fibrous tissue.

Holes are drilled into zones of relative avascularity down to areas of good bleeding bone, using a $\frac{1}{16}$-in drill. While healthy vascular bone throughout is desirable, it may be feasible to leave small, relatively dense areas of sclerotic bone as long as drill holes are placed into vascular bone. In some hips with osteonecrosis it may be necessary to shorten the head as much as 1.5 cm in order to have sufficient healthy bone before final implantation. A review of femoral head preparation is shown diagrammatically in Figure 9.8.

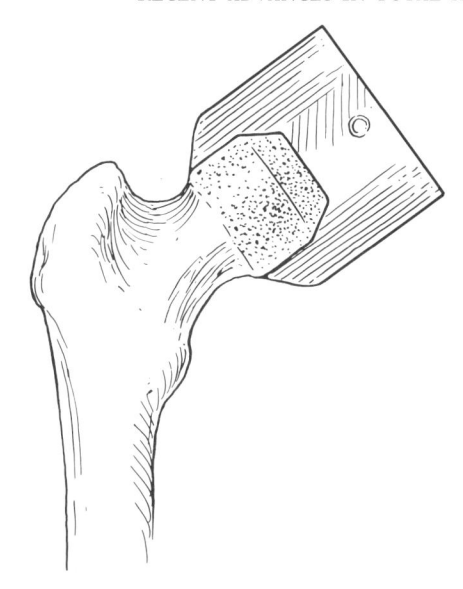

Fig. 9.7 Template replicates internal dimensions of prosthesis. The prosthesis should cover exposed cancellous bone

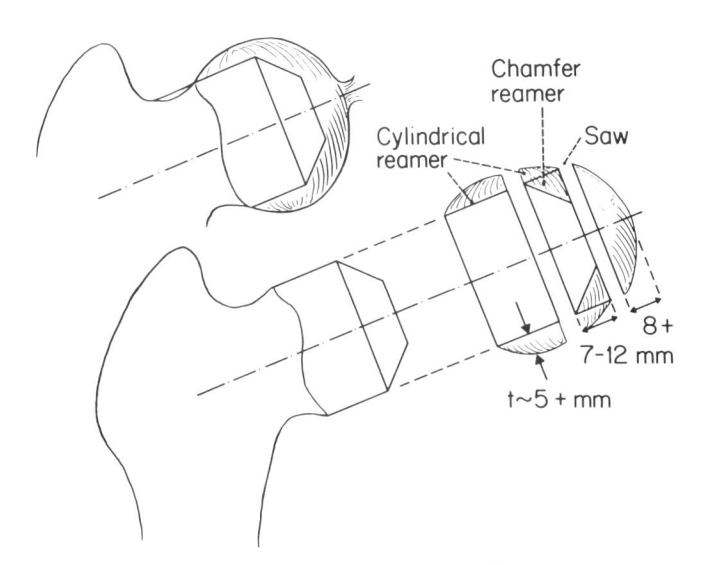

Fig. 9.8 Femoral head preparation

After the acetabulum and femoral head have been prepared, the shells are press-fitted into position, and a trial reduction and range-of-motion are performed. Measurement from the Steinmann pins retracting the trochanter to the base of the trochanter confirms that the leg length equality has been maintained. Final preparation of the bone bed of the acetabulum includes pulsating lavage of the cancellous surfaces to remove debris (Fig. 9.9). This technique permits better acrylic impaction, with smaller, less frequent radiolucent zones at the acrylic/bone junction immediately

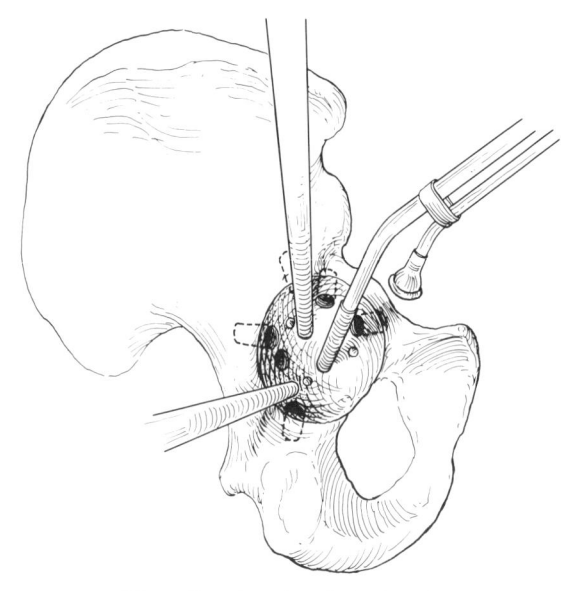

Fig. 9.9 Waterpik and suction. Irrigation of acetabulum

postoperatively. Prepolymerized spacers may be used to provide uniformly thick acrylic. The final position of the socket should be judged by the position of the socket shell gauge even if spacers are used. There should be space for at least 2 mm of acrylic all around and the rim of the gauge should be contained within the bony rim of the acetabulum.

The area is thoroughly cleansed of bone and clot by using pulsating lavage and then drying as completely as possible. Acrylic in a low-viscosity state is poured into a syringe and then injected under pressure into each of the fixation holes (Fig. 9.10).

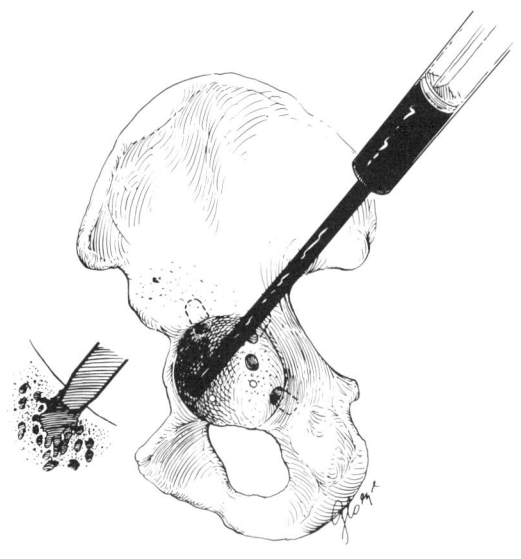

Fig. 9.10 Injection of acrylic

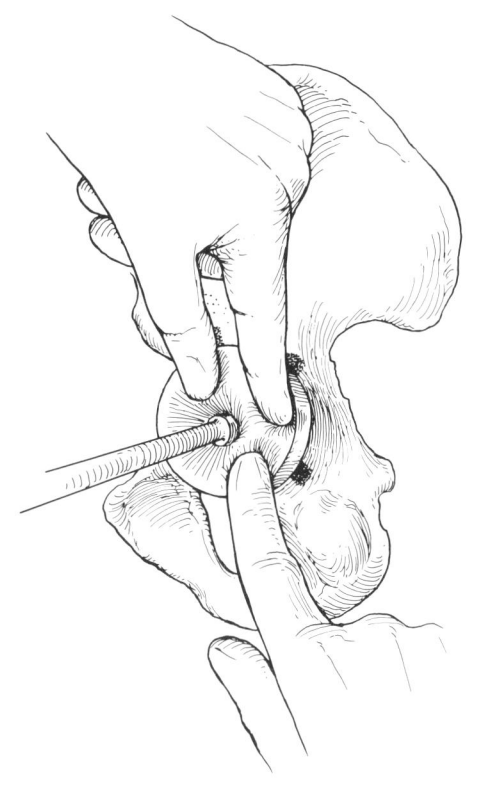

Fig. 9.11 Pressurization of acrylic with acetabulum compressor

Additional acrylic is then placed into the acetabulum and a flexible acrylic compressor (whose outside diameter is slightly larger than the acetabular opening) is applied, thereby forcing the acrylic into the cancellous bone (Fig. 9.11).

About four to five minutes before setting,* additional finger-packing of the fixation holes is performed. Acrylic is uniformly spread all around the acetabulum and the socket is carefully inserted. The acetabular margin is noted to avoid a 'bottom out' position with too thin an acrylic layer surrounding the cup and the acrylic spacers help to ensure a more uniform layer. The socket should be compressed into the acetabulum, guiding its direction by using the two handles of the inserter so that acrylic is expressed entirely around the rim (Fig. 9.12). Acrylic is trimmed from the edge of the socket with the sharp surface of a spatula or scalpel. The final socket position parallels the anatomical opening, which is about 45° lateral and 15–20° anterior.

The bone bed of the femoral head is similarly prepared with pulsating lavage, removing marrow, debris, and blood clots from the surfaces which are then thoroughly dried. A small gas-sterilized sausage-shaped balloon cut in half is filled with low-viscosity acrylic (Fig. 9.13), then applied over the femoral head while a wire is twisted at the neck base for containment (Fig. 9.14). The acrylic is finger-compressed into the interstices for several minutes, after which the wire is removed and

* Zimmer Bone Cement; setting time in our operating room 9–10 minutes.

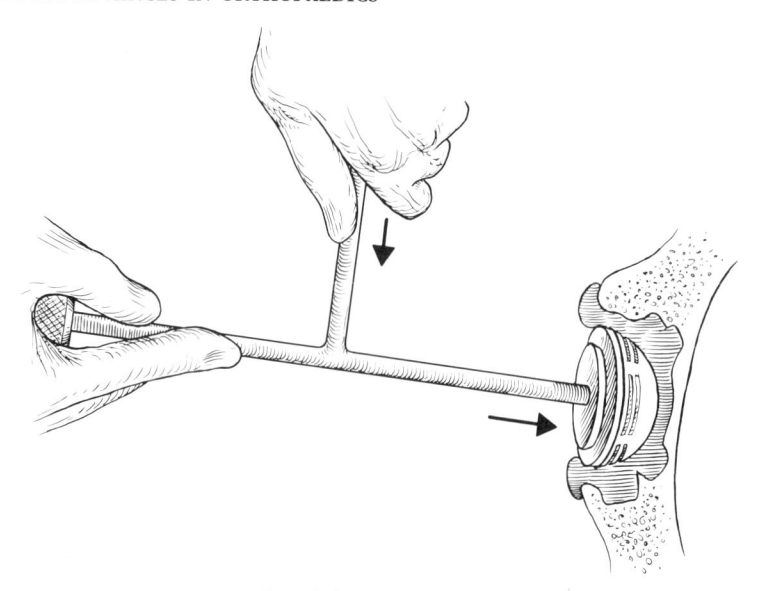

Fig. 9.12 Pressure triangulation to centralize socket within acetabulum

the ballooon cut free. Additional acrylic is further compressed by finger-packing. The component is filled circumferentially with remaining acrylic to avoid air spaces and is pressed onto the femoral head. After the component is positioned, the shell positioner is removed. Pressure is then applied with the shell pusher. The acrylic is continually trimmed, preferably with a blunt spatula, until the acrylic has polymerized. There should be no acrylic extending beyond the shell.

The greater trochanter is reattached with two cross-wires placed approximately 5–10 mm under the trochanteric base (10 mm are required if the bone is osteoporotic), as previously described (Amstutz & Graff-Radford, 1981). The vertical wire is then passed over the top of the trochanter through the abductor muscle mass. Three holes are drilled in the trochanter, using the trochanter holder as a guide. The distal

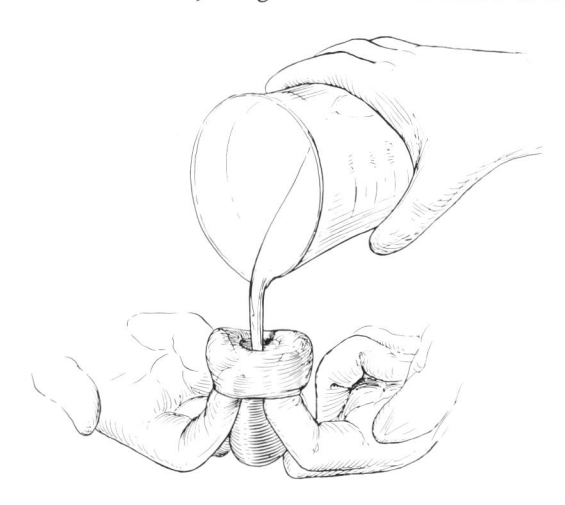

Fig. 9.13 Gas sterilized cut-off balloon filled with low-viscosity acrylic

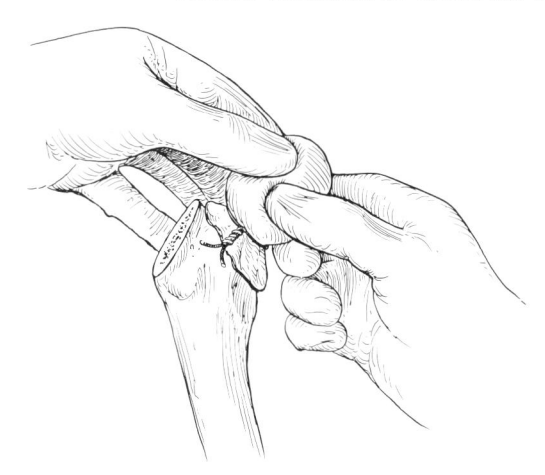

Fig. 9.14 Finger acrylic pressure contained by balloon and wire

hole is 1–2 cm from the distal tip, depending on the degree of advancement. The anterior and posterior holes are drilled as close to the bone margin as possible, to minimize the tendency to cause separation of the trochanter when the knots are pulled tight. The vertical wire is pulled tight to advance the trochanter over the vastus ridge after the vastus has been stripped with a periosteal elevator. A lap sponge applied to the slightly advanced trochanter is impacted with a mallet against the bed and the No. 18-gauge wires tightened with interlocked square knots (Fig. 9.15). The wires are cut about 1 cm long, bent at a right angle and impacted into the bone base. The trochanter must be rigid at the time of closure. The ends are individually turned into

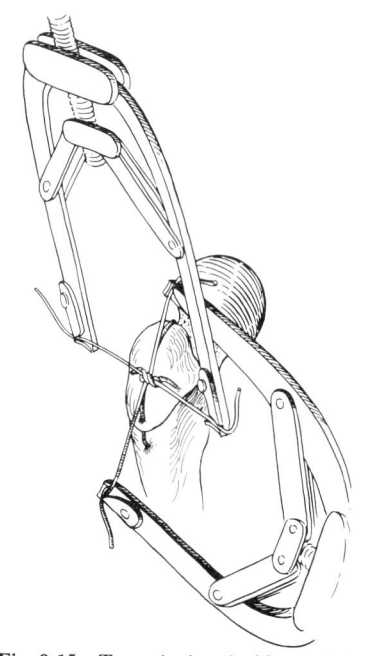

Fig. 9.15 Two-wire interlocking technique

the bone with needlenose pliers or Snowden wire Penzers and carefully flattened against the bone with a wire tamp to avoid nicking the underlying wire. The vastus lateralis is sutured with zero gauge suture material to assist trochanteric fixation. Wound drainage devices are inserted into the superficial and deep layers and the area is thoroughly irrigated to remove all debris and acrylic particles; closure is routine.

RESULTS

The first 350 of 500 THARIES replacements have been followed for periods ranging from one to six-and-a-half years. The primary etiology reflects a preponderance of osteoarthritis, but with a high incidence of osteonecrosis and dysplasia, the material encompasses nearly all diagnostic categories of hip disease (Table 9.2). The average age was 45.4 years among 21 patients with bilateral THARIES. An additional eight patients underwent contralateral conventional replacement.

Table 9.2 Etiology in population of 350 hips

Etiology	%
Osteoarthritis	41.8
Avascular necrosis	18.9
Rheumatoid arthritis	12.9
Congenital dislocation of the hip	7.5
Post-trauma	5.4
Slipped capital femoral epiphysis	2.6
Ankylosing spondylitis	2.6
Other	8.3

The average operating time was 171 minutes; although experience has enabled us gradually to reduce this, a hip replacement is rarely completed in less than two hours. The average blood loss at the time of surgery plus the suction drainage postoperatively averaged 1352 cc. The majority of procedures have been performed after an autologous blood protocol whereby patients bank three units preoperatively for use in the operative and postoperative periods. In later patients, greater use of hypotensive anaesthesia to achieve dryness at the interface for optimal fixation, blood loss has decreased on an average of approximately 500 cc. Only patients in good general health, without cardiac or renal medical problems, were considered for hypotensive anaesthesia. The hospital stay averaged 16.8 days (range 10–49 days); the standard deviation was 5.3 days. The distribution of SR sizes was skewed slightly to the left with a mode of SR-4 (Table 9.3). Although the small-thickness acetabular component was used in 57% of patients, now most components are of medium thickness.

Table 9.3 Frequency of component size

SR Size	1	2	3	4	5	6	Total
Surface — small	7	13	58	57	62	4	201 (57%)
Surface — medium	5	12	35	48	20	7	127 (36%)
Surface — large	2	3	0	1	1	0	7 (2%)
Protrusio	1	2	3	4	3	0	13 (4%)
Custom			2				2 (1%)
Total	15 (4%)	30 (9%)	98 (28%)	110 (32%)	86 (25%)	11 (3%)	350

The preoperative and postoperative results with respect to pain, walking, function, and range of motion have been entirely comparable with conventional replacement. Pain relief has been excellent, improving from an average of 4.2 to 8.5 on a 10.0 scale, similar to results obtained in our conventional hip replacement series. Moreover, there has been no deterioration since our early follow-up studies. Walking and function parameters both improved significantly from the preoperative status. Although on the average patients who underwent surface replacement were not as seriously disabled as those in our conventional hip replacement series, a continued improvement has been noted (Amstutz, 1980; Amstutz et al, 1981).

Table 9.4 Preoperative and Postoperative

	Preoperative	Postoperative
Pain	4.2 (1.5)	8.5 (1.7)
Walking	5.7 (1.5)	8.4 (1.9)
Function	5.6 (1.7)	8.1 (1.8)
Arc of flexion	82 (35)	106 (21)
Arc of rotation	24 (21)	61 (19)

The flexion arc improved from 82–106° and the rotation arc in extension from 24–61°. These latest postoperative values demonstrate improvement over our short-term follow-up study, in which the average postoperative flexion was 95° and rotation arc 52°. In general, flexion contractures have been substantially reduced or eliminated. There were nine hips in eight patients with less than 75° of flexion at follow-up, but this occurred in hips that were stiff to begin with or which developed Grade III or IV heterotopic bone.

COMPLICATIONS

Systemic

There have been relatively few systemic complications in this entire series. Two patients developed thrombophlebitis while in hospital on anticoagulation, and one had a non-fatal pulmonary embolus. Another patient required readmission for phlebitis. Eighteen patients required catheterization and seven had urinary tract infections. Six patients have had some cardiopulmonary complication, all of which resolved. Four patients died after less than one year of follow-up and two to four years of causes unrelated to their surgery. There have been six patients who developed postoperative peroneal nerve palsy, five in the first 200, and one in the next 150; of these, three recovered completely, but in the other three recovery has been incomplete.

'Minor' complications requiring surgery

Six patients who suffered trochanteric bursitis were temporarily relieved by injection but subsequently underwent trochanteric wire removal. Four of these patients achieved complete relief and are functioning normally; two others continue to be symptomatic, both having complex psychosocial histories. In two patients who had heterotopic bone excised, there was recurrence. Another 'minor' complication we encountered was in a patient who developed a femoral neck cyst which required bone grafting at 33 months postoperation. Seven months later this ossified although there is still some pain.

Dislocation

No dislocations have occurred in patients who have had normal or relatively normal bone stock and abductor musculature. Two dislocations have occurred in patients who have had major deficiencies of bone or muscle stock. Both were reduced and have experienced no further dislocation.

Loosening

In our first 350 THARIES there have been two septic and 19 aseptic loosenings of components that required revision surgery. Five of the aseptic patients had socket loosenings, two had femoral loosenings, and 12 had loosening in both the femoral and socket components. Of the 19 patients, five had congenitally dysplastic or dislocated hips, seven had osteonecrosis, three osteoarthritis, two had a slipped capital femoral epiphysis, one had osteochondritis dessicans, and one had congenital coxa vara. The average age of patients with loosening was 37 years at the time of revision.

Loosening has been related to diagnosis with particularly high complication rates in dysplasia, especially at the outset of our series. There was also an association with osteonecrosis, youth, high activity levels, length of follow-up and technique. All of these factors have been analyzed and a comparison made among our cases by cohorts of 150 hips.

There were 16 failures in the first series of 150 hips, including 14 aseptic loosenings (9.3%). Five of these occurred in dysplastic patients prior to the reduction in the socket depth to 3 mm under a hemisphere and 4 mm in osteonecrosis. In addition, there was one fracture and one infection. The second series of 150 hips have a one-and-three-quarter to three-year follow-up, and the loosening rate is 3.3%, with one neck fracture and one infection. The third series of 150 hips now have a six-month to one-and-three-quarter-year follow-up with no major complications.

Although no failures have occurred in post-traumatic osteonecrosis, our highest complication rate has been in non-traumatic osteonecrosis. In the first 150 it was 13% and in the next 150, 10%. In the more recent 150 there have been no failures. We recommend removal of most of the bone stock which is necrotic. Preservation of one-third of the reamed head circumference has allowed sufficient structural strength for the femoral component. Those with deficient bone stock and those who continue on steroids or alcohol remain at higher risk for loosening. Our recent results, however, are encouraging, especially with osteoarthritis. These patients, whose average age was 58 at surgery, have a 1% failure rate with only two loosenings in the first series of 150, 1.5% in the next 150 hips, and none in the most recent 150. Despite high activity levels, these patients have thrived regardless of imperfections in technique in our early series. We now regard THARIES as an excellent device for total hip replacement, even in the elderly, as long as bone preparation and fixation techniques are in accordance with current recommendations, 1981.

Rheumatoid hips in rheumatoid arthritis continue to have a low complication rate at UCLA Hospital; we have had no loosenings and only one neck fracture. To obviate the latter, we recommend approximately 1 cm shortening in cases with severe osteoporosis. In all THARIES we continue to reduce the femoral head size to that which will be just accommodated without notching the neck. This also enables us to save acetabular stock.

Although we have identified many etiologic factors in cases that loosened, the fact that those with longer follow-up have a higher failure rate deserves special analysis. How can we be assured that the more recent series of hips with shorter follow-up time will be better than the earlier group? While there are variations in age and etiology among the groups studied, the chief differences lie in the length of follow-up and the technique utilized. Is it possible to evaluate the improvement in technique in order to make valid comparisons? With the cylindrical chamferred prepared head of the THARIES, isolated femoral component loosening has been rare except in osteonecrosis. The major problem has been socket loosening, which if unrevised promptly will lead to femoral loosening. Therefore, the changes observed in the extent and width of socket radiolucencies may predict loosening and occur long before the onset of symptoms. We have correlated the extent, width, and progression of the X-ray radiolucency noted postoperatively at two months, at one year, and at three to six years. These were completed with the clinical results and complications. A similar study was made of the more recent group at the shorter follow-up time.

There has been a significant diminution in the extent and width of the radiolucency at the acrylic bone junction at comparable time periods. A majority of hips showed none or minor imperfection in technique sufficient to predict lower loosening rates at three to six years. In patients who follow the reduced weight-bearing policy postoperatively, most of the interfaces in the recent groups have retained their initial improved radiographic appearance when compared to the wider progressive zones of the first series of 150 hips. Although there are some exceptions, the worst results are in the group of young active patients.

Are there other factors which may adversely affect fixation compared to conventional replacements? We analysed the frictional torque of various-sized components in a simulator, and found that frictional torque was approximately proportional to the calculated value based on ball size. However, we observed rim contact with some of the large-sized components prior to 1981 which produced a higher initial torque. We do not know whether this has been influential in causing a higher loosening rate, but have worked with the manufacturer to rectify this problem. We recommend that all components be checked by using serum or saline lubrication in a rough spin test prior to insertion. Those that do not spin freely when matched should not be implanted. Even when optimal, the larger ball size of the resurfacing will have a higher frictional torque, and fixation should be optimized to prevent this increased interface stress.

Two neck fractures and two cases of sepsis have occurred in our entire series, including those in our overall failure rate.

Dislocation

The two patients who dislocated had gross muscle and bone stock deficiencies which probably could have been avoided if proper postoperative precautions had been followed. Both occurred with the current socket design, 3 mm under a hemisphere, which has provided ample stability under ordinary circumstances. However, we recommend trochanteric advancement in patients who require shortening, e.g., in cases of osteonecrosis or severe osteoporosis. Four patients with femoral loosenings, two from our own series, have undergone revision, and the femoral component was placed on the shortened femoral heads and extended down onto the neck in order to fix it on relatively good bone stock. All four patients had some restricted range of motion noted at the operating table which was improved considerably by sculpturing. Although at the conclusion there was slight restriction, this has not posed a problem postoperatively. The sculpturing in two patients required passing the cylindrical reamer down through the base of the trochanter, osteomizing and removing the lesser trochanter. We were careful not to violate medial calcar support. In these patients the greater trochanter was advanced to the lateral shaft.

Sepsis

We believe that the sepsis incidence is low because the intramedullary femoral canal is not violated. Many of our cases of haematogenous sepsis in conventional total hip replacement have occurred on the femoral side. Two cases of sepsis deserve special mention. One occurred in a 58-year-old man who sustained an open fracture dislocation of the right hip when hit by a speed boat while swimming. The area became septic, required six procedures for debridement and subsequent split-thickness grafts. The hip became ankylosed with severe myositis ossificans. No abductor muscles were found at surgery. In the postoperative period he was transferred to another hospital where a dislocation occurred which was unrecognized for several months. He then required an open reduction and did well for two years before the hip again became septic. Our other sepsis case was a 58-year-old man with bilateral osteonecrosis who developed culture-positive drainage during the postoperative period. In retrospect, this should have been debrided at the time. However, the wound healed but drainage recurred at eight months which was culture-positive for Streptococcus. At revision the loose acetabular component was removed and thoroughly debrided. The femoral component was tight and undisturbed, but three weeks after removal an acetabular penetration was bone grafted and the socket reinserted. The patient is now asymptomatic two years post-revision.

Heterotopic bone

The overall incidence of heterotopic ossification has been comparable to our conventional hip replacement series. There has been a 2% incidence of severe ossification but no ankylosis. While the cause of heterotopic ossification is unknown, we now place most high-risk male osteoarthritis patients on a diphosphonate protocol which includes 20 mg/kg of Didronel taken for two weeks prior to surgery and three months postoperatively. In addition, we carefully remove all accumulated debris by thorough cleansing at operation. We are also using radiotherapy at 2000 rads at 10 divided doses postoperation for exceptionally high-risk cases as described by Coventry et al, 1979.

Nerve palsy

The incidence of nerve palsy has been distressing despite a high percentage of recovery. We believe that this complication is due to stretching of the nerve during surgery. The operation is performed in the lateral decubitus position and palsy could stem from inadequate support of the leg when held by the assistant after the hip dislocation. When the hip is further externally rotated to deliver the femoral head for reaming, the leg should be supported by the assistant's leg and hands and the peroneal nerve at the knee protected from pressure against the operating table. Overzealous retraction should be avoided by carefully positioning of Homan retractors.

Trochanteric Bursitis
The incidence of trochanteric bursitis has been low despite the youth of our patient population and their high activity levels.

Neck fracture
Two fractures of the neck have occurred in our entire series of 500 patients. The first patient was a 52-year-old woman with rheumatoid arthritis who had suffered a fracture 12 months postoperatively which occurred through a portion of the head and not at the head–neck junction. There was no obvious cause other than the osteoporosis and the fact that the reconstruction had been performed with the normal femoral neck length. The second patient was a 29-year-old with osteonecrosis who fractured 41 months after replacement. Because not all of the necrotic bone had been resected in the initial procedure, this could be implicated.

In examining a large number of fractures in patients sent to us by other surgeons, we found etiologic factors in all but one. In three patients with osteonecrosis an inadequate resection of necrotic bone had resulted in fracture at the junction between necrotic and normal bone. In four others there was osteoporosis and a radiographically visible notch in the superolateral surface of the neck, suggesting that this was the initiating factor. In two hips a large intracapsular trochanteric osteotomy had been performed. Freeman has also observed fractures caused by large trochanteric osteotomies and stress risers owing to improperly located screws or holes. Notches due to femoral reaming or poor positioning can be avoided by carefully utilizing techniques available with the THARIES system.

WORLDWIDE RESULTS

Paltrinieri and Trentani, who were the first to implant acrylic fixed-hip surface-type replacements, recently reported a 46% failure rate in 60 hips followed for periods from four to eight years (Trentani & Vacarrino, 1981). A further 16% had sockets shown to have migrated on X-ray and would soon need revision. The average age of these patients at initial operation was 56 years. The 'average longevity' of the prosthesis was three years and four months in cases of rheumatoid arthritis, four years and eight months in osteonecrosis, six years and four months in patients with congenital dysplasias! These authors concluded that their procedure was contraindicated in severe rheumatoid arthritis, osteonecrosis involving more than one-third of the head, hips with marked dysplasia, and bilateral disease. Although few technique or design changes have been specified, they remain optimistic about their results achieved by using their new patient-selection criteria. Nevertheless, their complication incidence is indeed sobering.

The early Eicher (Indiana Conservative Hip, ICH) and Freeman (ICLH) series each reported 45% failures with their initial clinical trials followed two to five years. Even with his subsequent technique and design changes, Freeman reported a 35% failure figure in patients averaging 58 years at operation and followed up three to six years (Freeman, 1981). Although improvements in technique were made with the

ICH, as performed by Capello, 27% failed in patients averaging 49 years at three to six years (Capello & Trancik, 1981). Both reported high failure rates in the not-too-well-defined entity known as 'inflammatory arthritis'. Capello recently reported using metal backing as a solution for what was termed 'subchondral bone failure,' and Freeman is 'press-fitting' components without acrylic cement, but has also changed femoral component materials to a polymer. These reports indicate that further experimentation is proceeding in their clinical investigations.

Wagner has not presented recent, detailed statistics of his long-term patients. Always an advocate of osteotomy where possible for young patients, his resurfaced population averages 58 years. He previously reported a 5.3% failure rate in patients followed for periods from one to four years (Wagner, 1978). We do not know his comparative three- to six-year results, but he has reported a failure rate of 29% in inflammatory arthritis and now utilizes a ceramic femoral component exclusively.

All innovators agree that minor technical mistakes can cause early resurfacing failure. These include a poorly positioned trochanteric osteotomy or a faulty reattachment technique, neck notches during femoral head preparation leading to fracture, poor acrylic fixation and inadequate patient selection. In addition to the complications reported by innovators, comes news of high, short-term complication rates from other surgeons causing them to change prosthetic type or abandon the technique altogether.

Recently Head reported a 30% failure rate due to loosening, fracture, and necrosis in 41 patients followed one to four years using the Wagner prosthesis (Head, 1981). The average time to failure was 18 months, and he did not recommend the procedure. The TARA* prosthesis, which has a short curved stem, is now undergoing clinical trials, but it is not a true surface replacement because the stem enters the intramedullary canal. This obviates some of the potential biological and biomechanical advantages of surface replacement with respect to avoiding sepsis of the femur and transferring all stress to the prepared femoral head.

Townley has reported a 3.4% loosening failure rate in patients who had predominantly osteoarthritis at an average age of 58 years with a relatively short follow-up of only 19 months (Townley, 1981).

In view of all the statistical bad news and the large number of changes instituted in most reports, is it appropriate to ask about the future of resurfacing? We believe most affirmatively that the concept is sound and that at least the current THARIES (Total Hip Articular Replacement by Internal Eccentric Shells) resurfacing technique can produce good and durable results.

CONCLUSION

We have demonstrated that hip resurfacing can achieve results comparable to those of conventional total hip replacement in terms of pain relief, walking, function, and range of motion. Further, the enhanced stability and apparent lower risk of sepsis weigh in favour of its use for certain specific indications. There is an ongoing need to improve long-term interface durability to minimize and, it is hoped, to eliminate

---

* Total Articular Replacement Arthroplasty.

loosening. We are encouraged by our experimental results with the use of porous implants to obtain fixation, although we do not believe that the ultimate in materials and technique have yet been achieved by employing acrylic as the interface material.

Our series has encompassed the most difficult group of patients, i.e., the young and very active. However, it is doubtful that lifetime durability can be achieved for this group at the present time. Changes in component design, improvement in instrumentation, and, most importantly, in fixation technique, coupled with greater discretion in recommending the procedure for patients in whom other surgical procedures (i.e., pelvic shelving, rotational osteotomy or arthrodeses) would be preferable, should achieve improved long-term results.

The worldwide incidence of loosening subsequent to other types of surface replacement is of considerable concern. While there are many contributing factors, including prosthetic design, instrumentation and technique, we believe that the fixation technique is the single most important factor in the prevention of loosening. Moreover, fixation may be more critical than in the conventional procedure because of the large ball size and increased frictional torque.

Each surgical team engaging in surface replacement of any kind must focus on each complication and strive for prevention. For example, we believe that neck fractures are largely preventable. The THARIES range of components enables the surgeon to tailor the prosthesis to the hip, rather than the hip to the prosthesis. The instrumentation provides a useful guide to protect the neck, but the surgical team must be thoroughly versed in its advantages and its shortcomings. When bone stock is poor, such as in severe osteoporosis or necrosis, it is preferable to shorten the head so that the femoral component covers the head–neck junction.

While we understand the surgeon's preference for using a different surgical approach to the hip joint, we believe that at the outset, surgeons learning the technique should use a lateral, transtrochanteric approach because it provides wide exposure with a relatively low incidence of significant heterotopic bone formation. Surgeons should not compromise on bone preparation, cleansing and drying; exposure is most helpful in utilizing the new techniques of compression and containment for acetabular fixation. If the surgeon wishes to explore another approach, he should do so only after he can demonstrate to himself a consistent optimal interface without radiolucencies on a high-contrast postoperative X-ray. The fear of trochanteric migration can be minimized by concentrating on a technique proved to produce reliable results. We also believe that the surgeon must accept the considerable responsibility for obtaining the best possible fixation by using the known adjuncts for achieving this goal. These will be improved in the future, just as they have markedly improved in our own institution during the past six years. We agree with the concern regarding excessive sacrifice of acetabular bone stock, and believe that this can be minimized by utilizing our current technique.

There is no doubt that the time for optimizing fixation is at the initial surgery when maximal trabecular bone can be exposed by reaming. However, we also recommend that the hip should be protected from excessive stress during the postoperative period. The duration of protection or degree to which the surgeon and patient strive to achieve this goal has not yet been carefully defined. We advise a minimum of two months' non-weight bearing, partial-weight bearing with crutches for an additional month, and progressing to use of a cane in the fourth month.

Recently, preservation of subchondral bone plate has been recommended. While our own studies have demonstrated decreased bone strength and increased component micromovement with subchondral plate removal, we recommend its removal except in severe osteoporosis to maximize acrylic interdigitation with the exposed trabecular bone. In deciding for surface or conventional replacement, it is wise to consider need for restoration of biomechanics, bone stock available, risk of sepsis, possible need for revision, and the surgeon's confidence in fixation techniques. We do not generally recommend conventional replacement for patients younger than 60 years and believe there are significant advantages in our procedure for most older patients. Our follow-up suggests that the THARIES procedure is an effective method for the younger population preferably over 40 years who are at greater risk for complications with stem-type replacement when there is no good alternative. However, we are now more realistic concerning the considerably increased risk incurred by the even younger and active patient. As with patients who have conventional replacements, we observed that once a painless replacement is installed, it is easier for the young to forget precautions to avoid impact and protect the hip for long-term durability. We have also observed more complications and poorer results from unknown causes in patients with psychosocial abnormalities. Consequently, we must continue to evaluate the alternatives of osteotomy and arthrodesis. For many there is no urgency, and 'buying time' until improved technology is available could be the best choice for the very young.

The resurfacing procedure to achieve durability of fixation and absence of neck fractures requires exacting techniques. An entirely new technique has had to be developed and learned, particularly since we have challenged the procedure with the most difficult cases. While fellowships or apprenticeship arrangements are likely to improve the quality of surgery, it now is apparent that workshops and 'constant refreshers' with technique updates are essential if we are to achieve and provide the younger, high-risk patients with durable prosthetic reconstructions.

REFERENCES

Amstutz H C 1980 Surface replacement of the hip. In: Proceedings of the 8th open scientific meeting of the hip society. The Hip, C V Mosby, St. Louis, pp 47–67.

Amstutz H C, Graff-Radford A, Mai L, Thomas B J 1981 Surface replacement of the hip with the THARIES system. Journal of Bone & Joint Surgery vol. 63-A, 38: 1069

Amstutz H C, Graff-Radford A 1981 THARIES approach to surface replacement of the hip. In: Instructional course lectures (AAOS), Vol. 30, C V Mosby Co., St. Louis, pp 688–737

Capello W N, Trancik T M 1981 Indiana conservation hip-results, 2–4 1/2 years. AOA Second Annual International Symposium, Boston, Mass.

Clarke I C, Amstutz H C 1975 Human hip joint geometry and hemiarthroplasty selection. Proceedings of the 3rd Open Scientific Meeting of the Hip Society. St. Louis, The C V Mosby Co., pp 63–89

Clarke I, Amstutz H, Christie J, Graff-Radford A 1977 The John Charnley award paper: THARIES surface replacement arthroplasty for the arthritic hip: rebirth of an earlier concept: In: The hip, C V Mosby Co., St. Louis, pp 235–264

Coventry M D, Scanlon P W 1979 The use of radiation to discourage ectopic bone. Presented at the American Orthopaedic Association, Puerto Rico

Freeman M A R 1978 Some anatomical and mechanical consideration relevant to the surface replacement of the femoral head. Clinical Orthopaedics and Relative Research 134: 19–24

Freeman M A R 1981 ICLH surface replacement. Frontiers in total hip replacement. AOA Second Annual International Symposium, Boston, Mass.

Head W C 1981 Wagner surface replacement arthoplasty of the hip. Journal of Bone & Joint Surgery, 63-A: 420–427

Townley C O 1981 Conservative total articular replacement arthroplasty with the fixed femoral cup. Presented at American Academy of Orthopaedic Surgeons, 48th Annual Meeting, Las Vegas, Nevada
Trentani C, Vacarrino F 1981 Italian experience. Resurface arthroplasty utilizing the Paltrinier–Trentani resurface arthroplasty, 8 year assessment. AOA Second Annual International Symposium, Boston, Mass
Wagner H 1978 Surface replacement arthroplasty of the hip. Clinical Orthopaedics 134: 102

10. New materials in orthopaedics: carbon fibre

B. McKibbin

In reviewing the remarkable developments which have taken place in Orthopaedic Surgery over the past half Century it is impossible not to recognise that many of these have only become possible because of previous developments in the equally rapidly developing field of materials technology. There is perhaps no better example of this than that of joint replacement. Many of the ideas on which some of these are based are very old indeed but their realisation has had to await the coming of suitable implantable metals and plastics and similar considerations apply to many forms of fracture fixation. With these considerations in mind it must surely behove Orthopaedic Surgeons to be vigilant when confronted with still newer materials and to contemplate their possible use as surgical implants.

One such material is Carbon, which is capable of manufacture in a variety of physical forms, many of which have only recently been exploited commercially in such varied products as fishing rods and brake linings for aircraft.

Because it is an element and indeed one which is, by definition, an invariable component of every organic tissue it is doubly interesting since it would seem for these reasons, likely to be well tolerated by the tissues of the body (Benson, 1971).

There are two main forms of the material of current clinical interest, vitreous or 'glassy' carbon which is of course a solid, with many of the properties of glass, and filamentous carbon or 'carbon fibre' and while the former material has already found some biological applications it is with the latter that this article will be exclusively concerned. However, before going on to discuss its possible applications it is necessary to give some account of its manufacture and nature.

The manufacture of carbon fibre

Most man made fibres are produced by the extrusion of melted plastic materials through a fine orifice. This is obviously not possible in the case of Carbon whose melting point is around 3000°C and it is therefore necessary to make use of some intermediary or precursor material.

A wide variety of such are available but the one most commonly used is polyacrylonitrile which is the basis of the commercial fabric 'Acrilan'.* The starting material is illustrated in Figure 10.1 where it can be seen to be composed of comparatively thick filaments of a soft and pliable character and which have of course been produced by extrusion. This is then converted into what is effectively an 'ash' but the pyrolytic process is controlled in such a way that the molecular configuration of the original fibre is preserved. As a result its already high tensile strength is considerably enhanced.

* Registered trademark Courtaulds Ltd.

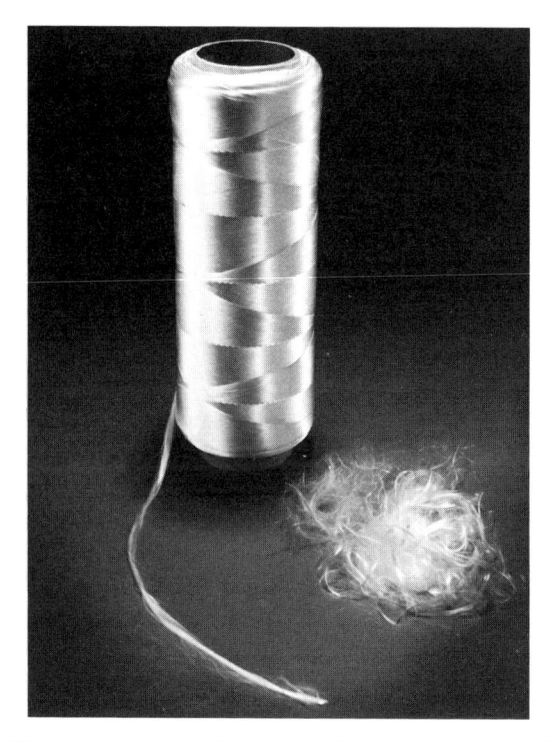

Fig. 10.1 Fibres of polyacrylonitrile prior to their conversion to carbon fibre 'ash'.

In the first stage of manufacture the polyacrilonitrile is oxidised in an oven at 220°C where it undergoes a series of colour changes before finally becoming its definitive black. In this process the fibres become narrower and their molecules tend to line up in an axial direction.

In the next stage, oxygen is excluded and usually replaced by Nitrogen so that further oxidation is prevented and volatile materials can be driven off by raising the temperature to 1500°C. In a further stage the temperature rises to 3000°C and tension is introduced in the fibre leading to crystallisation of the Carbon into a form of graphite. These fibres are then superficially oxidised by an electrolytic process to facilitate the subsequent adhesion of any materials with which the fibres may ultimately be coated. The end result therefore, in chemical terms, is a chain of six membered Carbon rings resulting in fibres which are approximately 8 microns in diameter compared with the 15 microns of the parent material and the physical appearance is, of course, greatly altered (Fig. 10.2).

Physical properties
In the course of this transformation the tensile strength of the fibres increases to about six times that of steel but at the same time there has been a considerable increase in stiffness so that they are easily broken if bent sharply.

These properties can actually be varied slightly by modifications in the manufacturing technique, and the less brittle forms are usually selected for clinical use. The

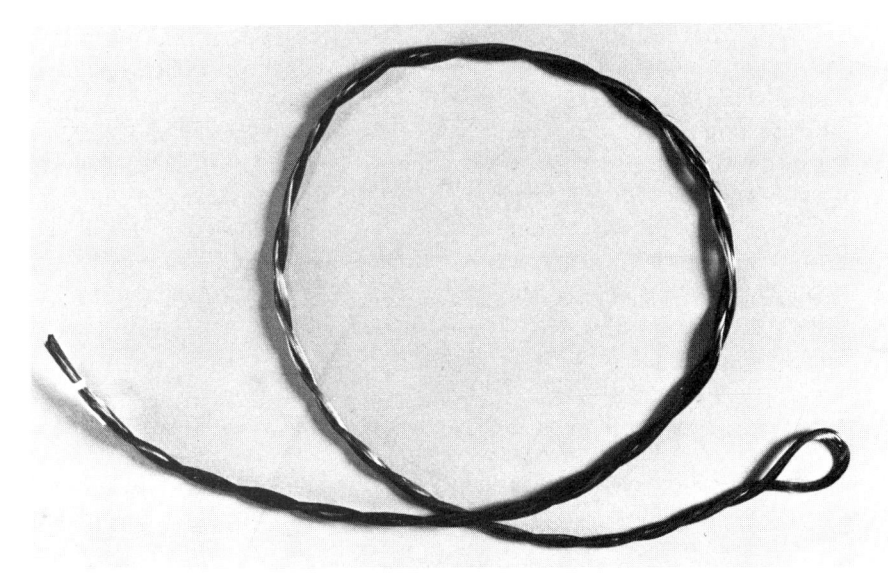

Fig. 10.2 Appearance of the fibres after the pyrolytic process. The resulting tow has been loosely braided to prepare it for clinical use.

fibres are elastic to their point of failure at approximately 140% extension but the great forces required to produce this are very unlikely to be met with in clinical use.

In spite of their great strength the fibres are extremely light (S.G. approx 1.8) and they enjoy good properties of both thermal and electrical conductivity with a low coefficient of thermal expansion, high resistance to chemical activity and a high fatigue life.

The brittleness of the fibres leads to some difficulties in handling and for that reason in most industrial uses the fibres are coated with a 'size' usually consisting of a resin but this stage may be omitted for clinical applications and more suitable materials substituted.

Biological properties

The expectation that carbon would prove to be inert in animal and human tissues appears to have been abundantly confirmed. This has been demonstrated for the material in its vitreous form (North American Rockwell Corporation, 1969; Jenkins & Kawamura, 1971; Mooney, Predecki, Renning & Gray, 1971; and others), and also as porous and solid carbon composites (Janake, Komorn & Cohn, 1974). In experiments conducted in our own Department using carbon/carbon composites (Hombal, Ralis & McKibbin, 1972) the reaction of solid rods of the material in rabbits was compared with that of similar rods made from a variety of contemporary metal surgical implants and found to provoke less reaction even than these extremely unreactive materials. However previous experience has shown that the reactivity of a material is dependent, not only on its chemical composition but also its physical form (Oppenheimer et al, 1958; Wroblewski, 1979). For that reason long term animal studies were set up using carbon fibre itself in a variety of forms (Tayton Phillips & Ralis, 1982) which fortunately produced reassuring results both in terms of tissue toxicity and carcinogenicity.

One of the early causes of concern was the fact that in the original sheep experiments deposits of carbon were found in the regional lymph nodes. There is of course no enzyme system in the body which can dissolve pure carbon so that these deposits must represent the scavinging activity by macrophages of small fragmented portions of the filaments and presumably therefore occurs only in the early stages. Nevertheless efforts have been made to locate the material elsewhere in the body (Jenkins, 1978) without success and it would seem that the fragments never pass beyond the first lymph node they encounter. Bearing in mind that most of us have large accumulations of carbon in the hilar glands of the lung throughout our lifetime there seems no reason to suspect that implantation of the material is likely to be harmful and the way to clinical trials seems clear.

USES OF CARBON FIBRE

For industrial purposes carbon fibres on their own are of comparatively little interest and their main applications lie in acting as reinforcing agents when incorporated in other materials. However when regarded as potential surgical implants a number of possibilities immediately suggest themselves.

The high tensile strength of the material has an obvious appeal as a tendon or a ligament substitute while the fact that the fibres can be woven means that the repair of larger tissue defects can be contemplated.

A quite different series of potential applications can be envisaged when it is realised that the material can be converted into solid form as in most of its industrial applications. The matrix material is usually some form of resin such as the familiar polymethyl-methacrylate or the even stronger Epoxy resins. Such composites, as they are usually called, do of course introduce additional potential problems in relation to possible unfavourable tissue reactions since we are now dealing with something other than simple elemental carbon.

Nevertheless a solid material can be manufactured which does in fact consist of nothing but the pure element. This is done by taking one of the resin composites, referred to above, and pyrolysing it in an oxygen free atmosphere in a similar manner to that employed for the carbon fibre itself in which the non-carbon constituents are again driven off. The result is an amorphous matrix of carbon whose physical strengths will be determined by the orientation of the carbon fibres embedded within it. However, as we shall see this carbon fibre reinforced carbon composite (CFRC) is by no means as strong as the carbon fibre reinforced polymer (CFRP) from which it derived.

It now remains to consider the specific applications and problems of these particular materials in detail dealing first with its use in purely filamentous form as a tendon or ligament substitute and then with applications in its solid form as a composite.

Carbon fibre as a tendon or ligament substitute

On more detailed inspection carbon fibre tow is not perhaps such an appealing material for clinical implantation as might at first appear. Its tensile strength is very evident but so also is its great brittleness. One has merely to twist it in the fingers a few times to produce a debris of small black individual filaments and it is so friable

NEW MATERIALS IN ORTHOPAEDICS: CARBON FIBRE   183

that if it is rubbed over a sharp corner a few times it will disintegrate altogether. It will not form knots readily, for unless under constant tension it tends to spring back into a loose fold. However its behaviour when actually implanted provides something of a surprise.

This was first reported from Cardiff in 1977 (Jenkins Forster McKibbin & Ralis) when it was used to replace the excised Achilles tendon in sheep and rabbits. In these experiments the entire tendon was excised and replaced with a loosely woven triple stand of the material produced by simple plaiting (Fig. 10.3). Its proximal end was interwoven into the remaining muscle of the triceps surae while the distal end was directly inserted into a drillhole in the os calcis.

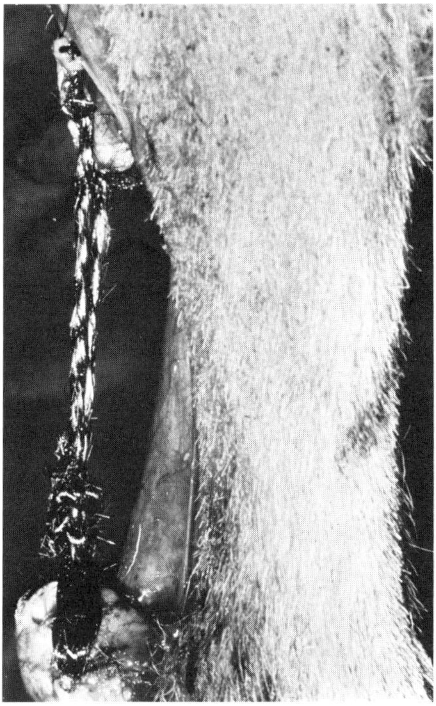

Fig. 10.3   Sheep: tendo calcaneus excised and replaced with a double stand of plaited carbon fibre.

It was found that not only did the implant survive and enable the animal to preserve normal function but by the end of three months the original black implant had become converted into a whitish cord which bore a close resemblance to the original tendon (Fig. 10.4). Subsequent histological examination revealed that this was due to the ingrowth into the implant of strong collagenous tissue whose fibres were predominantly orientated along its axis, in the direction of pull. The carbon fibres themselves had become widely separated by the ingrowth of the new tissue so that in section the appearances were not unlike that of the original tendon (Fig. 10.5). Similar changes were found in a further group of sheep where the material had been used as a substitute for the medial collateral ligament of the knee. The result is therefore something superior to a simple prosthetic replacement in that it is a living structure

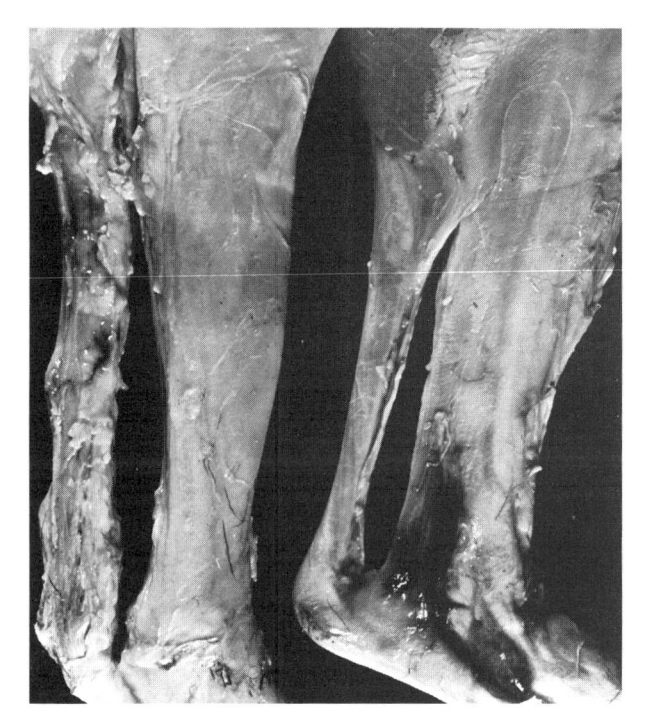

Fig. 10.4 The appearance of the new tendon in the sheep one year after its replacement by carbon fibre. Carbon left; normal right.

which actually becomes stronger with the passage of time and has the capacity to adapt to changing forces placed upon it.

These experiments have been repeated by other groups with similar results (Amis et al, 1981, Coombes et al, 1981) and in fact detailed studies of the new collagen formed has shown it to be remarkably similar in composition to that found in normal tendon and ligament. (Coombes et al, 1981.)

These surprise findings immediately prompt two further questions. The first, somewhat academic, concerns the biological mechanisms behind the phenomenon. It is, on the face of it, somewhat remarkable that a material whose initial attractiveness was its inertness as an implant should attract to itself a specific tissue, collagen, which is positively desirable for the purpose of a tendon or ligament implant. The second, more practical question which then arises is whether or not this reaction, whatever the reasons for its occurrence, can be exploited for clinical purposes. In short, there are both biological and clinical problems to consider.

Biological considerations
The inertness of carbon fibre when used as a simple subcutaneous or intramuscular implant has already been stressed. Forster et al (1978) confirmed this but also concluded that for significant collagenous infiltration to occur the implant had to be under a degree of tension as of course it was when used to replace the tendo achilles. When lying in the same anatomical situation without tension, on the other hand, the degree of infiltration was much less. They also found that even in the presence of

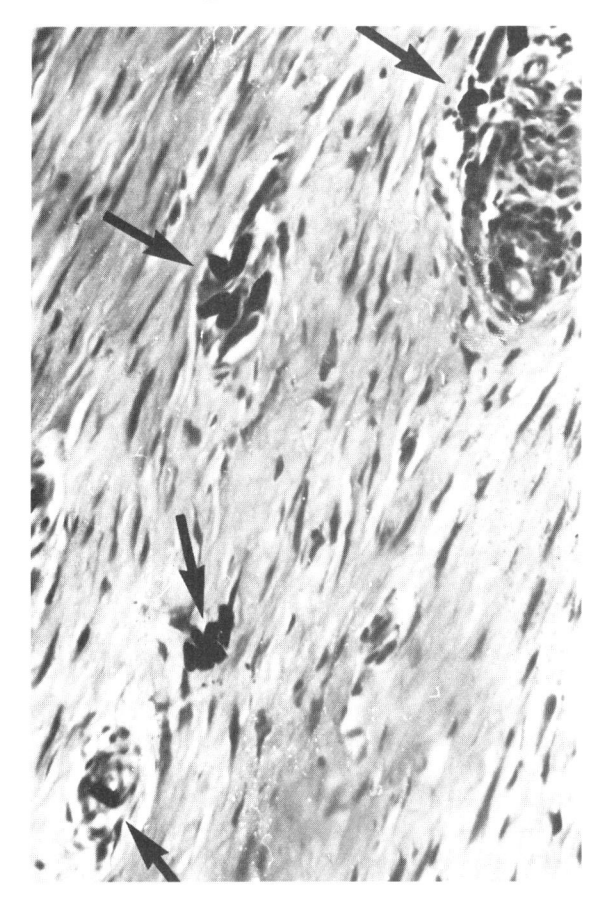

NEW MATERIALS IN ORTHOPAEDICS: CARBON FIBRE 185

Fig. 10.5 Carbon fibre replacing the calcaneal tendon. Although there is a mild foreign body histiocyte reaction, the individual carbon fibres (arrowed) are spread apart by masses of newly formed fibrous tissue, the cells and fibres of which resemble the structure of normal tendon.

tension the amount of new collagenous tissue depended on its anatomical situation and that for some reason close proximity to a neuovascular bundle produces an unusually good response.

Obviously the availability of a local blood supply to support the infiltration is important. Jenkins (1978) attempted to use the material experimentally to replace cruciate ligaments in sheep and found that while significant infiltration did occur this was by no means on the same scale as in the tendo achilles and indeed such a result might have been anticipated since the cruciate ligaments have to pass across a joint cavity and must presumably rely on deriving their blood supply from the bony attachments at either end.

The explanation for the biological behaviour of the material remains obscure. It may be that the infiltration process is simply related to fibre size which by a happy coincidence provided the ideal environment to encourage the process. There is some experimental evidence to support this idea which, if correct, would imply that other materials such as polyester might be equally effective (Amis et al, 1981) but the importance of tension in facilitating the process still has to be explained. Work is continuing in an attempt to elucidate this latter mechanism, but whatever the ultimate explanation the importance of maintaining tension must be born in mind if the material is used clinically.

Clinical considerations
From the foregoing it is apparent that we have a material which may be considered to be safe for use in the human as a long term implant and its most obvious applications would appear to be in the repair of deficiencies in tendons and ligaments.

Ligament repairs
It is in this field that the greatest need for the material has been found, with the knee joint, not surprisingly, providing the majority of the cases. The first clinical trials were undertaken by Jenkins in Cardiff and the first 60 cases reviewed independently by the present writer (Jenkins & McKibbin, 1980). In these early days it was not quite certain where the material would be most effective and it was used for a whole variety of indications, many being of a 'one off' nature. The results in general were extremely gratifying, the new ligaments developed as expected and the hypertrophy of the implant could often be confirmed by percutaneous palpation. A particularly successful group were the repairs of the lateral ligament of the ankle. The operation was quick and simple and by confining itself to a restoration of the calcaneo-fibular ligament avoided the restriction of subtalar movement associated with some repairs utilising the peroneal tendons. No late ruptures occurred nor were there any undesirable side effects. One lesson which did emerge in some of the early cases however was that the implant must not be allowed to 'bowstring' immediately under the skin otherwise ulceration of the latter may ensue. It is also essential that any anchoring knots should be countersunk for the same reason.

Similar satisfactory results attended the use of the material in the late repair of collateral ligament injuries of the knee. Technical considerations are obviously important here with regard to the exact placement and tension of the new ligament and it was felt that any deficiencies in the results arose from these factors rather than any failure of the material itself.

It should be stressed however that these early cases were in the nature of a clinical experiment whose chief object was to determine whether the material would behave in humans as in animals, and if it could be used safely at all. Fortunately no serious unforeseen complications were encountered. It was, of course, recognised that so far as collateral ligaments of the knee are concerned there already exist satisfactory techniques to deal with this problem, employing the patients own tissues, and the question inevitably arises as to whether this new material offers any advantage over these.

Over 400 such cases have now been operated upon in Cardiff and a more critical appraisal is now under way making a detailed comparison with the published results of these established techniques (Leyshon et al, 1982). Only preliminary results are yet available, but it would appear so far that the results stand up to the comparison surprisingly well and what is certainly obvious is that the surgical procedures themselves are very much simpler and quicker than when the patients own tissues are utilised.

However, undoubtedly the greatest clinical interest lies in the results of the repair of cruciate ligament injuries. Thirty three anterior cruciate repairs were reported in the original series, usually in combination with reinforcement of one or both collateral ligaments. As might have been expected the results were less impressive than in the other applications so far described and the result was very dependent on the exact placement of the new ligament. Nevertheless the majority of the patients (61%) reported an improvement in stability. It was obviously difficult to separate this from the effect of the improvement in collateral ligament stability, but objectively the anterior draw sign was reduced or eliminated in many.

A number of the patients complained of some residual discomfort in the knee while others reported some permanent loss of flexion movement. The explanation of the pain remains obscure, it was never severe and there were no instances of effusion or other signs of synovitis such as have been described by others (Dandy et al, 1982). These problems influenced the overall results to the extent that the most satisfied patients tended to be those who had had the most severe degree of instability preoperatively. Many of these were severely disabled and were perfectly willing to accept some degree of flexion loss together with some discomfort in return for improved stability while some of the less severely affected were understandably less satisfied with the exchange.

Others have reported their experience with cruciate ligament repair. Dandy et al (1982) reported 26 such cases in many of which the material had been inserted arthroscopically and reference to these is made elsewhere in this Volume. However he was disturbed by the development of synovitis in a number of his cases which in some circumstances was quite acute with the development of redness and effusion. He did not find the arthroscopic findings in these cases reassuring, with evidence of injection of the synovium and discoloration of the articular surface. He also observed evidence of small fragments of carbon fibre within the joint and suggested that the tissue reaction to carbon in joints was somehow less favourable than in other tissues. Similar observations of intra-articular fragmentation and cartilage discoloration have also been made by Aichroth (1981).

Dandy et al (loc. cit.) further pointed out that although the appearance of the new cruciate ligaments is often impressive, arthroscopic dissection sometimes reveals that this may be due to a very superficial covering of new tissue and the carbon fibre beneath is largely unchanged. This would of course fit in with experimental observations concerning the difficulties of vascularising the cruciates and suggests that the implant in this particular site might be acting as a prosthesis only, so that late failure might be anticipated.

In the most recent review in Cardiff (Leyshon et al, 1982), referred to earlier, 66 patients were recalled for reassessment at an average of $2\frac{1}{2}$ years after operation. The results confirmed the findings in the earlier smaller series with about 60% enjoying a significant improvement in stability, a figure which compares favourably with reports of some more established techniques.

Seventeen randomly selected cases were also subjected to arthroscopic inspection but here the findings were less reassuring. The amount of neotendon formation was much less than in extra-articular sites, as might have been expected, although contrary to expectation this did not appear to manifest itself in late re-ruptures. Only two such were identified even though some implants had been present for as long as 4 years. This suggests that either the amount of collagenous infiltrate needed to reinforce the implant is less than might have been expected or alternatively that much of the stabilising influence was due to the simultaneous reinforcement of extra-articular ligaments which had been carried out in the majority of instances.

However the biopsy specimens taken from these cases have provided some cause for concern with instances of villous synovitis and death of synovial cells and quite marked reaction to the carbon fibres with accumulations of small round cells (Fig. 10.6) in a way never seen in extra-articular sites. Animal experiments have also

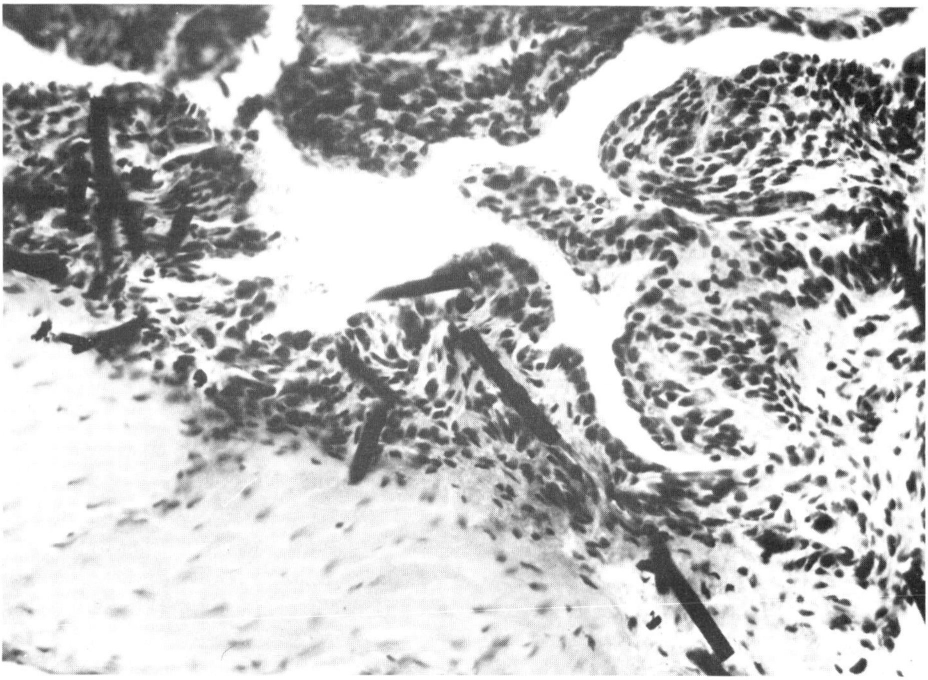

Fig. 10.6 Reaction of the synovial membrane in the knee joint of a man whose anterior cruciate ligament had been replaced 4 years earlier by carbon fibre. Inflammatory changes and villous formation are present. (Haematoxalin & eosin × 75 approx.)

suggested that the material is more reactive in joints than outside it (Phillips & Ralis, 1982). Nevertheless none of this appeared to manifest itself clinically. There were no cases of frank synovitis and the occasional feelings of discomfort in the knee reported in the original series appeared to have largely disappeared by the time of the later review.

There is some evidence from the most recent study to suggest that a synovial reaction is only seen where incorporation of the ligament has been slow suggesting that this may be a mechanical effect due to the free movement accorded to carbon fragments within a joint cavity which could possibly be controlled by some form of coating of the implant. However until this phenomenenon has been fully investigated it would seem prudent to restrict the intra-articular use of the material to very serious cases of instability where the alternatives are arthodesis or replacement surgery and to rely on its extrarticular use in less severely affected cases.

Tendon repairs

The most obvious use for the material is in the site where it was originally tested, the tendo achilles. In cases of long standing rupture where there is an unbridgeable gap the use of a few plainted strands of the material interwoven between the ends is a much simpler solution than the use of locally available natural tissues. Since the original report of its use for this purpose in 1980 (Jenkins & McKibbin, 1980) it has become standard practice in our Department with, so far, gratifying results. It has proved equally successful in a variety of other sites, particularly in late ruptures of the ligamentum patellae and in one case a late and disabling rupture of the tendon of insertion of the biceps.

However whenever its use for tendon replacement is considered the nature of the biological process must be kept in mind; a neotendon will only form if there is available an adjacent blood supply and the acquisition of this will inevitably mean adhesions. Where the surrounding tissues are mobile this is no problem, but obviously it has no part to play in the repair of tendons running in a sheath, an expectation which has been confirmed experimentally.

Even in apparently favourable anatomical sites adhesions can occasionally restrict movement. However once continuity has been established a secondary tenolysis can be followed by vigorous physiotherapy and this will usually restore movement.

Although not strictly a tendon repair an application which the writer has found useful is in the production of a tenodesis in front of the ankle to control dropfoot. This is a relatively minor procedure compared with the usually recommended bony operations. The material may also be conveniently used to extend the length of tendons in certain tendon transfers thus avoiding the necessity for separate incisions to obtain the patients own tissues such as facia lata.

Technical considerations

The difficulties in handling carbon fibre have already been referred to. It is particularly intolerant of being pulled across sharp bony edges which must therefore be rounded off and it is essential that when it is passed through a drillhole in bone for the purposes of attachment that the latter should be generous enough to accommodate it; a successful passage must be made at the first attempt otherwise a dismaying mass of frayed fragments will result.

It is important to stress that not all commercially available forms of carbon fibre are identical. The original implant used in Cardiff consisted of 10 000 filaments of industrial fibres (Courtaulds UK 'Grafil HMS') divided into three strands and loosely braided like a girls hair (Fig. 10.2) and the coating removed chemically, but latterly a commercially available surgical product has been used (Courtaulds 'Grafil AS', prepared by Johnson & Johnson Ltd) in which the fibres have never been coated and they are themselves of a less friable type. Earlier attempts were made to reduce the friability of the implant by using a tighter weave. This certainly produced a more easily handled material but experimental studies showed that this significantly reduced the degree of penetration by new collagen so that the modification was found to be self defeating and therefore abandoned.

Other workers have attempted to improve the handling properties by coating the implant either with polylactic acid or gelatine but no published results are yet available to assess the advantages of these modifications.

For all ligament repairs anchorage to bone is essential and this also presents problems. In Cardiff the solution generally adopted has been to make the initial anchorage with a knot and then rely on multiple passages of the material through drill holes across the entire diameter of the bone to hold it by friction. The final emerging strand is then oversewn along with any convenient locally available soft tissue.

Other techniques of fixation have been devised, Neugebauer (1980) raises a small osteoperiosteal flap of bone which he then clamps onto the filaments with a screw and a small plate which are removed later while Stover (1982) uses a specially designed carbon composite bollard which is driven into a drill hole together with the filaments. The relative merits of these techniques await evaluation and no doubt the ingenuity of surgeons will lead to the development of still better techniques. However whatever method of fixation is devised it should be realised that it is only required temporarily and will soon be greatly reinforced by tissue ingrowth, for that reason it is possible to accept a degree of fixation unthinkable in a pure prosthetic replacement.

Around the knee, collateral ligaments can be inserted through a series of very short incisions and the filament passed from one to the other by subcutaneous tunnelling or through the bone. If the cruciates are to be replaced, on the other hand, arthrotomy will be necessary although, as has already been mentioned even this may be avoided by the use of the arthroscope and indeed it can be argued that by this means a better view of the site of attachment of the original ligaments can be obtained leading to better placement (Dandy, 1981).

Post operatively, six weeks immobilisation has proved sufficient to allow tissue healing and stabilisation of the implant. However it should be remembered that full development of the new structure will probably take at least three months and only gradual resumption of activity can be permitted. Physiotherapists taking part in the post operative care should be made aware of the nature of the process with which they are dealing.

SUMMARY

What then is the clinical role of this new material? It appears from theoretical, experimental and clinical evidence that it may be safely implanted in bone and soft tissues although a doubt exists concerning its use within joint cavities.

It appears to be of unquestioned benefit when used to repair deficiencies in tendons provided that some adhesion formation can be accommodated; repairs of the tendon achilles, ligamentum patellae, biceps and peroneal tendons have been particularly successful and the technique offers an easier technical solution than alternatives which make use of the patients own tissues.

As a ligament substitute it also appears to offer the same advantages, at least when used extra-articularly and although the longest follow up available is 4 years there is no evidence that late stretching occurs, nor would one expect it from theoretical considerations.

The most common indications for its use in this capacity have proved to be the lateral ligament of the ankle and the collateral ligaments of the knee. In the opinion of the writer the former application is the procedure of choice since the results have been uniformly excellent but the verdict in the knee joint must await a more detailed comparison with other available techniques.

A great question mark hangs over the role of cruciate ligament replacement. There are theoretical objections here because of the difficulties of revascularisation and unquestionably the amount of collagenous infiltration is less here than in other sites. There is also undoubted evidence that the material behaves differently within joint cavities although this does not necessarily manifest itself clinically. Furthermore it remains to be established that its intra-articular application is any more effective in conferring stability than when used with complete safety outside the joint.

In the opinion of the writer it should only be used inside the joint at the present in cases of such severe instability that sacrifice of the joint may have to be considered in any case; its use in less severely affected joints should, at present, be regarded as experimental until it can be established that the inflammatory response has no serious long term effects, as the clinical evidence to date suggests.

However it would be a thousand pities if some unresolved questions concerning this particular use of the material should inhibit its use in other parts of the body where its value cannot be doubted.

USE OF CARBON FIBRE COMPOSITES — DEVELOPMENT OF PLATES FOR FRACTURE FIXATION

The development of Biomechanics as a science and its introduction into the field of fracture fixation has resulted in a virtual revolution in implant design. As recently as 1952 Watson Jones stated that 'there is no such thing as internal fixation, only internal suture' a point of view which can certainly not be sustained today when the object of such fixation is to give the patient freedom of movement of the injured limb with the minimum of external restraint.

This objective has only been achieved so far by the use of metal implants to provide the great strength which is necessary. Unfortunately most metals suitable for implantation suffer from the serious disadvantage that they are very prone to fatigue failure. This problem has been met with by increasing their strength and by applying them with due regard for mechanical considerations so that movement at the fracture site is virtually eliminated, at least when fixation by means of plates and screws is being considered.

Such rigidity clearly reduces the risk of fatigue failure but at the same time it causes profound modification to the biological process of fracture healing. In particular it results in the elimination of external callus formation so that union becomes dependent on the alternative process of so called 'direct' or remodelling reunion which is confined to the bone ends. This is a much slower process than external callus formation so that the patient is rendered dependent on his implant for a very long time (McKibbin, 1978) and in the case of plates, although modern designs and techniques of application can cope with this, undesirable secondary effects may be produced in the form of stress protection osteopaenia (Uhtoff & Dubuc, 1976). Thus in the case of tibial fractures it has been recommended that plate removal should not be performed earlier than 18 months since sound union cannot be reasonably expected before this time and even then a refracture rate of 1.5% may be expected (Muller et al, 1979). A further difficulty arises from technical considerations. If the aim of treatment is rigidity of fixation then there can be no compromise on this, the occurrence of even small amounts of movement will prevent direct bone union while at the same time they will conspire to produce fatigue failure of the plate. The amount of callus generated by such small movements will, on the other hand be insufficient to stabilise the fracture and the appearance of such callus is quite rightly regarded as a sign of failure rather than success. The surgical technique therefore is extremely exacting and unforgiving and this is reflected by the number of postgraduate courses currently available throughout the world in which these techniques have to be taught even to already well trained surgeons.

A further problem arises from the slowness in the healing process associated with rigid fixation if deep infection develops. This is usually manifest long before the fracture has united and leaves the surgeon with the unpleasant dilemma of whether or not to remove the implant in the interests of healing leaving him with the necessity of providing some other means of stabilising the fracture.

These problems have lead some surgeons to reconsider the desirability of total rigidity in the internal fixation of diaphyseal fractures in which cases it is necessary to contemplate the use of materials other than metals, possessed of greater elasticity and fatigue resistance. Here again carbon fibre has received a good deal of attention, this time in the role of a reinforcing agent in solid composites.

Development of carbon composite plates

The potential surgical use of these materials was pointed out as early as 1971 by Musicant and also by Benson (1971) and extensive animal experiments have been carried out by Woo and his group in San Diego (Woo et al, 1974; Akeson et al, 1975; Woo et al, 1976 and 1977). They used plates made from graphite fibre reinforced polymethyl-methacrylate on intact bones and on experimental fractures in the radius and femur of the dog. Rigid metal plates were used as controls and the healing process studied by mechanical strength testing and quantitative histology. They found that the speed of healing was roughly comparable in the two groups and was usually complete within a few months but where the plates were retained for longer they noted significant cortical atrophy under the metal plates but not with the CFRP plates. They therefore suggested that this might be of significant clinical advantage where prolonged plate retention was required but nevertheless identified an apparent dilemma.

By dividing the fracture healing process into two phases, a healing phase and a remodelling phase they foresaw a difficulty in achieving a balance between the *rigidity* which they saw as necessary during the healing phases and *reduced rigidity* during the remodelling phase and there certainly would appear to be problems in resolving this using a single material.

In our own laboratories similar experiments have been carried out with a variety of carbon fibre reinforced composites but with a rather different objective in view. Here the purpose was to permit such a degree of movement that not only would stress protection be avoided but external callus formation would still form in such quantities as to make a significant contribution to the healing of the fracture.

Initially attempts were made to avoid polymers and plates of pure carbon (CFRC) were used because of their undoubted biological compatability. Unfortunately even after many design changes a plate could not be constructed of sufficient strength to resist the torsional forces involved and this experience has been shared by others (Claes et al, 1980). As a result this material was abandoned and attention turned to the much stronger combination of carbon fibre reinforced polymer (CFPR). The polymer eventually selected was epoxy resin rather than polymethylmethacrylate because of its greater strength.

In conjunction with the Bioengineering Department of the North Staffordshire Polytechnic, a plate was developed for use on the tibia initially and later for the radius, ulna and femur which it was hoped would fulfil the conditions outlined above. The size of the plates were comparable with metal plates usually used for rigid fixation in these regions (Fig. 10.7) and the detailed design and physical characteristics for the

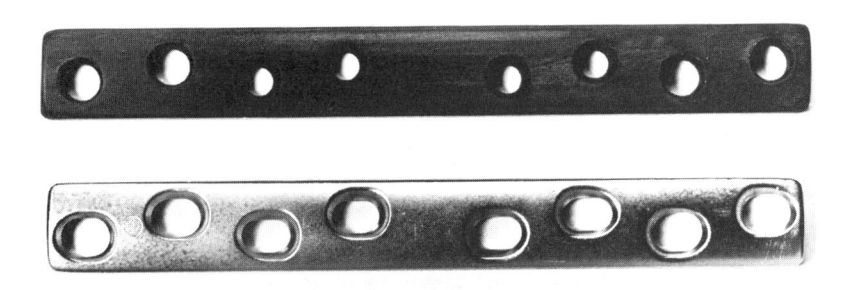

Fig. 10.7 The eight hole 'standard' design of CFRP plate shown above an eight-hole broad steel DCP of the AO design.

tibial plate have been described by Bradley, Hastings and Johnson-Nurse (1980). In summary they found that in four point bending tests, the ultimate strength of the plate (elastic limit) is comparable with that of a standard eight hole stainless steel A0 plate at levels far above anything one would expect clinically, the only difference being that at the elastic limit the CFRP plate broke while the steel plates merely bent. The elasticity of the CFRP was of course much greater, Youngs Modulus being approximately one third that of steel while the fatigue resistance was enormously increased. On the basis of these tests it was decided to embark upon animal, followed by clinical trials and the preliminary results of these have already been reported (Tayton et al, 1982). Long term tissue toxicity tests were also instituted.

Animal experiments
The basic design of the original experiments was similar to that of Woo and his colleagues except that the sheep tibia was used instead of the canine radius and femur. Transverse osteotomies were used and in the control animals standard eight hole DCP plates were used.

All the fractures where the fixation remained intact healed rapidly with direct union between the fragments occurring in both groups; there was however a striking difference in that with the composite plates where there was in addition a large accumulation of ensheathing callus (Fig. 10.8). Nevertheless since union was equally rapid in both groups this did not appear to confer any particular advantage although it was noted that the number of technical failures was less in this group.

However it has been pointed out before, notably by Olerud & Danckwardt-Lilliestrom (1971) that the healing of such simple osteotomies in animals has very

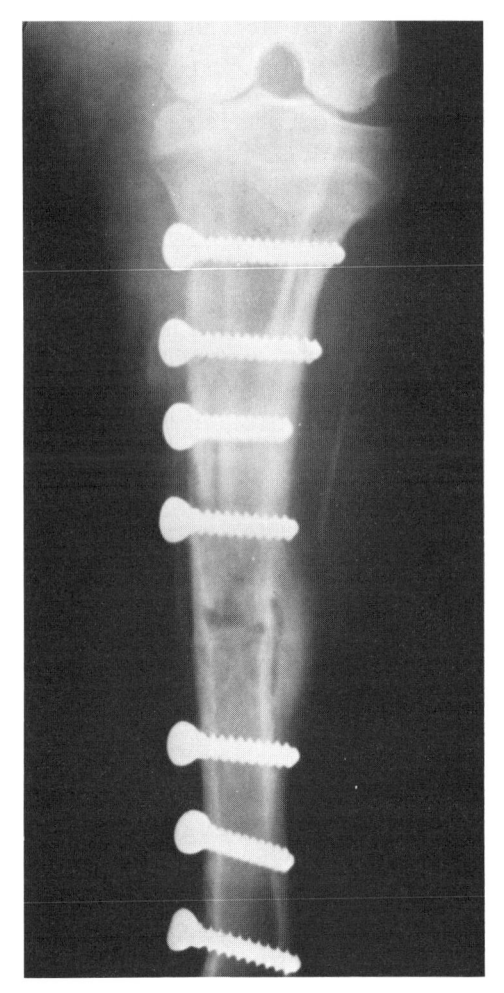

Fig. 10.8 Radiograph of a sheep's tibia eight weeks after a single osteotomy stabilised by a CFRP plate. (Note that the plate itself is radiolucent so that only the fixing screws can be seen.)

little relevance to the clinical situation. Such rapid healing is never seen in the human tibia where plate removal can seldom be contemplated before 18 months. The latter authors attributed this, in part, to the time taken to revascularise the dead bone ends and felt that a more realistic model was provided by a segmental osteotomy where the middle fragment was certainly dead and they succeeded in showing that the healing time of such fractures was very much greater.

Because of these considerations a second series of experiments was conducted using segmental fractures, again comparing metal with CFRP plates. Here a very striking difference was observed. With the latter, rapid healing again occurred due to the large sheath of callus which succeeded in bridging the entire dead segment and both osteotomy cuts (Fig. 10.9). Primary healing did not occur with the three months of the experiment and the bone segments could be removed from the main fragments by soft tissue dissection.

With the metal plates no healing had occurred at all by this time and the fractures

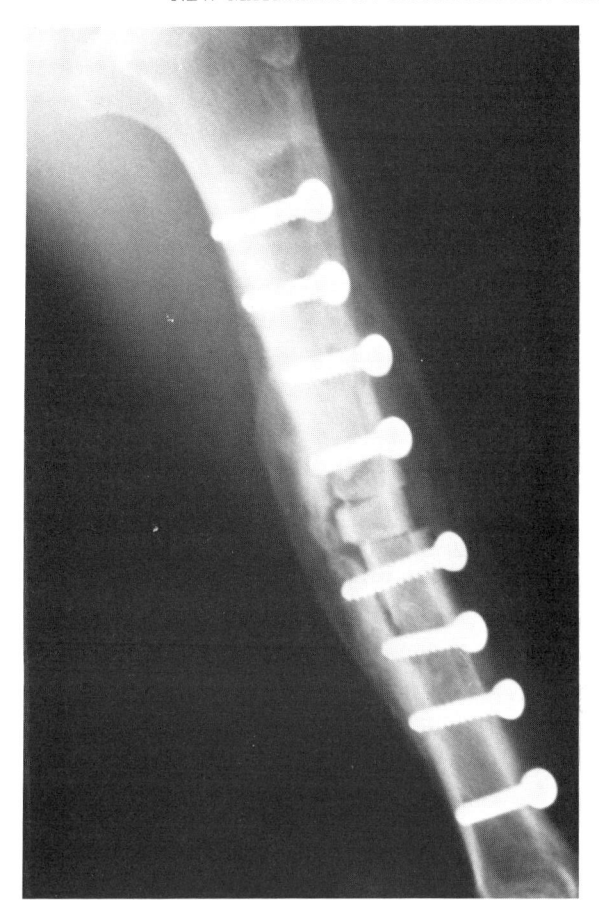

Fig. 10.9 Radiograph of a double osteotomy in a sheeps tibia eight weeks after it had been stabilised with a CFRP plate.

broke down when the plates were removed. Many actually failed mechanically before the three months was up, a phenomenon never seen with the CFRP plates presumably because they were assisted by the early support of the external callus.

It would appear therefore that the dilemma identified by Woo et al (1974) need not arise if the concept that healing must occur exclusively by direct union is abandoned. If healing by the 'natural' method of external callus is adopted instead, then rigidity is not required in the healing phase and indeed must be actively avoided. Thus the desirable mechanical environment of both the healing and the remodelling phases becomes identical. Such a policy therefore offers the possibility of more rapid healing by a method which is less technically demanding and on the basis of these experiments it was thought justified to embark on a trial in human subjects.

Clinical trials
The tibia was selected in the first instance because of the straightness of its shaft and initially the plates were applied to the lateral surface because of the muscle cover available. As confidence improved the medial subcutaneous border was used and this

is still current practice. All the subjects had either a transverse or short oblique fracture of the mid-shaft, some with a single butterfly fragment. Initially only closed fractures were treated but latterly the treatment of a small number of Group 1 and 2 compound fractures has been undertaken. Fixation was by eight 4.5 mm stainless steel AO cortical screws which were inserted with care to *avoid* crossing the fracture gap in order that interfragmentary movement should not be completely eliminated and thus inhibit the formation of external callus. For the same reason the plate was positioned subperiosteally if possible.

Post operatively, full weight bearing was permitted, initially with the assistance of a stick which the patient discarded when he chose. Union was assessed radiologically and the plates removed when consolidation was present beyond all doubt in order to study the reaction of the surrounding tissues. Once the plate had been removed unrestricted activities were permitted.

RESULTS

The clinical progress of the patients was encouraging. Many discarded their sticks within a matter of days and in some instances it was necessary to advise restraint of their activities. Many resumed work within two months of the injury in some cases to jobs involving standing. Early in the series a number of the patients with plates on the lateral border of the tibia experienced some discomfort on weight bearing and indeed, in some, movement of the fracture was apparent clinically. None of these problems has been encountered with the plate on the medial surface however. A single case of hypertrophic non-union was encountered in one of the early cases and exploration revealed that the plate had failed due to a serious manufacturing fault. Union was achieved subsequently following a sliding bone graft.

In all of the remainder union occurred through the medium of external callus (Fig. 10.10) which developed just as if the patients had been treated in plaster. The average time to plate removal was 44 weeks with a maximum of 54, but there is little doubt that because of initial caution many could have been removed much earlier. There have been no instances of refracture and all the patients have returned to their pre-accident activities.

A number of the cases showed interesting features which illustrate the great differences between fractures treated by elastic fixation as compared with rigid plating.

It has already been pointed out that the surgical technique is less demanding than with rigid fixation in that mistakes are less severely penalised, particularly if gaps are left between the ends of the fragments. The case illustrated in Figure 10.11 illustrates this point well and the reader is invited to consider how long a metal plate would have survived in this situation. With an elastic plate, on the other hand, the day was saved by the large amount of callus which came to the aid of the palpably inadequate fixation (Fig. 10.12). Poor technique is never to be recommended but when using this method it should be borne in mind that precise anatomical reduction is not essential any more than when closed techniques are used.

Infection is another problem which will inevitably develop if operative methods are used and in this series there have been unfortunately three such, constituting an uncomfortably high percentage. However the problem proved easier to solve than if rigid plates had been used, again because of the development of early callus which

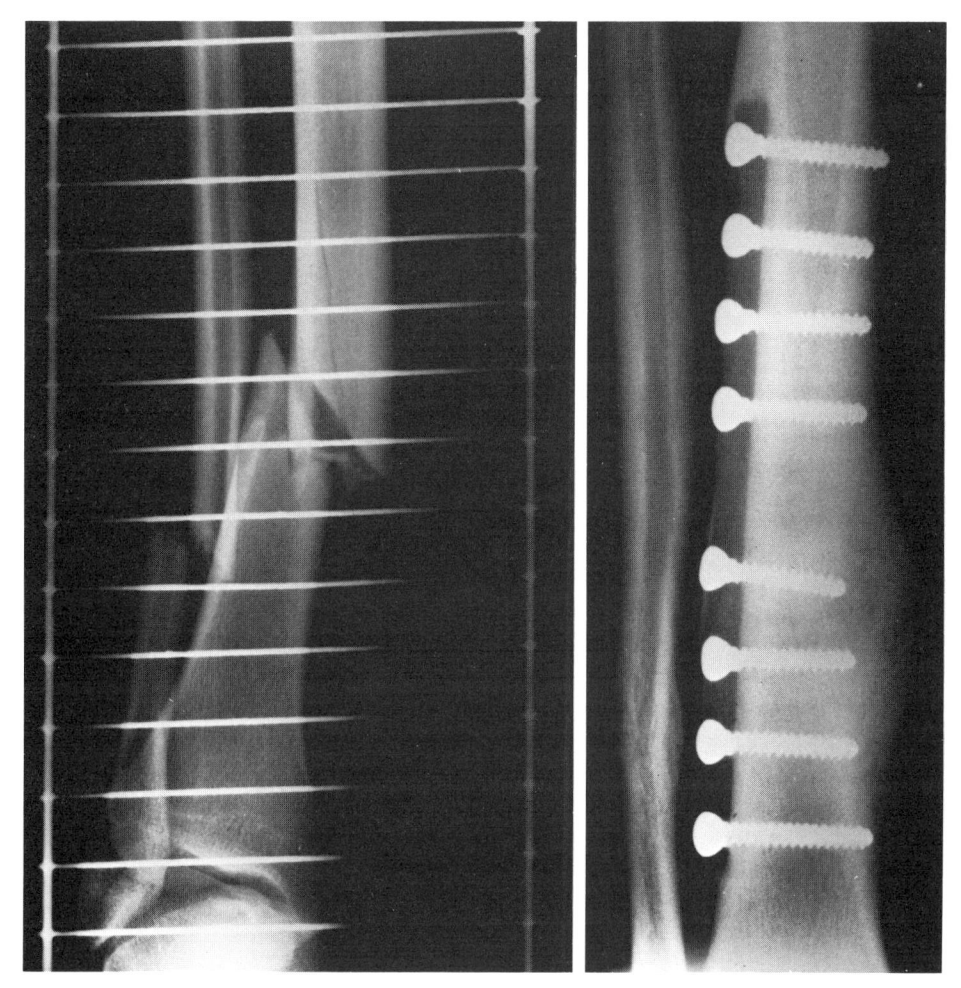

Fig. 10.10 Radiograph of a human fracture of the tibia and fibula. Left; initial injury, Right; appearance 54 weeks after fixation with a CFRP plate. Note there extensive formation of external callus and lack of evidence of bone atrophy.

made it possible to remove the plates at between 12 and 16 weeks because the fracture was already united. This, together with removal of some dead bone was sufficient to dry up the infection and the patients recovery was not significantly delayed.

Of the fractures treated in other bones it is too early to make but the most preliminary comments. However it would appear that it is in the radius and ulna that one of the most useful application of the plates is likely to be found since, unlike the tibia, there is a considerably consensus in favour of internal fixation for these fractures. It has been encouraging in that of the first 12 cases currently being reported (Tayton et al, 1982) all have united while the patients enjoyed a remarkable degree of freedom of use of the limb with no instances, as yet, of implant failure or refracture.

It has been noted that the amount of external callus formed has been more variable than in the tibia and subsequent mechanical testing of the plates after removal has shown that this correlates closely with their elasticity which varied considerably in

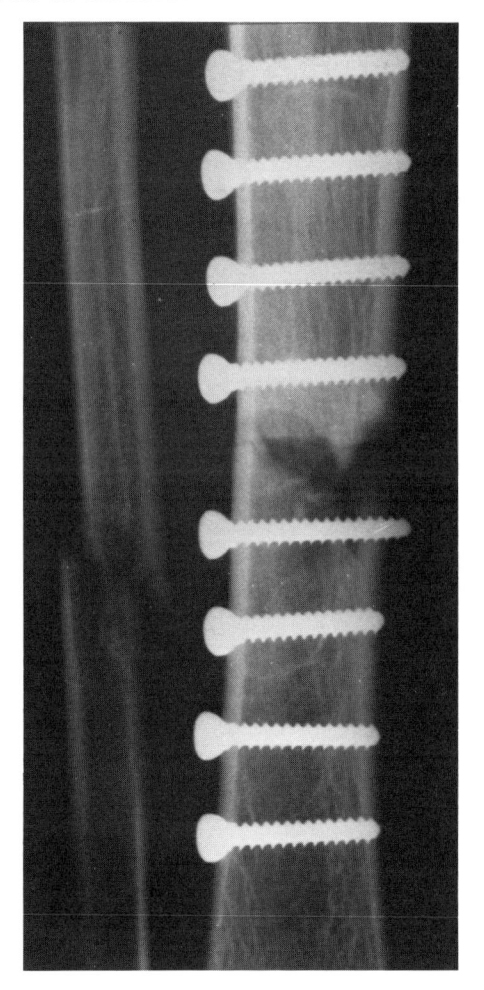

Fig. 10.11 Radiograph of a human fracture fixed with a CFRP plate. Due to a serious technical error a large bone defect was left of the medial side.

some instances. It is obvious that strict quality control and individual mechanical testing of each plate before insertion is essential at the moment since any excessive elasticity will inevitably lead to hypertrophic non-union. However given that these conditions are met the plates appear to offer the same advantages as when used in the tibia.

In the few cases of femoral fracture so far treated callus has been abundant, the fear here is obviously one of implant failure although so far there has been none.

Nevertheless the use of the plates for these fractures must still be regarded as being in the early experimental stages.

Disadvantages
In such a radical departure from conventional fracture plates it would be surprising if the new material did not present problems of its own. In the case of CFPR plates the

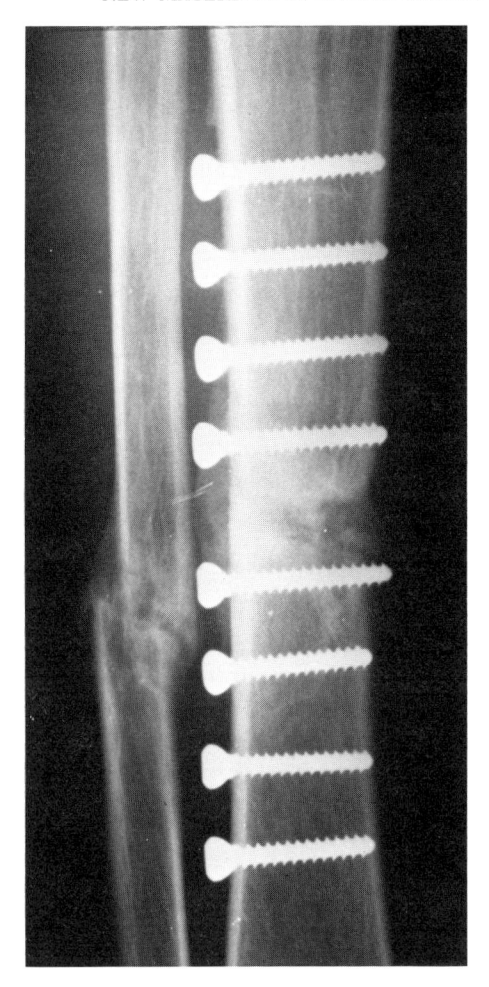

Fig. 10.12 Same fracture 23 weeks later showing bridging of the defect by external callus. The plate was eventually removed 47 weeks after fracture and there were no subsequent complications.

most serious difficulty lies in the very concept itself. If the plates are to be elastic then they cannot at the same time be bent and made to conform to the contour of the bone.

In practice this has been less of a problem than originally envisaged. Absolute anatomical reduction is not essential as in rigid plating techniques and mechanical considerations are less important in selecting a surface for application. For the majority of mid shaft fractures therefore straight plates have been satisfactory. However where the fracture is at the extremity of the bone there are obviously problems but it is believed that this can be met by providing a small selection of precontoured shapes so that a 'best fit' can be selected.

In the meantime the search continues for an alternative material which can be contoured at the table while preserving its elastic properties.

Naturally with any new material the question of biocompatability is paramount. Although it is present practice to remove the plates because of these fears inevitably small particles of detritus remain behind and indeed some blackening of the tissues can be observed. However animal tests have so far revealed no cause for concern and epoxy resin in its fully cured form has implanted in the form of cardiac pacemakers for many years without adverse reaction and the question of the biocompatability of the carbon fibre itself has already been dealt with. Nevertheless this is something which will have to be continually borne in mind for the present.

Miscellaneous uses of carbon fibre

In such a burgeoning field it is hardly surprising that new uses for the material are being described all the time and no claim is made in this review to be comprehensive. There are however one or two other applications of especial interest to Orthopaedic Surgeons which deserve mention.

Use of carbon fibre as a reinforcing agent in artificial joints

The incorporation of carbon fibres into polymers used as one of the bearing surfaces of an artificial joint was described as long ago as 1968 by Lancaster. In laboratory tests he found that using them as an additive to PTFE articulating with steel, wear was significantly reduced. The best results were obtained when the fibres were arranged at right angles to the articulating surface while random chopped fibres were the next best. Similar results were reported by Walker & Erkman (1974) for UHMWPE albeit with some increase of surface scratching, and also by Dumbleton et al (1974). Similar findings were reported using joint simulators (Ainsworth et al, 1976, and Greer, 1979). Already such reinforced components are available for hip knee and ankle although the writer is aware of no published clinical studies. From what we know of the behaviour of carbon there seems no particular reason to anticipate any problems from joint detritus but this is obviously a matter which should be investigated.

Use of carbon fibre for hernia repair

Stimulated by the phenomenon of neotendon formation with filamentous carbon Johnson-Nurse & Jenkins (1980) used a loose darn of the plaited fibre to repair large defects produced in the abdominal wall of sheep using a plastic mesh often used clinically for this purpose as a control. They found gradual invasion of the carbon by collagenous tissue which produced a sound repair in all cases while there were some recurrences in the control group. Such repairs are probably outside the normal range of practice of most specialist Orthopaedic Surgeons but they are sometimes called upon to repair large tissue defects e.g. in the fascia lata and these experiments suggest that carbon fibre would provide a simple and effective way of doing this.

Use of carbon fibre as a nerve graft

The ability of carbon filaments to attract collagen suggests that in other environments other tissues might be similarly induced. This was attempted using parallel strands of the fibre in large posterior tibial nerve defects in rabbits (Ralis et al, 1982). This provided technical problems of attachment which were eventually solved using the fibrin clot technique. Axons sprouts were found to be conducted between the carbon fibres within a few weeks (Fig. 10.13). However these eventually found themselves in competition with the inevitable ingrowth of non-neurological connective tissue and clinical recovery did not occur. In later experiments the graft and its suture lines was covered with a vein graft which not only assisted in creating the anastomosis but also

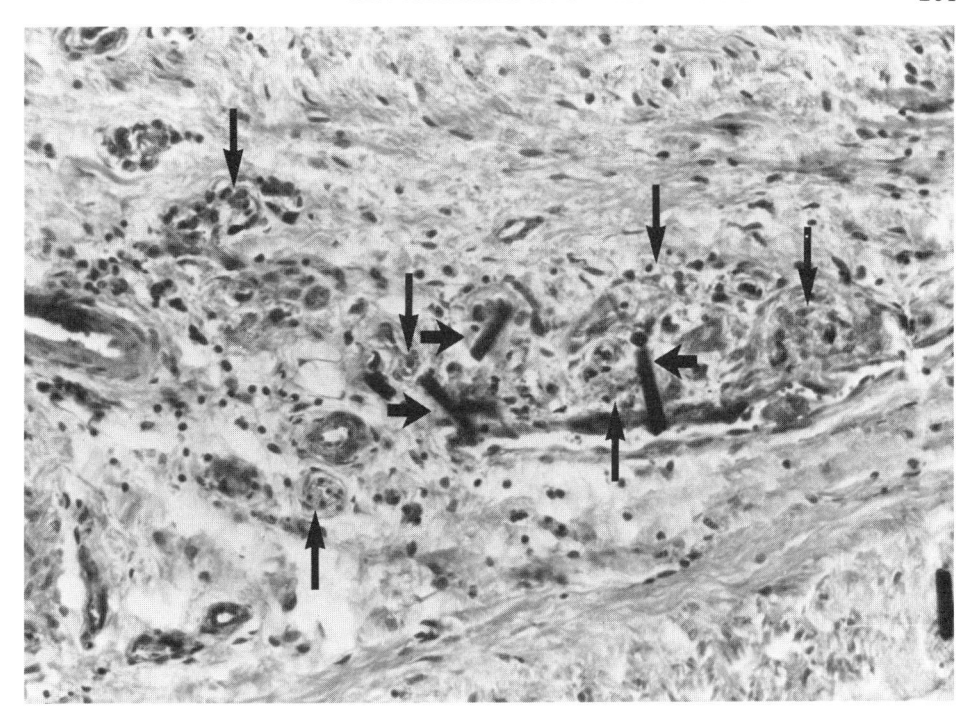

Fig. 10.13 Transverse section of a carbon fibre nerve bridge formed in a defect in the posterior tibial nerve of a rabbit 5 weeks earlier. The carbon fibres (horizontal arrows) are closely followed by sprouting regenerating nerve units (vertical arrows) on their way to the distal stump. (Haematoxalin & eosin × 75 approx.)

by preventing such ingrowth. Nevertheless although some clinical recovery did occur using this technique it was variable in extent and never complete.

Probably many factors were responsible for this, but no doubt the greatest problem is that of achieving bundle correspondence across such a large defect in a mixed nerve and it may well be that further investigations will have to involve the identification of individual bundles with the help of magnification as described elsewhere in this Volume. However the physiological potential for recovery does appear to be there raising the possibility of performing nerve grafts on a scale not previously attainable due to the lack of sufficient donor material.

Acknowledgements

Figures 10.3, 10.4, 10.5, 10.7, 10.8, 10.9, 10.10, 10.11, 10.12 are reproduced with permission from the editor of the Journal of Bone and Joint Surgery (British).

Figure 10.1 is reproduced by courtesy of Messrs Courtaulds Ltd.

REFERENCES

Aichroth P 1982 Personal communication
Ainsworth R D, Farling G M, Bardos D I 1976 Human surgical implant structural devices of carbon fibre reinforced ultra high molecular weight polyethylene. SPE National Technical Conference on 'High Performance plastics'
Akeson W H, Woo S L-Y, Coutts R D, Matthews J V, Gonsalves M, Amiel D 1975 Quantitative

histological evaluation of early fracture healing of cortical bones immobilised by stainless steel and composite plates. Calciferous Tissue Research 19: 27–37

Amis A A, Miller J H, Campbell J R, Kempson S, Wright V, Dowson D 1981 Filamentous implant reconstruction of tendon defects. Journal of Bone & Joint Surgery 63B: 296

Bader K F, Curtin J W 1968 A successful silicone tendon prosthesis. Archives of Surgery 97: 406–411

Benson J 1971 Elemental carbon as a biomaterial. Journal of Biomedical Materials Research 5 Symposium No. 2, Part 1, 41–47

Bradley J S, Hastings G W, Johnson-Nurse C 1980 Carbon fibre reinforced epoxy as a high strength low modulus material for internal fixation plates. Biomaterials 1: 38–40

Claes L, Burri C, Kinzl L, Fitzer E, Huttner W 1980 Less rigid fixation with carbon fibre reinforced materials: mechanical characteristics and behaviour in vivo. In: Uhtheff J D (ed) Current concepts of internal fixation of fractures. Springer-Verlag, Berlin, Heidelberg, New York

Coombs R R H, Graig-Gray J, Sayers D, Naveissi P, Nichols A, Pope F M Collagen typing in carbon fibre-induced tendon. Journal of Bone & Joint Surgery 63B: 296

Dandy D J 1981 Personal communication

Dandy D J, Flanagan J, Edixhoven P 1982 Clinical orthopaedics and related research (In press)

Dumbleton J H, Shen C, Miller E H 1974 A study of the wear of some materials in connection with total hip replacement. Wear 29: 163–171

Forster I W, Ralis Z A, McKibbin B, Jenkins D H R 1978 Biological reactions to carbon fibre implants. Clinical Orthopaedics and Related Research 131: 299

Greer K W 1979 Four years of wear testing experience on three joint simulators. Presented at 11th International biomaterials symposium, Clemson

Hombal J, Ralis Z A, McKibbin B 1972 Unpublished data

Janeke J B, Kmorn R M, Cohn A M 1974 Proplast in cavity obliteration and soft tissue augmentation. Archives of Otolaryngology 100: 24–27

Jenkins G M, Kawamura K 1971 Structure of glassy carbon. Nature 231: 175–176

Jenkins D H R, Forster I W, McKibbin B, Raliz Z A 1977 Induction of tendon and ligament formation by carbon implantation. Journal of Bone & Joint Surgery 59B: 53–57

Jenkins D H R 1978 The repair of cruciate ligaments with flexible carbon fibre. Journal of Bone & Joint Surgery 60B: 520–522

Jenkins D H R, McKibbin B 1980 The role of flexible carbon-fibre implants as tendon and ligament substitutes in clinical practice. Journal of Bone & Joint Surgery 62B: 497–499

Johnson-Nurse C, Jenkins D H R 1980 The use of flexible carbon fibre in the repair of experimental large abdominal incisional hernias. British Journal of Surgery 67: No. 2, 135–137

Leyshon R, Channon G W, Journal of Bone & Joint Surgery (In press)

Lancaster J K 1968 The effect of carbon fibre reinforcement on the friction and wear of polymers. British Journal of Applied Physics (J Phys D), Vol 1, Ser 2: 549–559

Leyshon R, Channon G W, Jenkins D H R J 1982 Journal of Bone & Joint Surgery (In press)

McKibbin B 1978 The biology of fracture healing in long bones. Journal of Bone & Joint Surgery 60B: 150–162

Mooney V, Predecki P K, Renning J, Gray J 1971 Skeletal extension of limb prosthetic attachments — problems in tissue reaction. Journal Biomedical Materials Research, Vol 5, Symposium No 2, Part 1, 143–159

Muller M E, Allgower M, Schneider R, Willenegger H 1979 Manual of internal fixation. Springer-Verlag, Berlin, Heidelberg, New York

Musicant S 1971 Journal of Biomedical Material Research 1: 225

Neugebaurer R 1980 The trapdoor. A possibility of fixation of carbon fibre strands into cancellous bone. First world biomaterials congress, Austria. Book of Abstracts 4, 7, 5

North American Rockwell Corporation 1969 Carbon for surgical implants. Production Engineer 40: 62

Olerud S, Danckwardt-Lilliestrom G 1971 Fracture healing in compression osteosynthesis. Acta Orthopedica Scandinavica, Supplement 137

Oppenheimer B S, Oppenheimer E J, Dantishetshy I, Stoutt A P, Eirich F R 1958 Further studies of polymers as carcinogenic agents in animals. Cancer research 15: 33–40

Ralis Z A, Forster I, Sozen J, McKibbin B 1982 The use of carbon fibre as a nerve graft (In preparation)

Strover A E 1981 Technical improvements in the use of carbon fibre for ligament repair. Proceedings South African Orthopaedic Association (In press)

Tayton K J, Bradley J S, Hastings G, McKibbin B 1982 The treatment of forearm fractures with carbon fibre reinforced epoxy plates (In preparation)

Tayton K J, Phillips G, Ralis Z A (1982) Long term effects of carbon fibre on soft tissues. Journal of Bone & Joint Surgery 64B: 112–114

Tayton K J, Johnson-Nurse C, McKibbin B, Bradley J, Hastings G 1982 The use of semi-rigid carbon-fibre-reinforced plastic plates for fixation of human fractures. Journal of Bone & Joint Surgery, 64B: 105–111

Uhthoff H K, Dubuc F L 1971 Bone structure in the dog under rigid internal fixation. Clinical orthopaedics and related research 81: 165–170
Walker P S, Erkman N J 1974 Variables affecting polymer wear in artificial human joints. In: Lieng-Huang Lee (ed) Advances in polymer friction and wear, Vol 5B Plennum Press, New York, 553–565
Watson-Jones R 1952 Fractures and joint injuries. E & S Livingstone Ltd, Edinburgh & London
Woo S L-Y, Akeson W J, Leventz B, Coutts R D, Matthews J V, Amiel D 1974 Potential application of graphite fiber and methyl methacrylate resin composites as internal fixation plates. Journal of Biomedical Material Research, 8: 321–338
Woo Savio L-Y, Akeson W H, Coutts R D, Rutherford L, Doty D, Jemmott G F, Amiel M S 1976 A comparison of cortical bone atrophy secondary to fixation with plates with large differences in bending stiffness. Journal of Bone & Joint Surgery 58A: 190–195
Woo S L-Y, Simon B R, Akeson W H, McCarty M P 1976 An interdisciplinary approach to evaluate the effect of internal fixation plate on long bone remodelling. Journal of Biomechanics 10: 87–95
Wrobleski B M 1979 Wear of high density polyethylene in bone and cartilage. Journal of Bone & Joint Surgery 61B: 498–500

Index

Angulation osteotomy, 24
Arthrodesis
  after failed knee replacement, 59
  chronic arthritis of knee, 48
Arthroscope
  diagnostic, 88
  operating, 91
  sterilisation, 88
Arthroscopic meniscectomy, 87, 96
  aftercare, 97
  checking meniscal rim, 97
  definition of lesion anatomy, 96–97
  removal of fragments, 97
  results, 98
Arthroscopic surgery of knee, 91–98
  adhesions, 93–94
  aftercare, 90–91
  carbon fibre repair of cruciate ligaments, 95, 187, 190
  complications, 99
  cutting instruments, 92
  drilling, articular cartilage healing and, 94–95
  equipment, 91–92
  fatpad lesions, 94
  ganglia removal, 94
  lateral release of extensor mechanism, 94
  learning techniques, 98–99
  ligament injuries, 95
  lipomata removal, 94
  loose bodies, removal, 94
  medico-legal problems, 99–100
  meniscal reattachment, 96
  meniscectomy *see* Arthroscopic meniscectomy
  osteophytes, 95
  percutaneous needle, diagnostic use, 90
  powered instruments, 91–92
  shaving patella/femoral condyles, 95
  synovectomy, 93
  synovial biopsy, 93
  synovial shelf syndrome, 93
  technique, 92
    triangulation, 92, 98
  workload and, 100–101
  see also Arthroscopy of knee
Arthroscopy of knee
  anaesthesia, 88
  diagnostic, 88–91
  examination of knee, 89–90
  historical aspects, 87–88
  insertion of arthroscope, 89, 90
  irrigation, 89
  preparation of leg, 88–89

Arthroscopy of knee (*cont'd*)
  probing hook, diagnostic use, 90
  tourniquet, 88
  see also Arthroscopic surgery
Attenborough knee replacement, 49, 58

Bone grafts
  osteomyelitis, 120, 122–124, 128
  THARIES replacement and, 157, 158

Carbon fibre, 179–201
  anchorage to bone, 189, 190
  biological properties, 181–182
  brittleness, 180, 181, 182–183, 189
  collagenous infiltration of implant, 183–185
    tension and, 184, 185–186
  deposits in regional lymph nodes, 182
  handling, improvements in, 189
  hernia repair and, 200
  intra-articular use, 187, 188, 190, 191
  ligament repair, 186–188, 190
    collateral knee, 183, 186, 190
    cruciate, 95, 187–188, 190, 191
    lateral of ankle, 186, 190
  manufacture from polyacrilonitrile, 179–180
  as nerve graft, 200–201
  physical properties, 180–181
  postoperative care and, 190
  as reinforcing agent in artificial joints, 200
  technical considerations, 189–190
  tendon repair, 189, 190
    achilles, 183, 189, 190
    biceps, 189, 190
    ligamentum patellae, 189, 190
    peroneal, 190
Carbon fibre composites, 182
  plates for fracture fixation, *see* Fracture fixation, carbon fibre-reinforced polymer (CFRP) plates and
Carpal tunnel syndrome, internal neurolysis and, 9
Chemonucleolysis, *see* Chymopapain chemonucleolysis
Chymopapain, 103
Chymopapain chemonucleolysis
  allergic reaction, 112–113, 114, 117
  CAT in diagnosis and, 108
  complications, 114
  contraindications, 106, 117
    absolute, 106, 108
    relative, 108

Chymopapain chemonucleolysis (cont'd)
  dissolution of nucleus pulposus, 103–104
  indications, 106
  narrowing/rewidening of disc space and, 103–104
  postoperative care, 113–114
  results, 113, 114–117
  reversibility of neurologic deficit, 114
  safety aspects, 105
  technique, 108–113
    anaesthesia, 108, 112
    anaphylaxis and, 112–113
    avoiding spinal nerves, 112
    discography, 111–112
  tolerance, 104
  toxicology, 104–105, 117
Congenital dislocation, hip, 23–43
  femoral side, reconstructive procedures, 23, 24, 39–43
    indications, 39
    rotational/angulation osteotomy, 24, 39
  pelvic reconstructive procedures, see Pelvic osteotomy
  salvage operations, 23
  THARIES replacement and, 157, 168, 170
  transfer of greater trochanter, 41–43
Coxa vara, 157, 170

DePuy Orthofuse, 138, 139
Dial osteotomy, 23, 37
Dwarfism, THARIES replacement and, 157

Electrical stimulation of bone healing, 131–151
  acceleration of normally-healing fractures and, 137, 138
  choice of method, 149–150
  current levels, 136
  distribution of current flow in living tissue, 131–132
  doubly-invasive procedures, 138–139, 149
    electromagnetic induction and, 147
  efficacy, 147–149
  electrical theory and, 131–135
  electrode positioning, 132, 136
  immobilization and, 150
  infection and, 137, 139, 141, 145, 147, 150
  magnetic induction of current, 132–135, 147, 150
  methods of applying current, 132
  non-invasive methods, 142–147, 150
    internal fixation and, 145, 147
    iron-core electromagnetic system, 145–147, 150
  piezoelectrical phenomena and, 135
  pseudoarthroses and, 141, 143, 145, 147
  safety, 150–151
  semi-invasive methods, 139–141, 150
    contraindications, 141
  streaming potentials and, 136
  stress-generated voltages, bone remodelling and, 136
  techniques, 137–147
  theoretical basis, 135–137
Electro-Biology Inc. Bi-Osteogen system, 142–145, 150

Femoral corrective osteotomy, 24, 39, 40
  prerequisites for reconstructive procedures, 40–41
Fracture fixation, carbon fibre reinforced polymer (CFRP) plates and, 191–192
  animal experiments, 193–195
  clinical trials, 195–196
    infection during, 196, 197
    results, 196–198
  contouring of plates to bone, 199
  development of plates, 192–193
  disadvantages, 198–200
  external callus in fracture healing and, 193, 194, 195, 196, 197
Freeman knee replacement, 49, 53–56, 59
Freeman-Samuelson knee replacement, 55, 60, 61

Greater trochanter, lateral displacement, 41, 43, 80–84

Hanging hip operation, 68–70
Hip joint, mechanical equilibrium analysis, 65–68

Insall knee replacement, 49, 56–57
Insall–Burstein knee replacement, 56, 61
Intertrochanteric osteotomy
  enlargement of weight-bearing surface of joint, 69
  osteoarthritis with protrusio acetabuli, 73
  postoperative aspects, 76–77
  preoperative X-rays, 74–75
  procedure, 75
  reappearance of joint space following, 73
  reduction of compressive stresses and, 78
  valgus with tenotomy, 72–73
  varus, 70–72

Knee replacements, 45–62
  age and, 48
  clinical assessment of, 46–47
  compartmental, 49–53, 61
  condylar, 49, 53–57, 60–61
  constrained hinges, 49, 58–59, 61
  coronal knee angle measurement and, 46–47
  deep infection following, 58, 59, 61
  failure
    management of, 59–60
    time since operation and, 47–48
  indications, 48–49
  patient activity and, 48
  radiographic assessment, 47
  semiconstrained linked, 49, 57–58, 61
  state of affected knee and, 48–49
  unicompartmental, 52–53

Legg-Calvé Perthes' disease, 157
Lumbar disc, chemonucleolysis treatment, see Chymopapain chemonucleolysis

Manchester knee replacement, 46, 49–50, 59, 61
Marmor knee replacement, 49, 50

INDEX 207

Nerve grafts, 4, 9, 10, 12, 13–16, 19
  block at distal suture site, 16
  compared with neurorraphy, 16
  distance to be bridged and, 13–14, 15, 16
  free cutaneous, 17, 18
  two suture sites and, 15, 16
  tension at suture sites and, 13, 14, 15
    graft length and, 16
  vascularised, 18
Nerve repair, 1–19
  adequate resection of stumps and, 3, 4
  collagen synthesis reduction and, 3
  connective tissue reduction and, 3–4
  entrapment syndromes, 9
  epifascicular epineurectomy, 9
  epifascicular epineurotomy, 8
  epineural, 1, 10, 11, 13
  epineural/endoneural fibrosis and, 8, 9
  external neurolysis, 8
  fascicular (perineural), 2, 10, 11
  grafts, *see* Nerve grafts
  healing after lesions and, 2–4
  implications of optical magnification, 2
    in internal neurolysis, 9
  interfascicular epineurectomy, 9
  internal neurolysis, 8, 19
  junctional scar tissue formation and, 3
  minimizing surgical trauma, 4
  neurolysis, 8–9
  neurorraphy, *see* Neurorraphy
  tension at suture site and, 3, 4, 10, 13
    joint fixation and, 13–14
    nerve grafting and, 15, 16
Neurorraphy, 10–13
  approximation of stumps, 12
  coaptation of stumps, 12
    maintenance of, 13
  compared to nerve grafting, 16
  fascicular pattern, technique selection and, 11–12
  orientation of stumps, 12
  preparation of stumps, 12
  primary versus secondary, 10
  tension at suture site and, 13
Non-union
  electrical stimulation of bone-healing and, 131–151
  in osteomyelitis
    bone grafts and, 125
    external fixation and, 126, 128

Osteoarthritis, hip
  articular pressure reduction, 65–84
  enlargement of load-bearing surface of joint, 68, 69–70, 72, 73, 79, 80, 81
  hanging hip operation, 68–70
  intertrochanteric osteotomy, 69, 70–73
    valgus with tenotomy, 72–73
    varus, 70–72
  lateral displacement of greater trochanter, 80–84
  with protrusion acetabuli, 67, 73
  reduction of load transmitted by joint, 68, 69, 70, 73, 80

Osteoarthritis, hip (*cont'd*)
  shortening of opposite leg, 79–80
  with subluxation, 67
  THARIES replacement and, 157–158, 168, 170
  uneven distribution of joint stresses and, 66, 67, 68
Osteoarthritis, knee
  arthrodesis and, 48
  arthroscopic removal of osteophytes, 95
  Manchester knee replacement and, 50
Osteomyelitis, 119–128
  antibacterial agents, 125–126, 128
  bone grafts to fill defect (Papineau procedure), 120, 122–124, 128
  classification, 119–120
  electrical stimulation of bone healing and, 141, 145, 147, 150
  fracture-associated, 119–120, 125, 126, 128
  free flap technique (composite graft and microsurgery), 122
  haematogenous, 119, 122, 125
  metal fixation in presence of infection, 126
  microbiology, 120
  muscle pedicle grafts, 122, 128
  with non-union
    bone grafting and, 125
    external fixation and, 126, 128
  obliteration of dead space, 120
  post-operative/post-traumatic chronic, 120, 125
  removal of dead bone, 120
  secondary intent, 124
  soft tissue coverage of exposed bone, 120
  split-thickness graft, 124
  suction irrigation and delayed closure, 120, 122
  surgical management, 120–124
Osteonecrosis, THARIES replacement and, 157, 168, 170
Oxford knee replacement, 49, 50–52, 61

Pauwels' osteotomy, *see* Intertrochanteric osteotomy
Pelvic osteotomy
  acetabular-femoral head relationship and, 25
    CAT scan, 27
    radiographic determination, 28–29
  arthrography of hip joint and, 25, 27
  'clear space' in hip joint and, 25
  dial (Eppright) osteotomy, 23, 37
  indications, 29–30, 33, 35, 37
  Pemberton pericapsular osteotomy, 30–33, 39
  preoperative radiography, 25, 27, 28
  prerequisites, 25–29
  range of hip motion and, 25
  Salter (redirectional) osteotomy, 33, 39
  spherical (Wagner) osteotomy, 37
  Steel (triple) innominate osteotomy, 35–37, 39
  Sutherland 'double' osteotomy, 23, 33–35
Pemberton 'pericapsular' osteotomy, 30–33, 39
Protrusio acetabuli, 67, 73
Pseudoarthroses, 143, 145, 147

Rheumatoid arthritis
  knee replacement and, 48, 50
  THARIES replacement and, 157, 168, 170
Rotational osteotomy, 24

Salter (redirectional) osteotomy, 33, 39
Sheehan knee replacement, 49, 57–58, 61
Shortening of leg, 79–80
Spherical osteotomy, 37
Spherocentric knee replacement, 49, 58
Stanmore knee replacement, 49, 59, 60, 61
Steel (triple) innominate osteotomy, 35–37, 39
Sutherland 'double' osteotomy, 33–35
Synovectomy, knee, 93
Synovial biopsy, knee, 93
Synovial shelf syndrome, knee, 93

Telectronics Osteostim, 138–139
Total Hip Articular Replacement by Eccentric Shells (THARIES) surface replacement system, 155–176
  age of patients and, 176
  complications, 169–173
    minor, requiring surgery, 169–170
    systemic, 169
  contraindications, 158
  design/development, 155–156
  dislocation following, 170, 171–172
  heterotopic ossification following, 172, 175

Total Hip Articular Replacement (cont'd)
  hypotensive anaesthesia, 157, 168
  indications, 157–158
  lateral transtrochanteric approach, 155, 158, 175
  loosening of components following, 170–171, 175
  minimal loss of bone stock, 155, 156, 175
  neck fracture following, 173, 175
  nerve palsey following, 172–173
  polyethylene sockets, 155–156
  postoperative peroneal nerve palsey following, 169
  postoperative protection from stress, 175
  reaming of femoral head, 155, 158, 161–162
  results, 168–169
    compared with other techniques, 173–174
  series following, 171, 172, 174
  surgical technique, 158–168
    injection of acrylic, 164–166
    reattachment of trochanter, 166–168
  trochanteric bursitis following, 169, 173
  use of eccentric shells, 155, 156
Total hip resurfacing, 173–174
  see also Total Hip Articular Replacement by Eccentric Shells (THARIES) surface replacement system

Walldius knee replacement, 46, 58, 59

Zimmer DCBGS Osteogenesis System, 139, 141

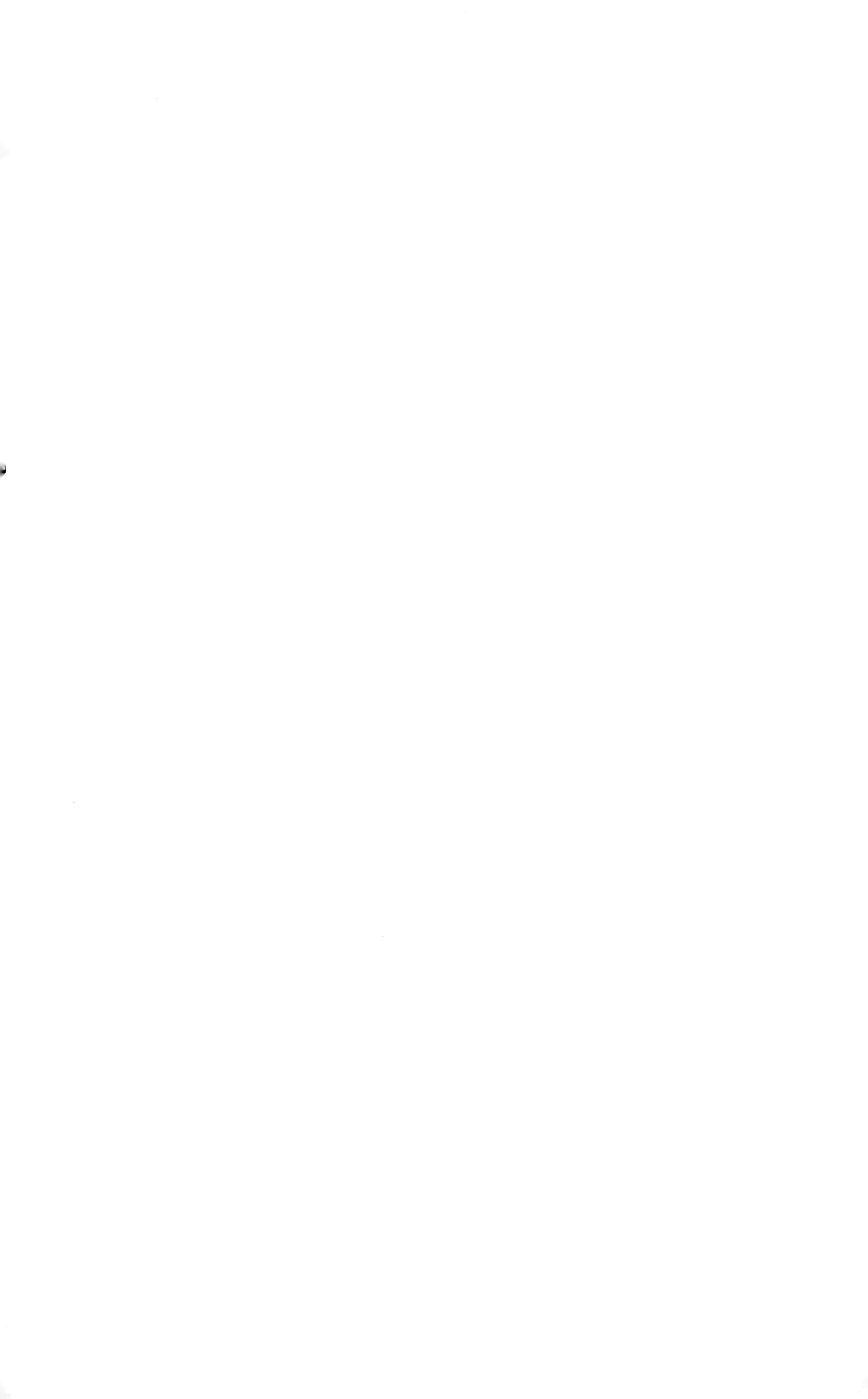

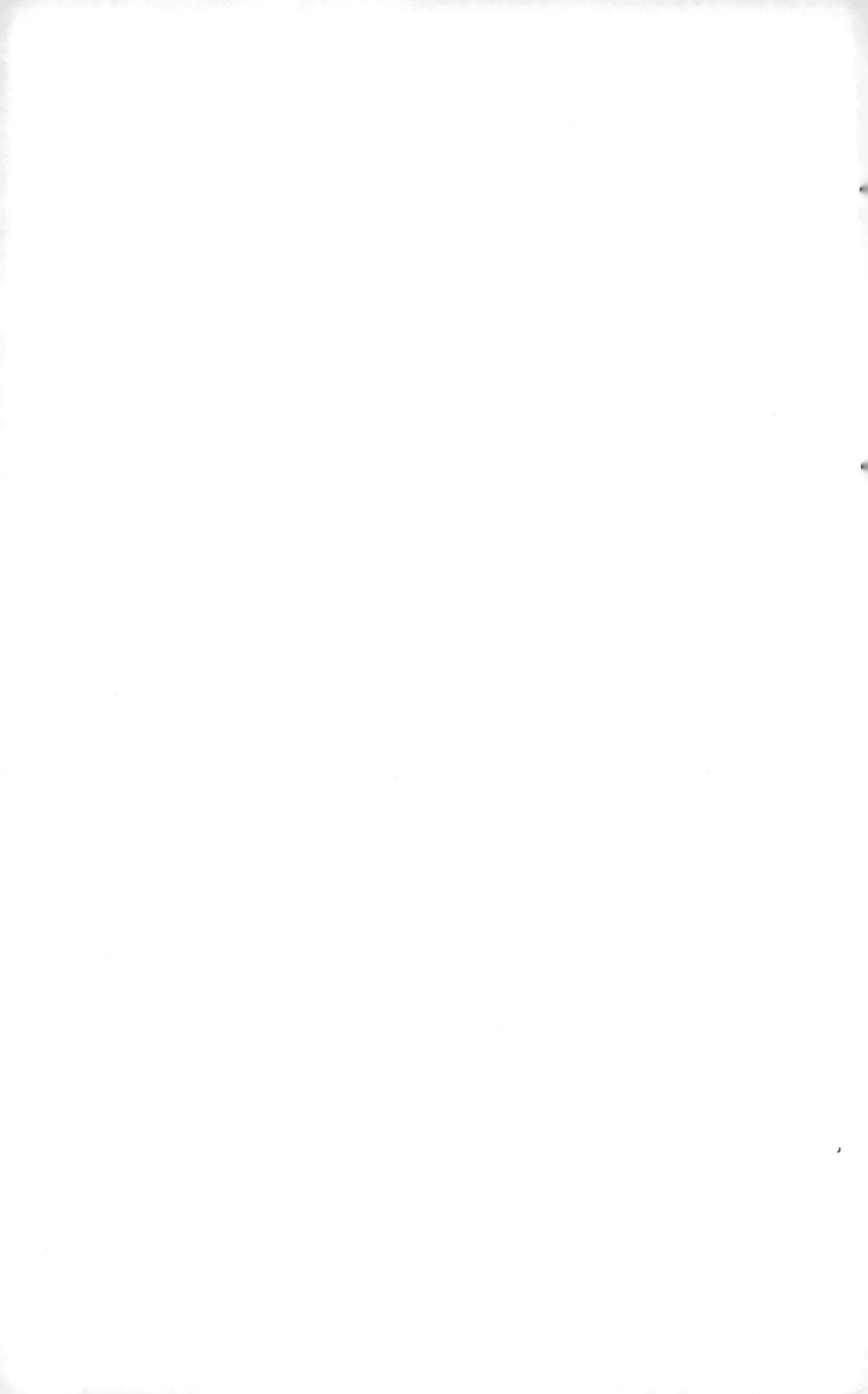

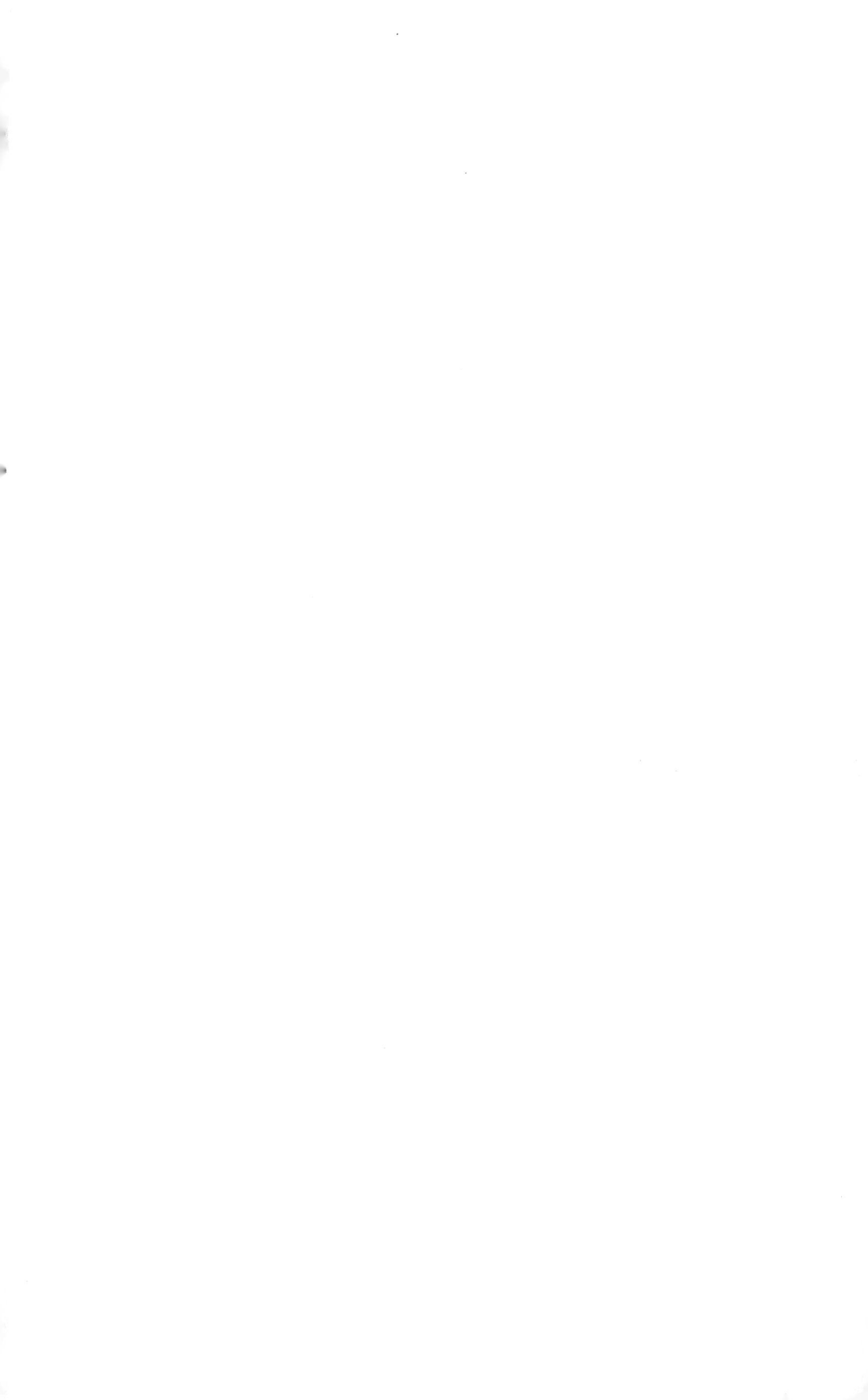

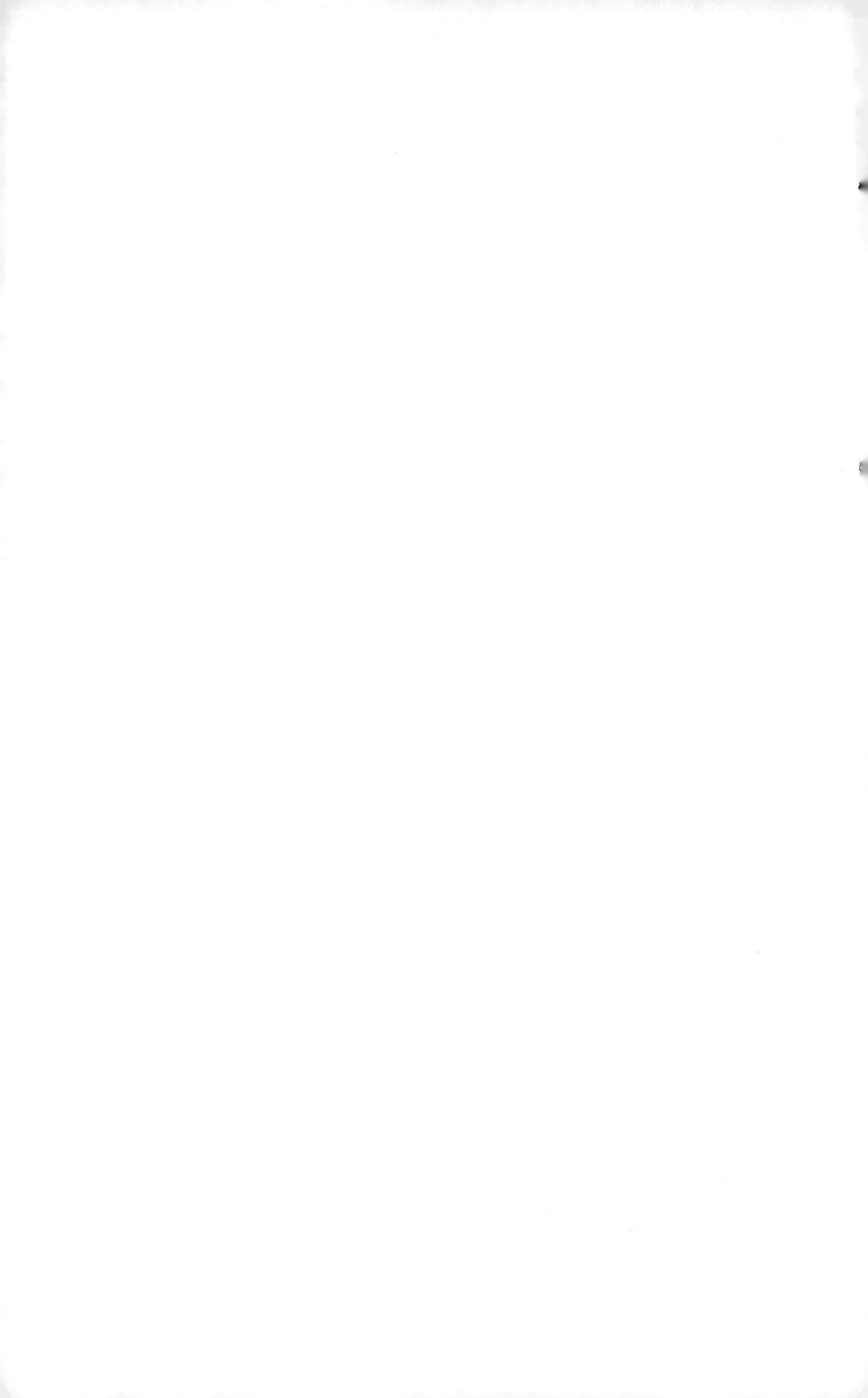

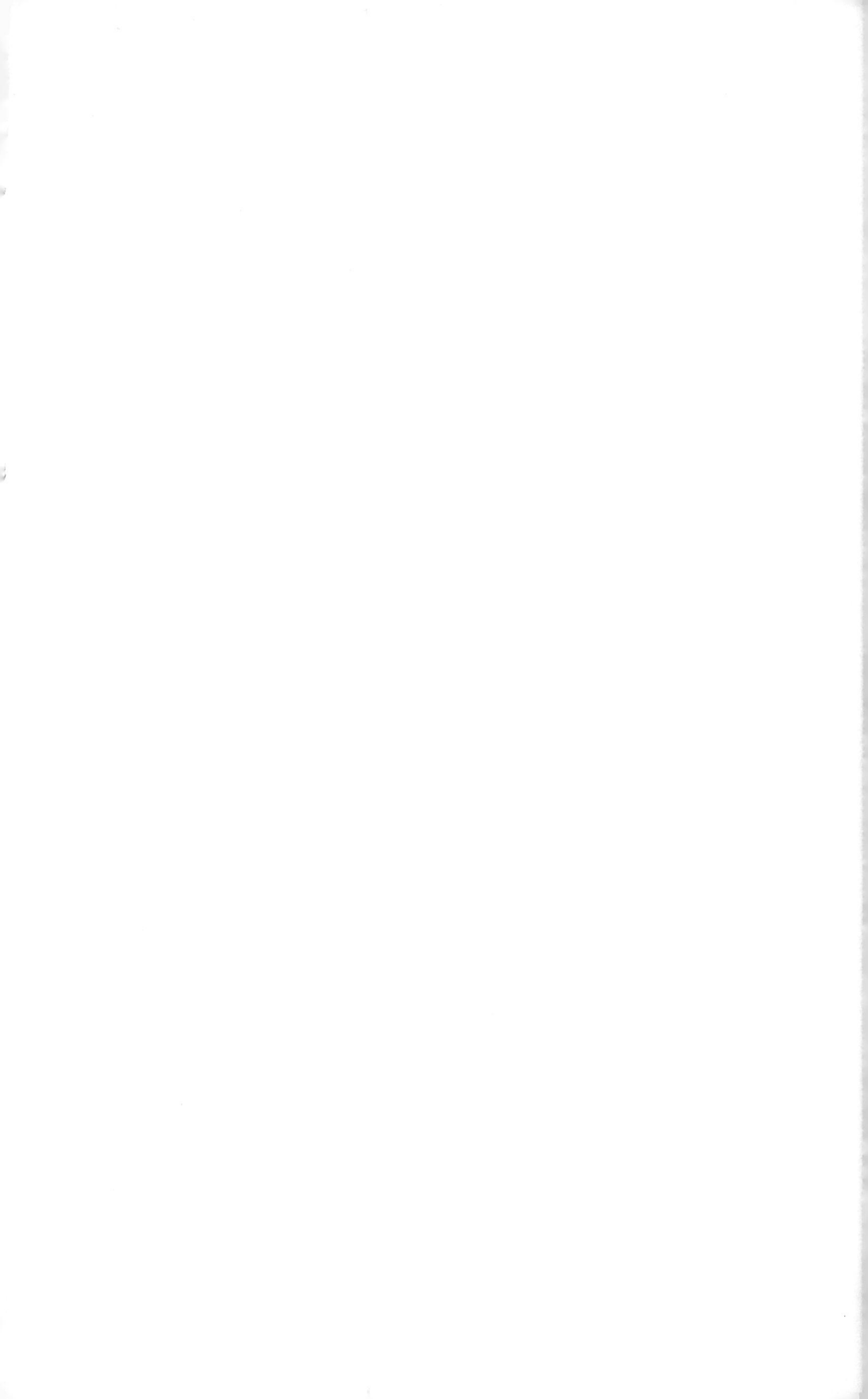